Clinical Paediatric Dietetics

Also of interest

Manual of Dietetic Practice
Second Edition
Edited by Briony Thomas
0–632–03003–8

Clinical Paediatric Dietetics

Edited by

Vanessa Shaw

and

Margaret Lawson

b

Blackwell
Science

© 1994 by
Blackwell Science Ltd
Editorial Offices:
Osney Mead, Oxford OX2 0EL
25 John Street, London WC1N 2BL
23 Ainslie Place, Edinburgh EH3 6AJ
238 Main Street, Cambridge,
   Massachusetts 02142, USA
54 University Street, Carlton,
   Victoria 3053, Australia

Other Editorial Offices:
Arnette Blackwell SA
1, rue de Lille
75007 Paris
France

Blackwell Wissenschafts-Verlag GmbH
Kurfürstendamm 57
10707 Berlin
Germany

Blackwell MZV
Feldgasse 13
A-1238 Wien
Austria

First published 1994
Reprinted 1995

Set by Best-set Typesetter Ltd., Hong Kong
Printed and bound in Great Britain at
the University Press, Cambridge

DISTRIBUTORS

Marston Book Services Ltd
PO Box 87
Oxford OX2 0DT
(*Orders*:   Tel: 01865 791155
            Fax: 01865 791927
            Telex: 837515)

North America
Blackwell Science, Inc.
238 Main Street,
Cambridge, MA 02142
(*Orders*:   Tel: 800 215-1000
            617 876-7000
            Fax: 617 492-5263)

Australia
Blackwell Science Pty Ltd
54 University Street,
Carlton, Victoria 3053
(*Orders*:   Tel: 03 347-5552)

A catalogue record for this book is
available from the British Library

ISBN 0-632-03683-4

Library of Congress
Cataloging-in-Publication Data
is available

Contents

Contributors

June Brown
Senior Dietitian
Westminster Hospital, Dean Ryle Street, London SW1P 2AP.

Christine Carter
Senior Dietitian
The Hospital for Sick Children, Great Ormond Street, London WC1N 3JH.

Christine Clothier
Former Chief Dietitian
Royal Liverpool Children's NHS Trust, Eaton Road, Liverpool L2 2AP.

Janet Coleman
Chief Paediatric Renal Dietitian
City Hospital, Hucknall Road, Nottingham NG5 1PB.

Mary Deane
Senior Dietitian
Royal Hospital for Sick Children, Sciennes Road, Edinburgh EH9 1LF.

Marjorie Dixon
Chief Dietitian
The Hospital for Sick Children, Great Ormond Street, London WC1N 3JH.

Jane Eaton
Chief Community Dietitian
Dorset Health Care NHS Trust, Bournemouth.

Jane Ely
Senior Paediatric Dietitian
Kings College Hospital, Denmark Hill, London SE5 9RS.

Lesley Haynes
Research Dietitian
Dystrophic Epidermolysis Bullosa Research Association, The Hospital for Sick Children, Great Ormond Street, London WC1N 3JH.

Karen Jeffereys
Chief Dietitian
Services for People with Learning Disabilities, PO Box 107, Southsea, Hants PO4 8NG.

Alison Johnstone
Senior Dietitian
Royal Hospital for Sick Children, Yorkhill, Glasgow G3 8SJ.

Sheena Laing
Chief Dietitian
Royal Hospital for Sick Children, Sciennes Road, Edinburgh EH9 1LF.

Bryan Lask
Consultant Psychiatrist
The Hospital for Sick Children, Great Ormond Street, London WC1N 3JH.

Margaret Lawson
Senior Lecturer in Paediatric Nutrition
Institute of Child Health, Guilford Street, London WC1N 1EH.

Anita MacDonald
Head of Dietetic Services
The Children's Hospital, Ladywood Middleway, Birmingham B16 8ET.

Anne Maclean
Senior Paediatric Dietitian
St George's Hospital, Blackshaw Road, London SW17 0QT.

Alison Macleod
Senior Dietitian
Royal Liverpool Children's NHS Trust
Eaton Road, Liverpool L12 2AP.

Judith Martin
Former Chief Dietitian
Whittington Hospital, Highgate Hill, London N19 5NF.

Marion Noble
Senior Dietitian
  The Hospital for Sick Children, Great Ormond Street, London WC1N 3JH.

Vanessa Shaw
Senior Dietitian
  The Hospital for Sick Children, Great Ormond Street, London WC1N 3JH.

Evelyn Ward
Senior Paediatric Dietitian
  St James University Hospital NHS Trust, Beckett Street, Leeds LS9 7TF.

Ruth Watling
Chief Dietitian
  Royal Liverpool Children's NHS Trust, Eaton Road, Liverpool L2 2AP.

Fiona White
Chief Dietitian
  Royal Manchester Children's Hospital, Hospital Road, Pendlebury, Manchester M27 1HA.

Sue Wolfe
Senior Paediatric Dietitian
  St James University Hospital NHS Trust, Beckett Street, Leeds LS9 7TF.

Debra Woodward
Former Senior Dietitian
  The Children's Hospital, Ladywood Middleway, Birmingham B16 8ET.

Bernadette Wren
Principal Clinical Psychologist
  The Hospital for Sick Children, Great Ormond Street, London WC1N 3JH.

Foreword

The role of nutrition in the prevention of ill-health, the promotion of health and the treatment of disease has become of ever-increasing importance. It is therefore a pleasure to write the Foreword to this new textbook on Paediatric Dietetics. It was preceded by four editions from the Hospitals for Sick Children of *Diets for Sick Children*, published from 1965 onwards, and the explosion of knowledge has been such that a multi-author publication from the Paediatric Group of the British Dietetic Association is most timely and essential.

Numerous experts including twenty-four dietitians have contributed to a wide range of topics covering enteral and parenteral feeding, the premature infant, inborn errors of many kinds, nutrition in cancer, abnormal eating behaviour and diets for children from ethnic groups, to name but a few of them. Each contributor brings to the subject not only expert knowledge but commonsense and a practical approach. The volume also includes an informative appendix, listing all the nutritional products mentioned and details of the manufacturers.

The authors, Vanessa Shaw and Margaret Lawson, have undertaken a monumental task in editing, and contributing to, this book. I congratulate them most warmly. They have made an outstanding contribution to the welfare of so many children, sick and well. It has been a privilege to write this Foreword and has given me much personal pleasure as Margaret undertook her postgraduate research under my supervision. I believe that she and Vanessa have just produced the first of a number of editions of this multi-author textbook!

Dame Barbara Clayton DBE, Hon DSc, MD, PhD, FRCP, FRCPE, FRCPath. *Honorary Research Professor in Metabolism, University of Southampton Honorary President, British Dietetic Association*

Preface

The aim of this manual is to provide a very practical approach to the nutritional management of a wide range of paediatric disorders that may benefit from nutritional support or be ameliorated or resolved by dietary manipulation. The text will be of particular relevance to professional dietitians, dietetic students and their tutors, paediatricians, paediatric nurses and members of the community health team involved with children requiring therapeutic diets.

The authors are largely drawn from experienced paediatric dietitians around the United Kingdom, with additional contributions from other specialized dietitians, a psychiatrist and a psychologist. The text does not attempt to discuss normal nutrition in healthy children (though references for this topic are addressed), but concentrates on the nutritional requirements of sick infants and children in a clinical setting. Normal dietary constituents are used alongside special dietetic products to provide a prescription that will control progression and symptoms of disease whilst maintaining the growth potential of the child.

Topics that have not been fully described in earlier texts include nutritional support in children with severe combined immune deficiency (SCID), acquired immune deficiency syndrome (AIDS) and anatomical abnormalities of the gut such as tracheo-oesophageal fistula (TOF). Arranged under headings of disorders of organ systems rather than type of diet, and with much information presented in tabular form, the manual is easy to use. Dietary restrictions due either to custom, religious beliefs or environmental conditions which may affect the nutritional adequacy of the diet of the growing child are also discussed.

Appendices list the many and varied special products described in the text, together with details of their manufacturers. The appendices are not exhaustive, but include the products most commonly used in the UK. The most recent data have been used in the preparation of this manual, but no guarantee can be given of validity or availability at the time of going to press.

Margaret Lawson
Vanessa Shaw
July 1994

SECTION 1

Introduction

CHAPTER 1

Principles of Paediatric Dietetics

This manual provides a practical approach to the dietary management of a range of paediatric disorders. The therapies describe dietetic manipulations and the nutritional requirements of the infant and child in a clinical setting. It does not attempt to address the nutrition of the healthy child in any detail (see Further Reading at end of this chapter), but illustrates how normal dietary constituents are used alongside special dietetic products to allow the continued growth of the child whilst controlling the progression and symptoms of disease. Dietary restrictions, due either to custom, religious beliefs or environmental conditions are also discussed.

DIETARY PRINCIPLES

The following principles are relevant to the treatment of all infants and children and provide the basis for many of the therapies described later in the text.

Nutritional assessment

Some form of assessing and monitoring nutritional status should be included in any dietary regimen or research protocol. There are a number of methods of assessing specific aspects of nutritional status, but no one measurement will give an overall picture of status for all nutrients. Table 1.1 summarizes the main methods available. Those listed as 'useful or routine' should be available in most centres. Those listed as 'less useful or research' may only be considered in special circumstances. Such measurements may be difficult to obtain in small children (e.g. skinfold thickness); there may be no standard or validated methodology for the paediatric age range (e.g. bio-electrical impedance measurements); the method may not be widely available or it may be expensive (e.g.

acute phase protein levels); the measurement may not yield a useful estimate of nutritional status (e.g. serum calcium); or the test may not be valid for children (e.g. immunological function).

Measurements of height/length and weight give the most useful assessment of overall status, although normal growth can still occur in marginally malnourished children. These measurements are relatively easy to make (although length is difficult to measure accurately in young children), and should be plotted on centile charts [1]. Weight and height should not differ from each other by more than two major centiles. Standards also exist for weight/height for age and weight for height [2] and weight and height velocity [1]. Measurement of head circumference may be useful in children under two years and mid arm circumference in under fives; standards exist for these [3,4].

Physiological tests such as developmental, intellectual and neurological function can be used for long term monitoring, but they are liable to bias and must be carried out within a standardized procedure.

Expected growth in childhood

Normal birthweight for infants in the United Kingdom varies between 3.3 and 3.5 kg for both sexes. There is some weight loss during the first five to seven days of life whilst feeding on full volumes of milk is established; birthweight is normally regained by the tenth to fourteenth day. Thereafter, average weight gain is as follows:

- 200 g per week for the first 3 months
- 150 g per week for the second 3 months
- 100 g per week for the third 3 months
- 50–75 g per week for the fourth 3 months.

Increase in length during the first year of life: 25 cm.

Table 1.1 Nutritional assessment in paediatrics

	Useful/routine data	Less useful/research data
Dietary intake	Recall Diet history Food diary	Duplicate diet analysis Weighed intake
Anthropometry	Weight Height/length Weight/height velocity Weight for height Weight/height for age Head circumference Mid upper arm circumference	Body mass index (BMI) Skinfold thickness Upper arm fat area Upper arm muscle area
Body composition		Total body water Total body potassium Bio-electrical impedance and body imaging methods for lean body mass etc.
Biochemistry – Serum/plasma blood levels – Other measurements	Albumin Trace metals Vitamins Haematological indices: haemoglobin, ferritin, total iron-binding capacity, red cell protoporphyrin Micronutrient-dependant enzyme functon: glutathione peroxidase, erythrocyte transketolase, glutathione reductase	Acute-phase proteins: retinol-binding-protein, transferrin, thyroxine-binding pre-albumin Serum calcium, phosphorus and magnesium Hair and nail trace element levels Saliva vitamin and trace element levels
Functional tests		Muscle strength Immunological function Developmental indices Neurological function

During the second year, the toddler following the 50th centile for growth velocity gains approximately 2.5 kg in weight and a further 12 cm in length. Average growth continues at a rate of approximately 2 kg per year and 10 cm, steadily declining to 6 cm, per year until the growth spurt at puberty.

Dietary Reference Values

The 1991 Department of Health Report on Dietary Reference Values [5] provides information and figures for requirements for a comprehensive range of nutrients and energy. The requirements are termed dietary reference values (DRV) and are for normal, healthy populations. It is important to remember that these are recommendations for groups, not for individuals; however they can be used as a basis for estimating suitable intakes for the individual, using the Reference Nutrient Intake. This level of intake should satisfy the requirements of 97.5% of healthy individuals in a population group. A summary of these DRVs for energy, protein, sodium, potassium, vitamin C, calcium and iron are given in Table 1.2. The DRVs for other nutrients may be found in the full report.

When estimating requirements for the individual sick child it is important to calculate energy and nutrient intakes based on actual body weight, and not expected body weight. The latter will lead to a proposed intake that is inappropriately high for the child who has an abnormally low body weight. In some instances it may be more appropriate to consider the child's height age rather than chronlogical age when comparing intakes with the DRVs as this is a more realistic measure of the child's body size and hence, nutrient requirement. An estimation of requirements for sick children is given in Table 1.3.

Table 1.2 Selected Dietary Reference Values

Age	Weight	Fluid	Energy (EAR)				RNI Protein		Sodium		Potassium		Vitamin C	Calcium	Iron
	kg	ml/kg	kJ/day	kJ/kg/day	kcal/day	kcal/kg/day	g/day	g/kg/day	mmol/day	mmol/kg/day	mmol/day	mmol/kg/day	mg/day	mmol/day	µmol/day
Males															
0–3 months	5.1	150	2 280	480–420	545	115–100	12.5	2.1	9	1.5	20	3.4	25	13.1	30
4–6	7.2	130	2 890	400	690	95	12.7	1.6	12	1.6	22	2.8	25	13.1	80
7–9	8.9	120	3 440	400	825	95	13.7	1.5	14	1.6	18	2.0	25	13.1	140
10–12	9.6	110	3 850	400	920	95	14.9	1.5	15	1.5	18	1.8	25	13.1	140
1–3 years	12.9	95	5 150	400	1230	95	14.5	1.1	22	1.7	20	1.6	30	8.8	120
4–6	19.0	85	7 160	380	1715	90	19.7	1.1	30	1.9	28	1.6	30	11.3	110
7–10	–	75	8 240	–	1970	–	28.3	–	50	–	50	–	30	13.8	160
11–14	–	55	9 270	–	2220	–	42.1	–	70	–	80	–	30	25.0	200
15–18	–	50	11 510	–	2755	–	55.2	–	70	–	90	–	40	25.0	200
Females															
0–3 months	4.8	150	2 160	480–420	515	115–100	12.5	2.1	9	1.5	20	3.4	25	13.1	30
4–6	6.8	130	2 690	400	645	95	12.7	1.6	12	1.6	22	2.8	25	13.1	80
7–9	8.1	120	3 200	400	765	95	13.7	1.5	14	1.6	18	2.0	25	13.1	140
10–12	9.1	110	3 610	400	865	95	14.9	1.5	15	1.5	18	1.8	25	13.1	140
1–3 years	12.3	95	4 860	400	1165	95	14.5	1.1	22	1.7	20	1.6	30	8.8	120
4–6	17.2	85	6 460	380	1545	90	19.7	1.1	30	1.7	28	1.6	30	11.3	110
7–10	–	75	7 280	–	1740	–	28.3	–	50	–	50	–	30	13.8	160
11–14	–	55	7 920	–	1845	–	42.1	–	70	–	70	–	35	20.0	260
15–18	–	50	8 830	–	2110	–	45.4	–	70	–	70	–	40	20.0	260

EAR Estimated Average Requirement
RNI Reference Nutrient Intake

Table 1.3 General guide to oral requirements in sick children

	Intants 0–1 year (based on actual weight, not expected weight)		Children
Energy	High: 130–150 kcals/kg/day (545–630 kJ/kg/day) Very high: 150–220 kcals/kg/day (630–920 kJ/kg/day)	**Energy**	High: 120% EAR for age Very high: 150% EAR for age
Protein	High: 3–4.5 g/kg/day Very high: 6 g/kg/day 0–6 months, increasing to maximum of 10 g/kg/day up to 1 year	**Protein**	High: 2 g/kg/day, actual body weight. It should be recognized that children may easily eat more than this
Sodium	High: 3.0 mmol/kg/day Very high: 4.5 mmol/kg/day a concentration > 7.7 mmolNa$^+$/100 ml of infant formula will have an emetic effect		For severely underweight children, initially an energy and protein intake based on weight, not age, is used
Potassium	High: 3.0 mmol/kg/day Very high: 4.5 mmol/kg/day		

Table 1.4 Infant milk formulas

Whey based	Casein based	Manufacturer
Aptamil	Milumil	Milupa Ltd
Cow & Gate Premium	Cow & Gate Plus	Cow & Gate Nutricia Ltd
Farley's First Milk	Farley's Second Milk	Farley Health Products Ltd
SMA Gold	SMA White	SMA Nutrition

Table 1.5 Follow-on milks

	Manufacturer
Farley's Follow-on Milk	Farley Healthcare Products Ltd
Progress	SMA Nutrition
Step-up	Cow & Gate Nutricia Ltd
Boots Follow-on Milk	Boots the Chemist PLC

Fluid requirements in the newborn

Breast feeding is the most appropriate method of feeding the normal infant and may be suitable for sick infants with a variety of clinical conditions. Demand breast feeding will automatically ensure that the healthy infant gets the right volume of milk and, hence, nutrients. If the infant is too ill or too immature to suckle, the mother may express her breast milk; expressed breast milk (EBM) may be modified to suit the sick infant's requirements. If EBM is unavailable or inappropriate to feed in certain circumstances, infant formula milks must be used (Table 1.4). After the age of six months a follow-on formula can be used (Table 1.5).

Infants over 2.5 kg birthweight

Fluid offered per 24 hours: 150–200 ml/kg. On the first day, if bottle fed, approximately one seventh of the total volume should be offered, divided into eight feeds and fed every two to three hours. The volume offered should be gradually increased over the following days to give full requirements by the seventh day of life, or sooner if the infant is feeding well. Breast fed infants will regulate their own intake of milk.

For infants under 2.5 kg, see page 51.

Fluid requirements in the first few weeks

The normal infant will tolerate four hourly feeds, six times daily once he is greater than a body weight of approximately 3.5 kg. By the age of three to six weeks (body weight approximately 4 kg) he may drop a night feed. A fluid intake of 150 ml/kg should be maintained. Infants should not normally be given more than 1200 ml of feed per 24 hours as this may induce vomiting and, in the long term, will lead to an inappropriately high energy intake. Sick infants may need smaller, more frequent feeds than the normal child and, according to the clinical condition, may have increased or decreased fluid requirements.

Once solids are introduced at four to six months of age the infant's appetite for milk will lessen. At six months, fluid requirements decrease to 120 ml/kg. At one year, the child's thirst will determine how much fluid is taken. Fluid requirements throughout childhood (if all fluid comes from feed and there is no significant contribution to fluid intake from foods) are given in Table 1.2.

Supplementing feeds for infants failing to thrive on normal strength feeds or who are fluid restricted

Supplements may be added to both EBM and to infant formula milks to achieve the necessary increase in energy and protein required by some infants. Care needs to be taken not to present an osmotic load of more than 500 mOsm/kg H_2O to the normal functioning gut, otherwise an osmotic diarrhoea will result. If the infant has malabsorption, an upper limit of 400 mOsm/kg H_2O may be necessary.

Carbohydrate

Carbohydrate provides 4 kcal/g (16 kJ/g). It is preferable to add carbohydrate to a feed in the form of glucose polymer, rather than using mono- or disaccharides, because they exert a lesser osmotic effect on the gut. Hence, a larger amount can be used per given volume of feed (Table 1.6). Glucose polymers should be added in 1% increments each 24 hours, i.e. 1 g per 100 ml feed per 24 hours. This will allow the point at which the infant becomes intolerant (i.e. has loose stools) to the concentration of the extra carbohydrate to be identified. Tolerance depends upon the age of the infant and the maturity and absorptive capacity of the gut. As a guideline the following percentage concentrations of carbohydrate (g total carbohydrate per 100 ml feed) will be tolerated if glucose polymer is used:

- 10–12% carbohydrate concentration in infants under 6 months (i.e. 7 g from formula, 3–5 g added)
- 12–15% in infants aged six months to one year
- 15–20% in toddlers aged one to two years
- 20–30% in older children.

If glucose or fructose needs to be added to a feed where there is an intolerance of glucose polymer, an upper limit of tolerance may be reached at a total carbohydrate concentration of 7 to 8% in infants and young children.

Fat

Fat provides 9 kcal/g (37 kJ/g). Long chain fat emulsions are favoured over medium chain fat emulsions because they have a lower osmotic effect on the gut and provide a source of essential fatty acids. Medium chain fats are incorporated where there is malabsorption of long chain fat (Table 1.6).

Fat emulsions should be added to feeds in 1% increments each 24 hours, so providing an increase of 0.5 g fat per 100 ml per 24 hours. Infants will tolerate a total fat concentration of 5 to 6% (i.e. 5 to 6 g fat per 100 ml feed) if the gut is functioning normally. Children over one year of age will tolerate more fat, though concentrations above 7% may induce a feeling of nausea and cause vomiting. Medium chain fat will not be tolerated at such high concentrations, and may be the cause of abdominal cramps and osmotic diarrhoea if not introduced slowly to the feed.

There are combined carbohydrate and fat supplements using both long and medium chain fats (Table 1.6). Again these must be introduced to feeds in 1% increments to determine the child's tolerance of the product. A schedule for the addition of energy supplements to infant formulas is given in Table 1.7.

Protein

Protein may be added to feeds in the form of whole protein, peptides or amino acids (Table 1.8). Protein supplementation is rarely required without an accompanying increase in energy consumption. The protein:energy ratio should be kept within the range 7.5%–12% for infants (i.e. 7.5%–12% energy from protein) and 5–15% in older children. In order for accelerated or 'catch-up' growth to occur it is probably necessary to provide about 9% energy from protein.

Protein supplements are added to feeds to provide a specific amount of protein per kg actual body weight of the child. It is rarely necessary to give intakes of greater than 6 g protein/kg; if intakes do approach this value, blood urea levels should be monitored twice weekly to avoid the danger of uraemia developing. Supplements should be added in small increments as they can very quickly and inappropriately increase the

Table 1.6 Energy supplements

a) Glucose polymers

Per 100 g	Ingredients	Energy* kcal	kJ	Na mmol	K mmol	PO4 mmol
Caloreen (Clintec Nutrition Ltd)	Hydrolysed corn starch	400	1674	<1.8	0.3	–
Super Soluble Maxijul (Scientific Hospital Supplies Group UK Ltd)	Hydrolysed corn starch	360	1500	2.0	0.1	0.16
Polycal (Cow & Gate Nutricia Ltd)	Hydrolysed corn starch	380	1610	2.2	1.3	2.3–4.2
Polycose (Abbott Laboratories Ltd)	Hydrolysed corn starch	380	1596	4.8	–	0.16
Vitajoule (Vitaflo Ltd)	Hydrolysed corn starch	385	1610	<1.9	<0.2	–

* As quoted by manufacturers

b) Fat emulsions

Per 100 g	Ingredients	Energy kcal	kJ	Na mmol	K mmol
Calogen (SHS)	Arachis oil	450	1850	0.9	0.5
Liquigen (SHS)	MCT oil	416	1740	1.7	0.7

c) Combined fat and carbohydrate supplements

Per 100 g	Ingredients	Energy kcal	kJ	Na mmol	K mmol
Duocal (SHS)	Cornstarch, maize oil, coconut oil	470	1988	<0.2	<0.1
MCT Duocal (SHS)	Cornstarch, coconut oil, sunflower oil	486	2042	1.3	0.09

child's intake of protein. The osmotic effect of whole protein products will be less than that of peptides, and peptides less than the effect of amino acids.

Concentrating infant formulas

Normally infant formula powders, whether whey and casein based formulas or specialized dietetic products, should be diluted according to the manufacturers' instructions as this provides the correct balance of energy, protein and nutrients when fed at the appropriate volume. However, there are occasions when to achieve a feed that is more dense in energy and protein it is easier to concentrate a formula than to add a series of separate supplements. Most normal baby milks in the United Kingdom are made up at a dilution of 13%. By making the baby milk up at a dilution of 15% (15 g powder per 100 ml water), more nutrition can be given in a given volume of feed e.g. energy content may be increased from 65 kcal (272 kJ)

Table 1.7 Schedule for the addition of energy supplements to infant formulas

Day	Energy source added	Additional CHO/Fat per 100 ml Feed	Energy Added per 100 ml (kcal)	(kJ)
1	1% Glucose Polymer	1 g CHO	4	17
2	2% Glucose Polymer	2 g CHO	8	33
3	3% Glucose Polymer	3 g CHO	12	50
4	3% Glucose Polymer +1% Fat Emulsion	3 g CHO 0.5 g Fat	16.5	69
5	3% Glucose Polymer +2% Fat Emulsion	3 g CHO 1 g Fat	21	88
6	4% Glucose Polymer +2% Fat Emulsion	4 g CHO 1 g Fat	25	105
7	5% Glucose Polymer +2% Fat Emulsion	5 g CHO 1 g Fat	29	121
8	5% Glucose Polymer +3% Fat Emulsion	5 g CHO 1.5 g Fat	33.5	140

Table 1.8 Protein supplements

Per 100 g	Energy kcal	kJ	Protein g	CHO g	Fat g	Na mmol	K mmol
Maxipro HBV whey protein (SHS)	393	1662	80	<5	6.0	5.6	12.0
Casilan caseinate (Farley Health Products Ltd)	373	1580	90	<0.5	1.3	1.1	0.3
Vitapro whole milk protein (Vitaflo Ltd)	388	1634	75	9.0	6.0	10.0	18.0
Code 767 peptides from hydrolysed meat and soya (SHS)	346	1469	86.4	–	–	–	–
Code 124 l-amino acids (SHS)	328	1374	82	–	–	–	–

per 100 ml to 75 kcal (314 kJ) per 100 ml and protein content from 1.5 g/100 ml to 1.7 g/100 ml. Carbohydrate and fat sources may still be added to the concentrated feed if necessary, following the above guidelines. This concentrating of feeds should only be performed as a therapeutic procedure and is not usual practice. Table 1.9 shows an example of a 15% feed.

If infants are to be discharged home on a concentrated feed the recipe may be translated into scoops for ease of use. This will mean that more scoops of milk powder will be added to a given volume of water than recommended by the manufacturer (15% dilution is equivalent to 4 scoops powder to 100 ml/3.5 oz water). As this is contrary to normal

Table 1.9 Examples of low birthweight formulas and supplemented infant milk formulas for preterm, low birthweight, failure to thrive or fluid restricted infants

	Energy kcal	kJ	Protein g	CHO g	Fat g	Per 100 ml Na+ mmol	K+ mmol	Osmolality mOsmol/kg
Low birthweight SMA	82	343	2.0	8.6	4.4	1.4	1.9	268
LBW SMA + Caloreen to 12% CHO	96	389	2.0	12.0	4.4	1.5	1.9	
13% SMA + Caloreen to 12% CHO + Calogen to 5% fat	98	403	1.6	12.0	5.0	0.7	1.5	
15% SMA	76	320	1.8	8.4	4.2	0.8	1.7	332
15% SMA + Caloreen to 12% CHO + Calogen to 5% fat	98	408	1.8	12.0	5.0	0.9	1.7	

Other Ready to Feed low birthweight/preterm formulas are: Cow & Gate Nutriprem, Milupa Prematil, Farley's Osterprem

Table 1.10 Supplemented expressed breast milk for preterm and low birthweight infants

100 ml mature human milk and either	Energy		Protein g	CHO g	Fat g	Na+ mmol	K+ mmol	Osmolality mOsmol/kg
	kcal	kJ						
3 g Pregestimil	82	345	1.7	9.0	4.6	0.9	1.9	
5 g Pregestimil	91	383	1.9	10.3	5.0	1.1	2.1	391
3 g SMA Gold	84	353	1.7	8.9	4.9	0.7	1.8	
5 g SMA Gold	94	396	1.9	10.0	5.5	0.9	2.1	
3 g Caloreen	81	339	1.3	10.2	4.1	0.6	1.5	348

Table 1.11 Vitamin supplements

Daily dose		Mother's & Children's Drops	Abidec	Ketovites
		5 drops recommended for all infants from 6 months of age	0.3 ml <1 yr 0.6 ml >1 yr*	5 ml liquid + 3 tablets
Thiamin (B1)	mg		1	3.0
Riboflavin (B2)	mg		0.4	3.0
Pyridoxine (B6)	mg		0.5	1.0
Nicotinamide	mg		5	9.9
Pantothenate				3.5
Ascorbic acid (C)	mg	20	50	49.8
Alpha-tocopherol (E)	mg			15.0
Inositol	mg			150
Biotin	mg			0.5
Folic acid	mg			0.8
Acetomenaphthone (K)	mg			1.5
Vitamin A	µg	200	1200	750
Vitamin D	µg	7.5	10	10
Choline chloride	mg			150
Cyanocobalamin (B12)	µg			12.5

* Values relate to 0.6 ml dose

practice the reasons for this deviation should be carefully explained to the parents and communicated to primary health care staff.

Low birthweight formulas are specifically designed for use in the premature infant (page 56). They may be a convenient way to provide an increased energy and protein intake in an infant who is fluid restricted, though the other nutrients provided by these formulas may not be appropriate for the term infant. Nutrient intake should be assessed for the individual. Low birthweight formulas can also be supplemented with additional energy (Table 1.9).

Milk base for supplemented feeds

The whey and casein based infant formulas (Table 1.4) are usually the feed base for infants under one year of age. These formulas do not provide adequate protein at the volumes fed to the toddler. The follow-on formulas, designed for normal infants to use rather than cows' milk as a drink from 6 months of age, are useful as a feed base as their protein contents are around 2 g/100 ml (Table 1.5). These follow-on formulas can be supplemented with fat and carbohydrate as described above.

Table 1.12 Mineral supplements

Daily dose		Aminogran Mineral Mixture	Metabolic Mineral Mixture
		1.5 g/kg/day up to full dose of 8 g/day*	
Sodium	mmol	14	14
Potassium	mmol	17	17
Chloride	mmol	–	4
Calcium	mmol	16	16
Phosphorus	mmol	15	15
Magnesium	mmol	3	3.2
Iron	mg	5	5
Zinc	mg	4	4
Iodine		trace	trace
Managanese	mg	0.4	0.4
Copper	mg	1	1
Molybdenum		trace	trace
Cobalt		trace	–
Aluminium		trace	trace

* Values relate to 8 g dose

Examples of supplemented feeds based on EBM, infant formula milks, low birthweight formulas and follow-on milks are given in Tables 1.9 and 1.10.

For the older child requiring fortified feeding there are a range of paediatric and adult enteral feeds and supplements available (Tables 3.2 and 3.3).

Vitamin and mineral requirements

Vitamin and mineral requirements for populations of normal children are provided by the DRVs. In disease states, requirements for certain vitamins and minerals will be different and are fully described in the dietary management of each clinical condition. The prescribable vitamin and mineral supplements that are most often used in paediatric practice are given in Tables 1.11, 1.12 and 1.13.

Prescribability of products for paediatric use

The majority of specialized formulas, supplements and special dietary foods are prescribable for specific conditions. The Advisory Committee on Borderline Substances of the Department of Health recommends suitable products and defines the conditions for which they can be used. Prescriptions from the general

Table 1.13 Vitamin and mineral supplements

Daily dose		Supplementary Vitamin Tablets for Infants (Cow & Gate)	Paediatric Seravit (powder) Unflavoured (SHS)	Forceval Junior Capsules (Unigreg)
		6 tablets	17 g powder	2 caps
Sodium	mmol	–	<0.09	–
Potassium	mmol	–	trace	–
Chloride	mmol	–	3.3	–
Calcium	mmol	–	10.9	–
Phosphorus	mmol	–	9.4	–
Magnesium	mmol	–	2.5	0.08
Iron	mg	5.1	11.7	10.0
Zinc	mg	3.7	7.8	10.0
Iodine	mg	0.07	0.06	0.15
Manganese	mg	0.03	0.78	2.5
Copper	mg	0.2	0.78	2.0
Molybdenum	mg	0.04	0.06	0.1
Selenium	mg	–	0.02	0.05
Chromium	mg	–	0.02	0.1
Vitamin A	µg	–	710	750
Vitamin E	mg	7.4	4.9	10.0
Vitamin C	mg	60	68	50
Thiamin	mg	1.5	0.54	3.0
Riboflavin	mg	1.5	0.75	2.0
Pyridoxine	mg	0.5	0.58	2.0
Nicotinamide	mg	5.0	5.95	15.0
Pantothenic acid	mg	3.0	2.89	4.0
Inositol	mg	–	119	–
Choline	mg	–	59.5	–
Vitamin D3	µg	–	9.44	10.0
Vitamin B12	µg	6.0	1.46	4.0
Folic acid	mg	0.4	0.05	0.2
Biotin	mg	0.05	0.04	0.1
Vitamin K	mg	0.8	0.03	50
Carbohydrate		sucrose	glucose polymer 75 g/100 g	
Osmolality			216 mOsm/kg H₂O at 10% dilution	

practitioner (FP10) should be marked 'ACBS' to indicate that the prescription complies with recommendations. A list of prescribable items appears in the *Monthly Index of Medical Specialities* (*MIMS*) and in the *British National Formulary* (*BNF*) under the Borderline Substances Appendix. Children under the age of 16 years in the UK are exempt from prescription charges.

REFERENCES

1 Tanner JM, Whitehouse RH, Takish M Standards from birth to maturity for height, weight, height velocity and weight velocity in British children. *Arch Dis Childh*, 1966, **41** 454–472 (Part I); 613–625 (Part II).
2 Waterlow JC *et al*. The presentation and use of height and weight data for comparing the nutritional status of children under the age of 10 years. *Bull of the WHO*, 1977, **55** 489–498.
3 Nelhaus G Head circumference from birth to 18 years. Practical composite international and interracial graphs. *Pediatr*, 1968, **41** 106–114.
4 Frisancho AR New norms of upper limb fat and muscle areas for assessment of nutritional status. *Amer J Clin Nutr*, 1981, **34** 2540–2545.
5 Department of Health Report on Health and Social Subjects No 41. *Dietary Reference Values for Food Energy and Nutrients for the United Kingdom*. London: HMSO, 1991.

FURTHER READING

Francis DEM (1986) *Nutrition for Children*. Blackwell Scientific Publications, Oxford.
Gibson RS (1990) *Principles of Nutritional Assessment*. Oxford University Press, Oxford.
Taitz LS, Wardley B (1989) *Handbook of Child Nutrition*. Oxford University Press, Oxford.
Talbot J (ed.) (1989) *Infant Feeding in the First Year*. Profile Productions Ltd., London.

CHAPTER 2

Provision of Nutrition in a Hospital Setting

The provision of an adequate nutritional service for the range of paediatric patients involves feed making, catering services and the close co-operation of medical and nursing staff, ward administrators, dietitians, caterers, portering staff, feed preparation staff, ward domestics and the child's carers.

Five types of provision are generally required: normal infant milks, usually in a Ready to Feed (RTF) form; specialized formulas or nutrient-dense formulas for infants who cannot tolerate or who cannot obtain sufficient nutrients from normal milks; enteral feeds for older children; a normal menu and the provision of special diets. Studies of children in hospital indicate a high prevalence of both acute and chronic malnutrition [1,2,3] and the dietitian has a pivotal role in the detection, prevention and correction of malnutrition by advising, liaising and training.

MILK FEEDS

Designated feed making areas

Wherever paediatric patients are cared for it is essential to have a designated feed making area. In large units this will normally be a separate feed making suite; in areas with few paediatric beds an area should be set aside specifically for feed preparation. The purpose of such areas is to provide hygienic and safe feeds which, because of their complexity, are not available commercially in RTF form. The area can also be used for the preparation or dispensing of paediatric enteral feeds. A number of children may be immunologically compromised and therefore have a poor tolerance to any microbiological challenge so hygiene is particularly important.

Legislative requirements

A feed making operation must comply with the requirements of the Food Safety Act 1990 [4]. The manager therefore has a legal obligation to ensure that it operates in accordance with acceptable standards of hygiene and practice. To establish such standards of quality assurance a Hazard Analysis and Critical Control Point (HACCP) concept should be implemented [5]. Such a policy requires that all aspects of production from the purchase of raw materials to the delivery of the finished product be subjected to a rigorous assessment for potential hazards and risks, and that adequate critical control points are incorporated into the process.

Structural design of feed making areas

A designated feed making area should be an independent unit or room whose access is restricted to authorised personnel. Designed to prevent the entrance and harbouring of vermin and pests and constructed to be easily cleaned, it must be operated to the highest standards of hygiene.

It is desirable to separate the unit into three areas:

A storage area, situated adjacent to the feed preparation area, where bulk goods are delivered, unpacked and stored. It should be large enough to accommodate adequate storage racks which are constructed and sited to permit segregation of commodities, stock rotation and effective cleaning. Items must be stored on racks or shelves, not directly on the floor. The temperature should be maintained between 10°C and 15°C and should be monitored daily. Entry to this area is restricted to unit and delivery staff.

A feed preparation area where very clean conditions prevail and access is only allowed to feed preparation staff who are suitably clothed (see later); entry should be via an anteroom containing a wash-hand basin and storage facilities for outer protective clothing. Bulk storage of items (e.g. large cardboard cartons) is not recommended. There should be sufficient space to allow clean equipment and small quantities of ingredients to be stored, preferably on wheel mounted stainless steel solid shelving, leaving worktops clear. During the preparation of feeds all other activities in the area should cease and the doors should be closed and secured against all staff (including dietitians) who are not involved in the manufacturing process. If it is necessary for staff to leave the preparation area they must, on re-entry, wash their hands again, according to the correct hand washing procedure.

A wash up area. A unit re-using feeding bottles will require a designated space, adjoining the feed preparation area, with a separate access for the delivery of dirty bottles. A unit using disposable bottles does not require such a wash-up room if a dishwasher is in operation for preparation equipment. Access to this area should be restricted to cleaning and delivery staff.

Storage of cleaning materials should be separated from ingredients and equipment and requires a designated clean, dry room or cupboard.

A cloakroom with a separate changing room for feed unit staff should be conveniently sited but segregated from the feed making area. The cloakroom should have a foot operated flush toilet, a wash-hand basin with foot or elbow operated taps; the changing room should contain secure lockers for storage of personal belongings and outdoor clothes and clean storage for protective clothing.

Recommendations for construction of feed units are as follows [6]:

Plant

Walls, floors and ceilings: hardwearing, impervious, free from cracks and open joints. Smooth surfaces to permit ease of cleaning and coved junctions between floors, walls and ceilings to prevent collection of dust and dirt. Light coloured sheen finish to reflect light and increase illumination.

Doors in the production area: self-closing with glass observation panel.

Windows: sealed to prevent opening.

Lighting level: to allow staff to work cleanly and safely without eye strain, and to expose dirt and dust. Light fixtures flush with wall or ceiling.

Ventilation in the production area: mechanical means; air supply filtered with temperature (and preferably humidity) control to give optimum working environment and control bacterial and dust contamination. Steam-producing equipment such as sterilizers, dishwashers and pasteurizers should be fitted with a canopy and exhaust fan system to draw off steam and fumes.

Wash-hand basins: one hand basin provided in each of the storage, wash-up and preparation areas. Hot and cold water with foot or elbow operated taps. Adjacent soap dispenser and either single use disposable towels or a hot air hand dryer.

Water supply: of potable quality from a rising main. Softened water supply to equipment is preferable, but water softened by ion exchange should not be used in feeds.

Hot water: provided from a fixed device such as a gas or electric water boiler to dispense water above 80°C.

Large equipment

- Large equipment such as shelving, tables and refrigerators should be castor mounted with wheel brakes to allow easy access for cleaning. Smooth impervious surfaces free from sharp internal corners, which may act as dirt traps, which can be easily cleaned and disinfected (e.g. stainless steel) are recommended.

- One or more refrigerators which operate at a temperature between 1–4°C is a necessity; the temperature should be monitored and recorded twice daily.

- A deep freeze which operates at −18°C will be necessary if feeds of expressed breast milk are to be stored for more than a few hours. Both the refrigerator and freezer should be self-defrosting and have shelves which are easy to clean. An alarm which is activated if the door is left open accidentally or the internal temperature rises is also useful.

- Pasteurization equipment which is suitable for the range of procedures carried out (see later) and which includes a method of monitoring and recording pasteurization cycles is desirable.

- Thermal sterilization or disinfection equipment is desirable in a small unit and essential in a large centralized unit. This can be a washer adapted for bottle and equipment washing, with a rinse cycle which holds a temperature of 85°C for two minutes. This ensures a surface temperature of 80°C for one minute, which is an effective disinfectant. A drying cycle is useful. For units with a very small workload, a domestic steam sterilzer is adequate for non-reusable bottles. Regulations affecting the use of autoclaves come into operation in 1994 [7] and units using autoclaves for bottles or equipment will need to comply with these.

- A feed delivery trolley, which may need to be refrigerated (see the section on Delivery).

Small equipment

- Mixing and measuring equipment including jugs, measures, cutlery, sieves and whisks should be made from plastic or stainless steel. It must be easily washed and cleaned.

- Electric whisks or liquidizers create large froth volumes in feeds, making accurate measurement difficult. They are also difficult to clean and, if used, the bowl and blades should be suitable for use in a washing machine, autoclave or chemical disinfectant.

- Weighing equipment should be easy to clean, easy to use and of the appropriate accuracy for the task. It may be battery or electrically operated but ideally computer linked and sensitive to product identity codes to aid in documentation and to help avoid mistakes in the formula.

- Feeding bottles are available in glass, polycarbonate or plastic polythene in 100, 120, 200 and 240 ml sizes. Glass is a hazardous material prone to cracking and chipping; polycarbonate shrinks if autoclaved at temperatures greater than 119°C and bottles become scratched or crazed after some time in use. Reusable bottles require washing, sanitizing by heat or chemical means; sealing discs or caps need to undergo a similar treatment and are likely to become lost or misshapen with continuous use. Disposable sterile polythene bottles (although apparently more expensive) reduce the workload in the unit as the responsibility for providing clean bottles is transferred to the manufacturer.

Staffing levels and staff procedures

Feed provision is usually required 365 days a year and staffing levels should take this fact and the workload into consideration. Part-time employment of some staff may be particularly appropriate.

In large units the dietitian may be managerially responsible for staff and feed preparation. In small areas attached to a ward the supervision and management may be the responsibility of the nursing staff with the dietitian acting in an advisory capacity. No specific qualifications are required for feed preparation staff, provided that adequate instruction and supervision is provided; in situations such as small units where this is difficult it is an advantage for staff to be trained nurses or nursery nurses.

Training should cover all areas of Good Manufacturing Practice [7,8], which includes personal hygiene, prevention of bacterial and foreign matter contamination, preparation procedures, cleaning procedures and documentation requirements. If staff numbers warrant, then a supervisor should be appointed. Regular meetings between the manager, supervisor, microbiologist and infection control officer will enhance communication and help ensure that standards are maintained.

Staff should be provided with an agreed job description suitable for their grade, a protective uniform fastened to the neck (changed daily) and a satisfactory laundry service. A disposable plastic apron should be worn during feed preparation and disposable head covering should completely cover the hair. Shoes should be flat-heeled and cover the foot; jewellery (with the exception of a wedding ring and stud type earrings) is not allowed.

Appointment of staff should be subject to a satisfactory medical examination; bacteriological screening of faecal specimens should take place prior to appointment, after a gastrointestinal upset and on return from a hot climate.

Feed preparation

A policy for documentation of raw materials should be implemented and goods received checked to ensure they meet the required standard and specification. Goods for storage should be marked and dated to aid identification and stock rotation. All raw materials should be dated when the packaging is opened and any surplus discarded after the recommended time or after one month.

Details of each feed to be prepared should be in a written or printed form and prepared by a responsible person such as the dietitian or senior nurse. These details should also be available at ward level. Prepared feeds should be cross-checked by staff to confirm that the ingredients and quantities are as intended. A further check by care staff at ward level at the time of delivery should confirm that the feeds received are those requested.

Feeds should be clearly identified by labels bearing the patient's name, hospital number, ward, feed ingredients and date of preparation. An instruction to 'store in a refrigerator' and 'discard after 24 hours' or a use-by date should be included. A polysaccharide backed peelable label is essential for non-disposable bottles.

Feed ingredients

Only unopened tins and packets of milk powder or feed ingredients should be allowed into the preparation area. Bulk goods (e.g. glucose polymer) should be decanted into a disinfected container prior to entry. Ultra heat treated (UHT) cows' milk is recommended as it does not need to be refrigerated until opened. If pasteurized milk is used, its storage conditions and shelf life need to be carefully controlled; pasteurized cows' milk that has not been used should be discarded at the end of each working day.

Expressed breast milk (EBM) should be handled carefully and a procedure adopted for its use on the wards and milk room. The Department of Health and Social Security Report No 22 [9] makes recommendations for the handling and storage of human milk. More recent recommendations regarding the microbiological safety of EBM are given on page 25.

A mother whose infant is too sick to feed at the breast should be encouraged to provide expressed breast milk for her own infant providing there are no contraindications to milk feeding. Milk can be expressed by manual massage, but if expression is needed for several days a manual or electric breast pump makes the process easier. Expression of milk can be carried out in a designated room, but may be done more succesfully at home (where the mother is more relaxed) or by the infant's cotside (where the sight or sound of the baby aids the let-down reflex). Portable electric pumps should be available on neonatal units; the National Childbirth Trust (NCT) loans portable pumps for home use.

Pumps should be capable of easy disassembly for thorough cleaning and disinfection. Autoclaved or disposable pre-sterilized connections should be supplied to the mother, and she should be taught the correct method of use of the pump. Basic hygiene, such as hand washing, frequent changing of breast pads and underwear and the importance of a daily bath or shower should be emphasized.

Milk should be expressed into pre-sterilized bottles; it should be labelled with the infant's details, the date and time of expressing and the name of any drug being taken by the mother. Expressed milk should be immediately placed into a designated refrigerator if it is expressed in the hospital, or into a domestic refrigerator if at home. Milk should be delivered to the hospital in insulated containers at least once daily; if such frequent deliveries are not possible, milk should be frozen at home rather than refrigerated.

If the milk is to be fed to the infant within a few hours of expressing and hygienic precautions have been taken, microbiological examination or pasteurization of milk should not be necessary. A container of expressed milk should be opened once only in a clean feed preparation area and aliquots of volumes suitable for the infant's requirements should be decanted into sterile feeding bottles (or sterile syringes if bolus feeding by tube). Where milk is decanted it should undergo microbiological examination. Criteria used to establish the safety of untreated milk should be formulated with the microbiology department. If the milk is unlikely to be fed within 48 hours it should be stored frozen after microbiological sampling.

Pasteurization

The type of feeds prepared in the milk room will readily support the growth of harmful micro-organisms and it is therefore recommended that they are end-stage pasteurized. A pasteurizer built to the specifications of the unit should be equipped with a computer printout to show the temperature and process time for each batch of feeds.

There are two methods of pasteurization:

- *holder method for breastmilk only*: the temperature is raised to 62.5°C for 30 minutes, followed by rapid cooling to less than 10°C
- *flash method for milk formulas, modular feeds and supplements*: The temperature is raised to 67.5°C for 4 minutes followed by rapid cooling to less than 10°C.

After pasteurization feed should be stored in a suitable refrigerator (see above) until delivery.

Delivery

Feed delivery to wards should be compatible with food safety requirements of being refrigerated to 4°C or less without avoidable delay. If the preparation unit is some distance from wards this requires a refrigerated trolley. Feeds should be checked and placed in a designated refrigerator at ward level; this refrigerator should be reserved for milk feeds and should not contain items of food. The temperature of ward refrigerators should be between 1–4°C and should be checked twice daily.

Cleaning procedures

Sterilization (the destruction of all micro-organisms and their spores) is not attainable in a Special Feeds Unit. Sanitation or disinfection of small equipment can be achieved by autoclaving, a dishwasher or by chemical means.

Autoclaving, although effective, has a number of disadvantages: equipment first has to be washed, dried, packed and sealed; this is costly and time consuming. In addition water condensation forms and remains in feeding bottles, where it can induce bacterial activity. Regulations affecting the use of autoclaves will come into operation in 1994 (see above).

Thermal disinfection in a dishwasher requires less time and the inclusion of a drying cycle will ensure that all equipment is dry and ready for storage. To achieve thermal disinfection the water in the dishwasher should reach a minimum temperature of 85°C for two minutes (page 15, Large Equipment).

Chemical disinfection (e.g. hypochlorite) reduces levels of harmful bacteria to acceptable levels and is also satisfactory for small (non-metallic) equipment provided recommendations are followed, although heat sanitization is the preferred method. Disinfection will only be effective if:

- the equipment is adequately cleaned; residual organic matter inactivates the chlorine content of the disinfectant
- the disinfectant is freshly and correctly prepared with all air bubbles removed to ensure the solution reaches each surface of the equipment

- the equipment remains in the disinfectant for the recommended length of time.

After disinfection the equipment should be rinsed free of contaminated hypochlorite with clean water. Feed equipment should be covered with sterile paper or drape and used within 24 hours of disinfection. Equipment which is stored for longer than this should be re-disinfected before use.

Walls of a Special Feed Unit should be washed every six months, floors cleaned daily and all cleaning procedures documented. Separate, clearly indentified cleaning equipment should be used for the 'clean' and 'dirty' areas of the unit.

Microbiological surveillance

To ensure satisfactory standards of working practice a microbiological surveillance policy should be implemented and monitored. The following samples should be sent for microbiological analysis once each month: each type of feed (both freshly prepared and after storage); water from boiler, tap and pasteurizer; a swab from work surfaces, sinks, shelving, mixing equipment and feeding bottles. An air sample should be taken if *Staphylococcus aureus* is identified.

Procedures and documentation

To comply with legislative requirements, standards for all procedures within the feed preparation area should be set, implemented, monitored and recorded. To increase staff awareness and to aid training a 'Procedure Manual' should be drawn up which should be available to all staff. It should contain staff job descriptions, guidelines for personal hygiene and prevention of cross-infection, procedures for ordering supplies, feed preparation, instructions for pasteurization, cleaning and disinfection, procedures for microbiological surveillance and accident procedures. Information about equipment maintenance and emergency telephone numbers in case of breakdown should also be displayed.

Currently there are no accepted published standards for the preparation of enteral feeds for the paediatric age range. Operational practices should be based on standards identified for food products, medical devices and pharmaceuticals as appropriate [7,8,10].

NORMAL DIET IN A HOSPITAL SETTING

In the provision of normal diet it is the role of the dietitian to advise the caterer of the nutritional requirements of the paediatric age groups and to assist the caterer in menu planning. If appropriate, training of catering staff should also be undertaken to ensure a basic nutritional knowledge and the preservation of nutrients through good catering practice [11].

A hospital menu should, over a period of days, provide the minimum nutritional requirements [12]. Whilst a nutritionally sound diet incorporating appropriate nutrition education messages may be desirable, it is vital to encourage children to eat something when they are in unfamiliar surroundings with feelings of anxiety and depression. It is most important, therefore, that familiar foods are included on the menu and that healthy eating guidelines are applied with caution. Where there are paediatric wards in a general hospital a separate children's menu should be available and food items such as full-fat milk provided for the paediatric wards. Patient choice of food is generally recommended [13] and where practically possible choice should also be offered to paediatric patients. Caterers should also be aware of the wide age range encountered in a paediatric setting and provide an appropriate selection of food choices and portion sizes (Table 2.1). At ward level food should be attractively presented with crockery and utensils appropriate to the age range.

If possible children should be encouraged to eat together and they should be adequately supervized. Accurate charting of food and fluid intake in combination with mealtime supervision greatly assists the detection of patients at risk from a poor food intake [14]. Where such a problem does occur, it may be simply solved by increased supervision at mealtimes, use of favourite foods, inclusion of regular snacks and the availability of nutritious supplements such as milk-based drinks.

It is important that all hospital patients are provided with food which is acceptable to them. Choices

Table 2.1 Portion sizes for different age groups

	1 Year	2–3 Years	3–5 Years	10 Years
Meal pattern	3 small meals and 3 snacks plus milk	3 meals and 2–3 snacks or milky drinks	3 meals and 1–2 snacks or milky drinks	3 meals and 1–2 snacks or milky drinks
Meat, fish etc.	½–1 tablespoon – 20–30 g minced/finely chopped, with gravy/sauce; ½–1 hard cooked egg	1½ tablespoons – 20–30 g chopped; 1 fish finger; 1 sausage; 1 egg	2–3 tablespoons – 40–80 g; 1–2 fish fingers/sausages	90–120 g meat; 3–4 fish fingers/sausages
Cheese	20 g grated	25–30 g cubed or grated	30–40 g	50–60 g
Potato	1 tablespoon – 30 g mashed	1–2 tablespoons – 30–60 g; 6 smallish chips	2–3 tablespoons – 60–80 g; 8–10 chips	4–6 tablespoons – 100–180 g; 100–150 g chips
Vegetables	1 tablespoon – 30 g soft or mashed	1–2 tablespoons – 30–60 g or small chopped salad	2–3 tablespoons – 60–80 g	3–4 tablespoons – 100–120 g
Fruit	½–1 piece – 40–80 g	1 piece – 80–100 g	1 piece – 100 g	1 piece – 100 g
Dessert (e.g. custard/yoghurt)	2 tablespoons – 60 g	2–3 tablespoons – 60–80 g	4 tablespoons – 120 g; 1 carton yoghurt – 150 g	6 tablespoons – 180 g
Bread	½–1 slice – 20–30 g	1 large slice – 40 g	1–2 large slices – 40–80 g	2–4 large slices – 80–160 g
Breakfast cereal	1 tablespoon – 15 g; ½ Weetabix	1–1½ tablespoons – 15–20 g; 1 Weetabix	2–3 tablespoons – 20–30 g; 1 Weetabix	3–4 tablespoons – 30–40 g; 2 Weetabix
Drinks	¾ teacup – 100 ml	1 teacup – 150 ml	1 teacup – 150 ml	1 mug – 200 ml
Milk	500 ml whole milk/day	350 ml whole or semi-skimmed/day	350 ml whole or semi-skimmed/day	350 ml whole, semi-skimmed or skimmed/day

should be available for vegetarians, vegans and those whose eating habits are based on religious and cultural beliefs.

MODIFIED DIET IN A HOSPITAL SETTING

The major role of the dietitian is to liaise with the medical and nursing staff and to advise on the appropriate therapeutic regimen. The advice and education given to children requiring modified diets and to their carers is the responsibility of the dietitian. In addition to this the dietitian assists in the provision of modified diets within the hospital. Usually this is in a supervisory and advisory capacity to diet cooks employed by the caterer, but rarely dietitians may also be managerially responsible for the diet kitchen. In the majority of cases design and maintenance of the diet preparation area, staff management, supply of provisions and responsibility for hygiene will rest with the catering manager. If these are the responsibility of the dietitian the same principles apply as previously described for feed making areas [4].

Staff involved in the preparation of modified diets must be aware of the need for accuracy, appropriate portion size for age, consistency of nutrient content and variety. For those on a modified diet the food provided in hospital is taken as an example and must therefore be correct. It is advisable that staff employed to prepare modified diets should have as a minimum qualification City and Guilds 706/2 and have attended a diet cookery course. In-service training of diet cooks should be undertaken by the dietitian particularly to ensure that staff are kept up-to-date with changes to dietary treatment.

The dietitian should specify to the caterer standards of quality and suitability of provisions for use in the diet preparation area. Stocks of specific dietary products such as gluten-free and low protein products should be available and those working in the area should be familiar with the use of these products.

Appropriate equipment for preparation of small quantities of food must be available for the diet cooks. Specifically a sturdy industrial liquidizer, small pots and pans and accurate scales are all essential items. Freezer space is also required, as it is useful to keep frozen portions of rarely used items, e.g. vegetable casserole for low protein diets, low protein bread.

A suitable plating system for diets must be used. Where a bulk catering system is operated, individual foil containers, clearly labelled, are suitable for diet meals. If a plated system is in use the diet meals should be clearly labelled.

The dietitian should always provide the diet cooks with clear written and verbal instructions for each individual diet being prepared. The written information should include the patient's name, age and ward, the diet required and specific instructions regarding the composition of the diet.

Within the diet preparation area there should be a diet manual. This should include instructions regarding commonly requested modified diets and appropriate recipes. It is also useful to include details of any patients on unusual diets if they are likely to be admitted. This manual should be regularly updated.

To ensure consistency and accuracy, the provision of modified diets should be monitored regularly. The following should all be considered: the quality, freshness and suitability of the provisions; the storage methods; the preparation of raw ingredients; and the presentation to the patient. Regular monitoring should ensure a high quality product. Additionally, where the dietitian is responsible for the management of the diet preparation area, then the legal obligations of the Food Safety Act 1990 [4] should be fulfilled.

IMMUNOSUPPRESSION AND 'CLEAN' MEAL PROVISION

Children with a number of conditions (including acute megaloblastic leukaemia, Stage IV neuroblastoma, relapsed acute lymphoblastic leukaemia and immunodeficiency syndromes) requiring a bone marrow transplant or autograft, and children undergoing heart-lung transplantation receive drug therapy which causes severe immunosuppression and neutropenia. They require protective isolation in the immediate post-transplant period and, since they are highly susceptible to food-borne pathogens, must be protected from gastrointestinal infection [15]. In immunosuppressed patients even normally non-pathogenic organisms may cause problems. Particular attention should be paid to personal hygiene in the food handler, and to food purchase, storage and preparation.

Sterile meals

In some units food production may be a sterile or near-sterile method incorporating the use of gamma-

Table 2.2 Foods for a 'clean' diet

Food	Allowed	Not allowed
Water	Sterile water Boiled tap water	Mineral water Unboiled water
Drinks	Fruit juice and soft drinks – individual cartons or cans Ice cubes and ice lollies – made with sterile water High energy packaged drinks (e.g. Hycal, Polycal Liquid) Tea, coffee, cocoa etc. – individual sachets	Squashes unless repacked and pasteurized
Milk and dairy products	Milk – UHT, pasteurised, condensed or sterilized in individual portions Cheeses – individually vacuum wrapped portions; cheese spread portions; processed cheese Yoghurt – pasteurized Butter/margarine – individual portions Cream – UHT or sterilized Ice cream – individually wrapped portions	Unpasteurized milk Soft cheeses Unwrapped hard cheese Blue cheeses Unpasteurized or 'live' yoghurt Fresh cream
Cereals	Breakfast cereals – individual packets Bread from newly opened loaf Biscuits and cakes – individual portions Rice – well cooked Pasta – tinned or dried	Cereals with added milk powder; sugar coated cereals Unwrapped bread Cream cakes Slow-cooked rice (e.g. rice pudding) Fresh pasta
Meat and poultry	Pork, lamb, beef, veal – fresh or frozen, well cooked Tinned meats: chicken, sausages, ham, corned beef Meat paste in individual jars	Chicken, turkey – fresh or frozen Sausages Pies (unless home made) Take away meals (e.g. hamburgers) Salami Liver pâté, liver sausage
Fish	Freshly-cooked fresh or frozen fish Tinned fish Fish fingers, fish paste	Shellfish

Table 2.2 *Continued*

Food	Allowed	Not allowed
Eggs	Hard boiled egg Fried egg	Raw egg, soft-cooked egg
Vegetables	Fresh leafy vegetables – well washed and cooked Root vegetables, washed, peeled and cooked Jacket potato; oven chips Beans and lentils – well cooked or tinned Tomato and cucumber – raw, peeled Tinned and frozen vegetables	Salad vegetables which cannot be peeled (e.g. lettuce, radish) Raw root vegetables
Fruit	Fresh fruit that can be peeled Tinned fruit	Unpeeled fruit Dried fruit
Snacks and Soups	Crisps, sweets etc. – individual packets Tinned soups, packet soups – made with boiled water	Unwrapped sweets
Miscellaneous	Cooking oils Puddings, pies, custards – freshly made Jelly – made with sterile/boiled water Salt, salad cream, sauces – individual portions Pepper – gamma irradiated	Instant puddings made with cold water Herbs and spices

irradiated and canned foods prepared in a filtered laminar airflow system. Such a system requires specialized facilities and equipment and is labour-intensive and costly. Irradiation adversely affects food flavour and texture and consequently patient acceptability of food [16].

'Clean' meals

A practical and acceptable alternative is the use of a reduced bacterial diet or 'very clean food regimen'. Such regimens avoid the use of raw foods, reheated dishes and foods known to contain high levels of pathogenic and non-pathogenic bacteria, such as soft cheese, chicken and pâté. Details of foods allowed and forbidden are given in Table 2.2.

Purchasing

(1) Many chilled and frozen foods contain unacceptably high levels of organisms for the immunosuppressed patient. Before allowing them to be included a sample of the product should be tested. Canned and sterilized products are generally suitable.
(2) The 'Best Before' date should be checked on manufactured foods.
(3) Individual portions of foods (e.g. jams, butter/margarine, breakfast cereals, juices, sugar) should be purchased where these are available.
(4) Foods should be purchased as fresh as possible and cooked shortly after purchase.

Storage

(1) Check temperatures of refrigerators and freezers regularly.
(2) Ideally food for 'clean' meals should be stored in a separate refrigerator; where this is not practical, the top shelf should be used.
(3) Transfer food that is to be eaten cold to the refrigerator as quickly as possible; cover or wrap all foods stored in the refrigerator. Leftover food should be disposed of quickly; leftovers and re-heated foods should not be used.

Preparation

(1) Wash hands thoroughly with soap and water and dry with a hand drier or a clean paper towel before handling food.
(2) In the hospital setting the food handler should wear a fresh plastic apron over the usual kitchen dress.
(3) Use clean utensils, containers and chopping boards which have been through a dishwasher.
(4) In a hospital kitchen, work surfaces should be wiped with a suitable disinfectant solution before 'clean' meals are prepared. This precaution should be unnecessary at home.
(5) Do not use wooden utensils (e.g. chopping boards).
(6) A fresh packet or tin should be used for each meal to avoid re-opening containers. Large packets (e.g. a loaf of bread, a pint of milk etc.) can be divided into convenient size portions and individually wrapped at the beginning of each day.

(7) Before opening packages such as tins the top should be wiped with a clean cloth or paper towel.
(8) Tin openers should be washed daily, preferably in a dishwasher.
(9) Cooking methods employed should ensure a minimum core temperature of 70°C, and this temperature should be maintained until the food is eaten.
(10) There should be minimum delay between food being cooked and consumed.

Acceptable bacterial levels should be determined in consultation with the microbiologist and haematologist/immunologist. There are a few guidelines to assist with this [17]. Additionally guidelines on the bacteriology of enteral feeds may be a useful starting point [10].

The 'very clean food regimen' should be fully explained to the patient and carers prior to transplant as it should be commenced as soon as the patient is able to take anything orally. Prior discussion also allows time to obtain supplies of favourite or unusual foods and to liaise with the catering department regarding provision of supplies.

The diet can be relaxed after discharge, but care must still be taken to avoid take away meals, delicatessen foods, ice cream from ice cream vans, ready-cooked chicken, soft cheeses, pâté, shellfish and damaged fruit and vegetables. These precautions may be necessary for approximately six months post-transplant.

REFERENCES

1 Moy RJD, Smallman S, Booth IW Malnutrition in a UK children's hospital. *J Hum Nutr Diet*, 1990, **3** 93–100.
2 Merritt RJ, Suskind RM Nutritional survey of the hospitalised paediatric patient. *Am J Clin Nutr*, 1979, **32** 1320–1325.
3 Parsons HG *et al.* The nutritional status of hospitalised children. *Am J Clin Nutr*, 1980, **33** 1140–1146.
4 *The Food Safety Act.* London: HMSO, 1990.
5 Eardley G (personal communication) 1992.
6 Sprenger RA *Hygiene for Management*. Doncaster: Highfield Publications, 1991.
7 *Guide to Good Manufacturing Practice for Sterile Medical Devices and Clean Products.* London: HMSO, 1981.
8 Sharpe JR *Guide to Good Pharmaceutical Manufacturing Practice.* London: HMSO, 1983.
9 Department of Health and Social Security Report on

Health and Social Subjects No 22. *The Collection and Storage of Human Milk.* London: HMSO, 1981.

10 Parenteral and Enteral Feeding Group of the British Dietetic Association *Microbiological Control in Enteral Feeding – a guidance document.* Birmingham: BDA, 1986.

11 *Health Service Catering: Nutrition and Modified Diets.* Third Edition. 1986. Department of Health London.

12 Department of Health Report on Health and Social Subjects No 41. *Dietary Reference Values for Food, Energy and Nutrients for the United Kingdom.* London: HMSO, 1991.

13 King's Fund *A Review of Hospital Catering.* London: King Edward's Hospital Fund for London, 1986.

14 Todd EA *et al.* What do patients eat in hospital? *Hum Nutr: Appl Nutr,* 1984, **38A** 294–297.

15 Dezenhall A *et al.* Food and nutrition services in bone marrow transplant centres. *J Am Diet Assoc,* **87** 1351–1353.

16 Aker SN, Cheney CU The use of sterile and low microbial diets in ultra isolation environments. *J Parent Ent Nutr,* 1983, **7** 390.

17 Pizzo PA, Purvis DS, Waters C Microbiological evaluation of food items. *J Am Diet Assoc,* 1982, **81** 272.

SECTION 2

Enteral and Parenteral Nutrition

CHAPTER 3

Enteral Feeding

Enteral feeding is the method of supplying nutrients via the alimentary tract. It includes the intake of oral food and fluids, but usually indicates the use of naso-gastric, gastrostomy or jejunostomy feeding.

Enteral feeding of all patients has changed markedly over the last few years and both feeds and equipment are now being developed specifically for the paediatric age range. Until recently, enteral feeds for children had to be modified by the dietitian using an 'adult' feed as a base, with the addition of extra energy, fluid, vitamins and minerals as necessary to meet the requirements of the individual child. There were many concerns over the adequacy of this practice: time spent in calculations, possible microbial contamination, accuracy of measurement of ingredients and the suitability of the area in which the feed was prepared. This led to the formation of a working party between two of the special groups of the British Dietetic Association: the Paediatric Group and the Parenteral and Enteral Nutrition Group (PENG). They have laid down nutritional guidelines for the use of manufacturers for the production of both whole protein and hydrolysed protein feeds specifically for the 1–5 year age range, weighing 8–20 kg [1]. Despite these recommendations and subsequent production of whole protein paediatric enteral feeds, tube feeding children still requires the knowledge and expertise of the paediatric dietitian and nurse in using both feeds and feeding equipment which relate to the individual requirements and clinical condition of the patient.

ENTERAL FEEDS FOR INFANTS UNDER 12 MONTHS

Breast milk

A mother's breast milk may be given to her own baby. Microbial analysis may be undertaken to assess the bacterial safety (and hence the cleanliness of the collection technique) of the milk and a decision then made as to whether the milk can be used raw or whether it needs to be pasteurized.

Criteria for pasteurizing milk are [2]:

- total count of bacteria exceeding 1×10^5 cfu per ml
- counts of *Staph. aureus*, Streptococci, Lactose fermenting gram negative rods and Pseudomonas species exceeding 1×10^3 cfu per ml.

In the early 1980s the human immunodeficiency virus (HIV) was found to be excreted in breast milk and many milk banks closed. In 1981 the Department of Health and Social Security (DHSS) listed 15 milk banks; now only six are functioning [3]. Pasteurization has now been shown to inactivate the virus [4] and in 1988 the DHSS published specific advice on protecting babies from the accidental transmission of HIV in donated human milk [5]. Pasteurization, however, will also destroy a percentage of the anti-microbial, hormonal and enzymatic factors within the milk [6,7]. Should donor breast milk be given to an infant, records are required to be kept indicating to which patients banked breast milk has been given.

The principal benefits of using breast milk are the presence of immunoglobulins, antimicrobial factors and lipase activity. In addition, there is a psychological benefit to the mother if the only care she can give to her sick child is to provide breast milk. These benefits are counteracted by the possible poorer nutritional quality of the milk, particularly energy density, if there is an inadequate quantity of fat present, which is in higher proportion in the latter part of a breast feed (hind milk). If the child fails to gain weight, breast milk can be supplemented either with energy, in the form of a glucose polymer and fat emulsion, or fortified using infant formula, either cows' milk or peptide based. 'Human milk fortifiers' are also available. In the majority of cases, however, a decision will be made to substitute some or all of the breast milk with a preterm formula (page 57).

Infant milks

Normal infant formulas are suitable for use from birth and during the first 12 months and meet the DHSS guidelines on Artificial Feeds for the Young Infant [8]. They provide an energy density of approximately 65 kcal/100 ml (272 kJ/100 ml) and will be adequate to feed an infant who does not have increased requirements up to 4–6 months of age. However, most infants requiring enteral feeding do have increased needs, for energy at least, in which case they can be supplemented with both carbohydrate and fat. Glucose polymer powders are easier to incorporate into feeds than the liquid preparations available and are not flavoured (Table 1.6). An example of a supplemented infant formula providing 1 kcal/ml (4.2 kJ/ml) is given in Table 3.1.

Table 3.1 Increasing the energy density of an infant formula for enteral feeding

a) Separate energy sources

	Protein g	Fat g	CHO g	Energy kcal	kJ
12.9 g Cow & Gate Premium (3 level scoops)	1.4	3.6	7.5	66	276
5 g Glucose Polymer	–		5.0	20	84
3 ml Calogen + water to a total of 100 ml	–	1.5	–	14	58
Total	1.4	5.1	12.5	100	418

b) Dual energy source

	Protein g	Fat g	CHO g	Energy kcal	kJ
12.9 g Cow & Gate Premium (3 level scoops)	1.4	3.6	7.5	66	276
7 g Duocal powder + water to a total of 100 ml	–	1.6	5.2	34	142
Total	1.4	5.2	12.7	100	418

If an infant requires a feed based on soya protein, a follow-on formula (not before 6 months) or a hydrolysed protein feed, then the same principles apply for the addition of energy supplements. The dual energy source Duocal can also be used to supplement feeds, and should be introduced gradually to tolerance.

Hydrolysed protein/elemental feeds

These are used when an infant does not tolerate the whole protein source in a standard infant milk and requires its provision either in the form of peptides or amino acids (Table 6.13). In addition there may be associated fat malabsorption requiring the use of medium chain triglycerides (MCT) in the feed and a number of these feeds have a proportion of their fat as MCT (Table 6.16).

The energy density of these feeds is between 66–75 kcal/100 ml (276–314 kJ/100 ml) and although their fat and carbohydrate concentrations may differ from a standard infant milk the same general principles apply for energy supplementation of the feed. However, depending on the clinical state of the patient, energy supplements may require introduction at a slower rate.

Modular feeds

Comminuted chicken

This feed is predominantly used in patients with protracted diarrhoea and short gut syndrome where an infant does not tolerate a hydrolysed protein feed. It consists of finely ground chicken meat in water and allows for individual protein, fat and carbohydrate sources to be used. It is not a complete feed and must be both diluted and supplemented with carbohydrate, fat vitamins and minerals. It will take several days to establish a child on a full strength comminuted chicken feed (Table 6.14).

Protein sources

Where a modular type feed is indicated or desirable, other protein sources, such as Maxipro (Table 1.8) or Generaid (page 83), may be used depending on the clinical requirements of the patient. They have the same flexibility in choice of added carbohydrate, fat and vitamin and mineral sources as the comminuted chicken feed.

ENTERAL FEEDS FOR CHILDREN OVER 12 MONTHS

Whole protein

It is feeding the patient in the 1–5 year (8–20 kg) group which, until recently, has required the most significant modifications of feeds because of the lack of a standard paediatric whole protein feed. Previously an adult feed had to be modified (Table 3.2). Initially the protein requirement of a child needs to be established to calculate the amount of the adult feed which is to be used as a base. Then, to obtain the correct energy to protein ratio, additional energy and fluid need to be added to achieve a 1 kcal/ml (4.2 kJ/ml) density. As the adult feed used as a base is effectively diluted, the vitamin and mineral profile will alter depending on the volume used. Supplements therefore need to be given. The nutrients usually affected are vitamin D, the B group of vitamins, sodium, calcium, and zinc. The requirements of the individual child should always be compared with the nutrients provided by the adapted adult feed.

Not only is this adaptation time consuming it also introduces other risks to the sick child. Firstly the use of several components to prepare a suitable feed will increase its osmolality. Secondly most hospitals do not have designated milk rooms or feed preparation areas, the usual area being either the diet kitchen or ward kitchen – neither environment is microbiologically ideal. There is more likelihood of bacterial contamination [9] due to the number of necessary ingredients, the preparation area used and the fact that there may be several individuals involved in feed preparation [10] (especially in a ward kitchen, where it is unlikely that there is one designated nurse involved). Regular microbiological monitoring of feeds should occur as a matter of course, wherever feeds are produced [11].

Following the publication of guidelines for paediatric enteral feeds [1], two feeds were specifically introduced to the United Kingdom market, Nutrison Paediatric and Paediasure. Both feeds are based on cows' milk for their protein source and provide 1 kcal/ml (4.2 kJ/ml) (Table 3.3).

As yet, there have been no recommendations for the child between 5–10 years and this may be addressed now that suitable feeds have been produced for the 1–5 year age group. The requirements of a child over 10 years should be met by the range of adult feeds available [1].

Hydrolysed protein/elemental feeds

These are used when a child does not tolerate a whole protein source, usually cows' milk protein. Guidelines have also been laid down for the approximate composition of a peptide-based feed [1]. Some feeds currently available are Pepdite 2+, MCT Pepdite 2+, Flexical, Peptamen and Elemental 028 (Table 6.15).

FEED TOLERANCE AND ADMINISTRATION

This ultimately depends on the clinical condition of the individual child. Nasogastric, gastrostomy and jejunostomy feeds are usually started at full strength, but commencing with a low rate of infusion and gradually increasing the rate in stages. There is no set starting rate for a paediatric enteral feed as it would depend upon many factors:

- the age and weight of the child
- the child's clinical condition
- the amount of oral intake prior to enteral feeding
- any other fluid infusion, i.e. intravenous hydration or parenteral nutrition
- total fluid requirement and any fluid restrictions.

Table 3.2 Adaptation of adult enteral feed to conform to guidelines from the Joint Working Party of the Paediatric and PEN Groups of the BDA *per 100 ml*

	Protein g	Fat g	CHO g	Energy kcal	kJ	Na mmol	K mmol
65 ml Standard Adult Feed	2.6	2.5	8.0	65	272	2.3	2.3
5.5 g Glucose Polymer	–	–	5.5	21	88	0.1	–
3 ml Fat emulsion + Water to 100 ml	–	1.5	–	14	58	–	–
Total	2.6	4.0	13.5	100	418	2.4	2.3
1988 Guidelines [1]	2.6	4.0	13.5	100	418	2.5	2.5

Plus vitamins and minerals to requirements

Occasionally, a child with persistent diarrhoea may need to be regraded back onto feeds starting with quarter or half strength.

Continuous *vs* bolus feeding

Generally, children will tolerate continuous feeds better than bolus feeds. Continuous feeds will also involve a smaller time commitment for staff and parents. Neonates requiring small volumes may need to be given their feed by hourly bolus because the length of tubing between the reservoir and child creates a 'dead space' holding feed. This is particularly relevant if the baby is being fed expressed breast milk (EBM) as some fat can be lost due to adherence to the sides of the burette and tubing. Essentially, the milk fat separates out rapidly after the infusion is set up so that if the burette is infrequently agitated the infant receives feed with lower energy content initially, which then increases as the upper fatty layer passes through the tubing [12].

A jejunostomy feed must always be given by continuous infusion because of the effect of dumping a bolus within the jejunum. A feed delivered into the stomach utilizes the holding and regulatory function of the stomach which will control the amount of fluid which passes on through the pylorus and into the small bowel. As the jejunum cannot act as a reservoir, jejunostomy feeding must always be regulated by an enteral feeding pump which can continuously deliver the prescribed volume of feed. Complications of abdominal distension, dumping syndrome (which can cause a drop in blood sugar levels and blood pressure, dizziness and tachycardia) and diarrhoea will occur if bolus feeds are given or gravity used, which will not maintain an accurate or slow enough delivery.

Certain feeds are not recommended to be administered by continuous infusion as the feed is not held in suspension. An example would be comminuted chicken as the chicken meat, although finely ground, separates out from the rest of the feed when left to stand and can therefore block the tube. Some other powder based feeds do not remain in solution very well and, although they can be used in tube feeding, the reservoir bag or bottle requires regular agitation to maintain the solution. These feeds tend to be the hypoallergenic feeds where stabilizers have not been added to the formulation since this would limit their clinical use.

A thickener, Nestargel at dilution of 0.5%, has

Table 3.3 Comparison of the two paediatric feeds and the Paediatric and PEN Group Joint Working Party Guidelines [1] per 100 ml

		1988 Guidelines	Nutrison Paediatric (Cow & Gate Nutricia Ltd)	Paediasure (Ross Laboratories, Abbott)
Energy	(kJ)	418	418	418
	(kcal)	100	100	100
Protein	(g)	2.6	2.7	3.0
Fat	(g)	4.0	4.5	5.0
CHO	(g)	13.5	12.2	11.0
Vitamins				
Vit A	(µg)	35	40	77
Vit D	(µg)	0.7	1.0	1.3
Vit C	(mg)	3.0	4.5	10
Riboflavin	(mg)	0.2	0.2	0.2
Thiamin	(mg)	0.15	0.2	0.3
Niacin	(mg)	0.8	0.9	1.7
Pantothenate	(mg)	0.3	0.3	1.0
Vit B6	(mg)	0.09	0.1	0.3
Folic acid	(µg)	12.0	15.0	37
Biotin	(µg)	6.0	7.0	32
Vit B12	(µg)	0.2	0.2	0.6
Vit E	(mg)	0.4	0.6	2.3
Vit K	(µg)	2.0	2.0	3.8
Minerals				
Sodium	(mmol)	2.5	2.5	2.0
Potassium	(mmol)	2.5	2.0	3.3
Phosphorous	(mmol)	1.7	1.8	2.0
Iron	(mg)	0.7	1.0	1.4
Calcium	(mg)	55.0	80.0	98
Magnesium	(mg)	15.0	15.0	20
Iodine	(µg)	6.0	6.0	9.6
Zinc	(mg)	0.7	1.0	1.2
Copper	(mg)	0.1	0.1	0.1
Chromium	(µg)	4.0	1.9	3.0
Manganese	(mg)	0.1	0.1	0.3
Selenium	(µg)	4.0	2.5	2.3
Inositol	(mg)	15.0	–	8
Choline	(mg)	15.0	–	30
Molybdenum	(µg)	5.0	1.5	3.6
Osmolality	(mOsm/kg H₂O)	isotonic	297	320

been used to make a thin gel which can hold a comminuted chicken feed in suspension. In this way it can then be fed continuously using an enteral feeding pump via nasogastric, gastrostomy or, rarely, a jejunostomy tube. Great care needs to be taken with all tubes and regular flushing to avoid blocking is imperative, especially with jejunostomy tubes which tend to be a finer gauge; they have to be surgically inserted and cannot be easily repassed if blocked.

Nasogastric feeding

This is the most common route for enteral feeding and, unless prolonged enteral nutrition is expected, with a normally functioning upper gastrointestinal tract it would be the route of choice [13] (see Fig. 3.1).

All children should have the process of feeding explained to them and there are now a number of booklets which can help [14,15]. Dolls fitted with enteral feeding tubes can also help in a child's understanding. Older children and teenagers are naturally sensitive about their body image and are likely to be reluctant to start long term nasogastric feeding at home. If feasible, however, they may be receptive to a regimen where they can be taught to place their own nasogastric tube each evening to start feeding and to remove it each morning before going to school [13]. In addition to the help of an experienced nurse, it may be of value to introduce the child to another who is using

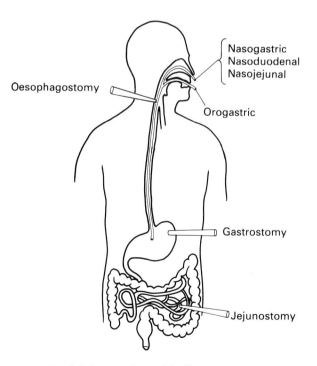

Fig. 3.1 Routes of enteral feeding

this method successfully to enable discussion of concerns and practicalities.

Long term nasogastric feeding in some children may cause inflammation or irritation of the skin on the face where the nasogastric tube is secured with tape. Use of Granuflex (Convalex) or Comfeel (Coloplast) placed onto the skin so that the sticking plaster then secures against it can improve this.

It is essential to ascertain before commencing any nasogastric infusion that the tube is situated in the stomach. The easiest and most common method is to aspirate a small quantity of gastric juice which will turn litmus paper red indicating acidic fluid. Under no circumstances should feeding commence before the tube position has been checked as it is quite possible that the tube could be sited or have re-sited into the bronchus. If ascertaining position by litmus test is unsuccessful, the tube should be withdrawn and repassed and the procedure repeated.

Gastrostomy feeding

This is becoming a more widely used route, especially when long term enteral feeding is required [16,17]. Gastrostomy feeding is generally well accepted with children because it is more comfortable, obviates the need for frequent tube changes and the tube can be hidden by clothes. It also still allows them to take part in normal physical activities such as swimming and sports.

Indications for gastrostomy feeding include children who require extensive, prolonged feeding or have undesirable side effects from nasogastric feeding. This includes children with the following:

- upper gastrointestinal tract abnormalities
- inability to suck or swallow, e.g. developmentally delayed children
- congenital abnormalities such as oesophageal atresia or tracheo-oesophageal fistula
- oesophageal injuries, e.g. following ingestion of caustic soda or chemicals.

Contraindications include children with severe gastro-oesophageal reflux, intractable vomiting or delayed gastric emptying, where gastrostomy feeding would not be of benefit over nasogastric feeding.

Gastrostomy catheters need to be surgically placed and depending on the type used may be secured by a deflatable balloon (which tends to be a simpler procedure when tubes need replacing) or an internal disc or buffer (which may require endoscopic or surgical replacement). If a catheter is inadvertently removed, it should be replaced within 6–8 hours or the tract will start to close.

The main complication of gastrostomy feeding is leakage from around the gastrostomy site. This can cause severe inflammation and time should be spent teaching both parents and child, if appropriate, to care for the site [18].

The percutaneous endoscopic gastrostomy (PEG) method is gaining popularity as a quicker technique with fewer complications, as a general anaesthetic is not necessarily required for its insertion. Once the tract has formed (after about three months) the child may be fitted with a gastrostomy button, which sits almost flush against the skin. This is more popular, particularly with teenagers, as it is far more discreet than the tubing associated with a conventional gastrostomy catheter. The button will need replacing every 9–12 months. Conventional gastrostomy tubes need to be replaced every 6–8 weeks.

Jejunostomy feeding

Indications for jejunostomy feeding include:

- congenital gastrointestinal anomalies
- inadequate gastric motility

- following upper gastrointestinal surgery.

Complications can include bacterial overgrowth, malabsorption, bowel perforation and a blocked tube. Sterile water must be used for flushing the tube as the stomach has been bypassed and great care must be taken with regular flushing to ensure patency of the tube, especially if there is a break in the feeding regimen.

Whole protein feeds may be used, but if there is any degree of malabsorption due to inadequate mixing of the feed with bile and pancreatic juices, a change to a hydrolysed feed will be required.

Table 3.4 summarizes the advantages and disadvantages associated with nasogastric, gastrostomy and jejunostomy feeding.

Nasojejunal feeding

This route is chosen when there is a risk of aspirating gastric contents or the stomach function is inadequate, e.g. poor gastric emptying. Placement of a tube is difficult, having to wait until it passes out of the stomach. Maintaining the position of the tube causes numerous problems as it can often spontaneously re-site into the stomach or be inadvertently pulled back by the patient. Weighted tubes do not seem to be of much value in preventing this occurrence [19]. If nasojejunal feeding is required and the patient is undergoing a surgical procedure, then a jejunostomy

Table 3.4 Advantages and disadvantages of various routes of feed administration

Nasogastric feeds	Gastrostomy feeds	Jejunostomy feeds
Advantages	*Advantages*	*Advantages*
• no surgical procedure required	• percutaneous gastrostomy tubes can be inserted without a general anaesthetic	• no possibility of aspiration
• procedure can be easily taught	• no nightly insertion of tube	• no nightly insertion of tube
• non-invasive		
Disadvantages	*Disadvantages*	*Disadvantages*
• nausea	• nausea	• nausea
• dislodgement of the tubes with coughing	• vomiting associated with coughing and reflux	• tube blockage
• vomiting associated with coughing and reflux	• feeling full	• placed under general anaesthesia
• feeling full	• local infection	• increase risk of nutrient malabsorption
• difficulty in inserting nasogastric tube	• leakage around the tube causing granuloma formation	• leakage around the tube causing granuloma formation
• irritation to the nose and throat	• possibility of aspiration	• local infection
• possibility of aspiration	• tube blockage	• tube dislodgement

By kind permission of A. MacDonald

tube is likely to be placed which is a much easier route of feeding.

Orogastric feeding

This route is not necessarily used in all hospitals. It is principally used for feeding neonates where nasal access is not feasible or respiration would be compromised, e.g. use of nasal oxygen. The tube is passed via the mouth into the stomach either at each feed if infrequent orogastric feeds are given, i.e. the infant is taking breast or bottle at some feeds, or taped in place if all feeds are given via the orogastric tube.

Gastrostomy coupled with oesophagostomy

Patients with tracheo-oesophageal fistulas may, following surgery, be left with a feeding gastrostomy and an oesophagostomy. Whilst the child is then being nutritionally fed via the gastrostomy, he or she can be fed a small amount by mouth to both maintain stimulation and develop oral techniques at normal developmental stages (i.e. milk, purée, lumps, minced). The small amounts given orally are collected at the oesophagostomy site. The child will be assessed surgically as he or she grows with a view to reconnecting the oesophagus and stomach at a later date.

ENTERAL FEEDING EQUIPMENT

Nasogastric enteral feeding tubes

These differ in length and gauge to allow for the different sizes of children, and also in the material from which they are manufactured. They should have a male luer connection to avoid confusion with intravenous connections. They will also have a syringe adapter to use for flushing, aspirating or administering drugs. Some tubes may have separate side ports.

Polyvinylchloride (PVC) tubes

These are used for short term enteral feeding. They should be changed every week as the plasticizers in them leak out and cause the tube to stiffen. They may be changed more frequently when used with neonates. This type of tube is less likely to be displaced than a polyurethane tube.

The patients most suited to this type of tube include:

- children who vomit repeatedly e.g. patients with reflux or receiving chemotherapy
- children with swallowing difficulties
- unconscious patients.

Polyurethane and silicone tubes

These are designed for longer term nasogastric feeding and are very much softer and more comfortable than PVC tubes. Each tube comes with its own guidewire or stylet to allow it to be positioned. These tubes can remain in place for a month before resiting. They can also be used for overnight feeding, removed during the day and repassed again as long as storage and cleaning instructions are adhered to.

Enteral feeding pumps

When enterally feeding adult patients, it is often good enough to administer the feed by gravity as they have larger stomachs in which to hold the feed. Paediatric patients, however, require much closer attention to fluid volume delivered and, therefore, they should be routinely fed using an enteral feeding pump. Use of an enteral feeding pump can also offer other safety features such as alarm systems which can include:

- occlusion alarm – this will detect a lack of flow of feed through the drip chamber and relates either to an obstruction in the feeding tube or completion of feed in the reservoir
- low battery alarm – will indicate when a battery requires charging, for those pumps which can be both mains and battery operated
- alarms indicating inappropriate fitting of the infusion set or inappropriate setting of the feeding rate.

There are a number of enteral feeding pumps on the market which offer different features. Choice of the pump system will depend upon requirements within the hospital or unit or an individual patient. Points to consider include:

- what type of flow rates and increments will be required?

- which alarm systems are essential and which desirable?
- does the patient require the pump to be portable?
- how easy is the pump to operate?

All enteral feeding pumps claim to work within ±10% accuracy of flow rate setting. Pumps should be checked with the medical physics or biomedical engineering department in the hospital initially and then monitored under a regular programme of servicing. Pumps purchased by the community for the long term feeding of patients at home should come under the same system of servicing, either centrally through the hospital or the company from whom it was purchased.

The main advantages of enteral pump feeding are that a feed can be delivered over 24 hours if necessary to achieve tolerance in the individual. During that time more of the prescribed feed is likely to be delivered safely when compared with gravity or bolus feeding, which increase the amount of nursing time involved in either checking or giving the feed. The disadvantage is mobility, even with a battery operated pump, and can be especially difficult in the young child. The cost of purchasing and servicing the pumps is an important consideration.

Reservoirs

There are a number of different reservoirs on the market; glass and plastic bottles, rigid containers which may be pre-filled with a standard feed, plastic bags and burettes. The choice of reservoir will depend upon:

- the feed given – if not a standard feed it will require preparation and then decanting into the reservoir
- the environment – hospital/home; glass bottles are both heavy and dangerous and not advisable for a protable system
- volume required – neonates may only require a few millilitres of feed per hour whereas an older child may need at least 1 litre for the overnight feed.

Glass bottles   these contain a standard feed. They may be suitable for hanging on a hospital ward if no adjustments need to be made to the feed and the child is not mobile.

Plastic bottles   those pre-filled with a standard feed reduce the weight and danger of glass, but still only allow for patients on standard feeds.

Empty rigid bottles   these have more flexibility for using the modified and modular feeds frequently used in paediatrics and may have the flexibility of different sizes. However, they do require an air inlet with a microbial filter.

Plastic bags   these also have more flexibility for modular feeds. Air inlet valves are not required with bags as they collapse as the feed is pumped out. They can be difficult to fill unless they have a rigid neck to help with the procedure. It is also preferable to be able to fill the bag from the top to avoid breaking the connection between reservoir and giving set.

Burettes   these have small capacity and are principally for hospital use, for example in a post-surgical neonate on a small amount of enteral feeds which are complementing a parenteral infusion.

Generally, children tend to require smaller reservoirs than adults, especially when using a portable system. The reservoir and giving set should always be changed every 24 hours and discarded. Any practice of sterilization and re-use potentially leads to infection and is not to be encouraged.

Some units, particularly those caring for immuno-compromised patients may recommend more frequent change of both reservoir and giving set.

Administration sets

Enteral and intravenous systems should be incompatible because of the potential fatal consequence of inadvertent connection of an enteral feed to an intravenous line [20]. Therefore the nasogastric tube should have a male luer end and the administration set a female luer end. As an added safety feature, enteral and intravenous lines should be labelled as such. A drip chamber in line is preferable, otherwise there is the possibility of retrograde bacterial contamination [21].

FEED ADMINISTRATION AT HOME

Continuous, or intermittent continuous feeding of the paediatric patient at home is safe and increasingly used [13]. It can, however, present many practical problems if the child is to continue with long term home feeding. Whilst the young infant is effectively stationary, i.e. in a cot or pushchair, the problems are relatively few as the pump and stand can be placed nearby. However, between the time when the child starts to crawl until he is about 4–5 years old, it is very difficult to continue enteral feeding through the day at home because the child cannot carry any system currently available and certainly will not keep still. One way in which this dilemma can be resolved is to give an extended night feed, so that feeding starts at about 4 PM (whilst the child is occupied with children's television) and continues until 8–10 am, depending on whether there are siblings who need to be taken to school. If the child is established on enteral feeding in hospital, it is usually relatively simple to commence taking him off the feed for a short period during the day and at the same time increasing the feed rate over the remaining hours, until the required regimen is achieved, for example:

Child on 1200 ml total feed/24 hours = 50 ml/hour.

To change over to give 6 hours off during the day:

Day 1 – 55 ml/hour over 22 hours
Day 2 – 60 ml/hour over 20 hours
Day 3 – 65 ml/hour over 18 hours.

Occasionally, children will not tolerate the increased rate required to allow enough time free from the pump, or a longer time off is required for domestic reasons. In these instances, it may be feasible to arrange for 2–3 bolus feeds to be given through the day, with the continuous feed running overnight. Bolus feeding does, however, involve a much greater time commitment from the parents and it is advisable to attempt a break in such feeding initially.

A break in feeding can also help to encourage the child to join in the normal family mealtimes to gain benefit from the socializing that takes place at these times.

It is advisable that any child to be started on home enteral feeding be admitted to hospital for the feed to be initiated [22]. It is most important that the parents be taught how to look after their child safely, the equipment and feed [23]. Correct procedures and adherence to safety is paramount and all parents will require help and supervision to become familiar with the techniques involved.

When the decision has been made that a child will continue with enteral feeding at home it is essential to identify and contact the key community personnel who will be sharing care; general practitioner, paediatric district nurse/district nurse, health visitor, social worker. Early notification will allow community staff to come into the hospital to familiarize themselves with the regimen and equipment and to meet patient, parents and hospital staff. Joint discussions can then also take place on the practicalities of supply and funding of equipment in the community [23].

Home enteral feeding services

These have now been set up for the supply of both feeds and equipment. They will help patients by delivering supplies direct to their homes. Dietitians and nursing staff should also benefit from a reduction in time spent organizing the supplies either from hospital or community budgets, as the delivery systems are still not prescribable by the general practitioner [8]. Use of these services should ensure regular servicing of equipment supplied and also, back-up cover in the event of breakdown and should therefore be considered for those patients on long term home enteral feeding.

REFERENCES

1 Russell C *et al. Paediatric Enteral Feeding Solutions and Systems*. A Report by the joint Working Party of the Paediatric Group and Parenteral and Enteral Group of the British Dietetic Association. Birmingham: BDA, 1988.

2 Sorrento Milk Bank *Protocol for Collection and Processing of Human Milk*. Birmingham: Birmingham Maternity Hospital, Revised 1992.

3 Balmer SE, Wharton BA Human milk banking at Sorrento Maternity Hospital, Birmingham. *Arch Dis Childh*, 1992, **67** 556–559.

4 Eglin RP, Wilkinson AR HIV infection and pasteurisation of breast milk. *Lancet*, 1987, **i** 1093.

5 Department of Health and Social Security *HIV infection, breast feeding and human milk banking*. DH Circular PL/CMO (88)13. London: HMSO, 1988.

6 Evans TJ, Ryley HC, Neace LM *et al*. Effect of storage and heat on antimicrobial proteins in human milk. *Arch Dis Childh*, 1978, **53** 239–241.

7 Department of Health and Social Security Report on Health and Social Subjects No 22. *The Collection and Storage of Human Milk*. London: HMSO, 1981.

8 Department of Health and Social Security Report on Health and Social Subjects No 18. *Artificial Feeds for the Young Infant*. London: HMSO, 1980.

9 Anderton A, Howard JP, Scott DW *Microbiological Control in Enteral Feeding*: A guidance document.

Birmingham: Parenteral and Enteral Nutrition Group of the British Dietetic Association, 1986.

10 Hobbs P Enteral feeds. *Nursing Times*, 1989, 85(9) 71–73.

11 Payne-James JJ Enteral nutrition and the critically ill: infection risk minimisation. *Brit J Intensive Care*, 1991, 1(4) 135–140.

12 Brook OG, Barley J Loss of energy during continuous infusions of breast milk. *Arch Dis Childh*, 1978, 53 344–345.

13 Puntis JWL, Holden CE Home enteral nutrition in paediatric practice. *Brit J Hospital Med*, 1991, 45 104–107.

14 Holden C *et al. Feeding Time with Roo and Joe.* Crawley, Sussex: Sherwood Medical Industries Ltd, 1987.

15 Holden C *et al. Tube Feeding At Home: A Parents' Guide.* Crawley, Sussex: Sherwood Medical Industries Ltd, 1990.

16 Taylor E, Watson A Supplementary feeding using a gastrostomy button. *Paediatric Nursing*, 1990, Dec 16–19.

17 Sidey A The management of gastrostomies. *Paediatric Nursing*, 1991, Sept 24–26.

18 Holden C, Fitzpatrick G *Gastrostomy Care: A Parents' Guide.* Birmingham: Birmingham Childrens Hospital, 1992.

19 Rees RGP *et al.* Spontaneous transpyloric passage and performance of 'fine-bore' polyurethane feeding tubes. A controlled clinical trial. *J Parent Ent Nutr*, 1988, 12 469–472.

20 Ulicny KS, Korelitz UL Multiorgan failure from inadvertent intravenous administration of enteral feeding. *J Parent Ent Nutr*, 1989, 13 658–660.

21 Payne-James JJ *et al.* Retrograde spread of bacteria from enteral tube to diet container. *J Parent Ent Nutr*, 1990, Suppl 14 18S.

22 Lennard-Jones, JE *et al. A Positive Approach to Nutrition as Treatment* London: Kings Fund Centre, 1992.

23 Holden CE *et al.* Nasogastric feeding at home: acceptability and safety. *Arch Dis Childh*, 1991, 66 148–151.

FURTHER READING

Lennard-Jones JE *et al. A Positive Approach to Nutrition as Treatment.* London: Kings Fund Centre, 1992.

Taylor S, Goodinson-McLaren S *Nutritional Support: A Team Approach.* London: Wolfe Publishing Ltd, 1992.

Holden C, Handy D, MacDonald A *Enteral Feeding Protocol*, Birmingham: Birmingham Childrens Hospital, 1991.

Evans-Morris S, Khein M *Pre-feeding Skills.* Tucson, Arizona: Therapy Skill Builders, 1987.

Poskitt EME *Practical Paediatric Nutrition.* London: Butterworth, 1988.

CHAPTER 4

Parenteral Nutrition

There has been little critical assessment of the need for total parenteral nutrition (TPN) or of its advantages over enteral feeding when this is an option [1]. The aims of TPN are to provide all the nutrients required for normal growth and development and to maintain a body composition similar to that of the enterally fed child. Adequate fluid, energy, protein, vitamins, minerals, electrolytes and trace elements should be provided, in an appropriate form to facilitate the aseptic delivery of sterile solutions directly into a vein. TPN is required only when a child is unable to tolerate any enteral nutrition. Improvements in specialized enteral feeds and delivery methods have reduced the need for long term TPN. However, TPN remains a potentially life saving therapy, particularly for infants during intractable diarrhoea or following major gastrointestinal surgery. Major advances in the composition [2,3] of products, techniques of venous access and equipment for the administration of solutions have greatly reduced the incidence of complications. Nevertheless, metabolic, vascular and septic complications still occur in 5–10% of patients, so candidates for TPN should be carefully selected and the indications for parenteral feeding should be clear.

TPN is necessary when:

- The gut is inaccessible, e.g. in tracheo-oesophageal fistula.
- Although accessible, the gut canot be used due to a functional derangement, e.g. an obstruction.
- Complete rest of the gut is indicated, e.g. in necrotizing enterocolitis.

Parenteral nutrition may also be used to provide single or selected nutrients when total requirements cannot be met by enteral feeding alone, due to limited gut function – for example in short gut syndrome.

INDICATIONS FOR PARENTERAL NUTRITION

The most common indications for parenteral nutrition are:

- Major gastrointestinal surgery, e.g. tracheo-oesophageal fistulas, multiple intestinal atresias, malrotation and volvulus, gastroschisis, Hirschprung's disease, short bowel syndrome.
- Low birthweight infants.
- Protracted diarrhoea of infancy and idiopathic failure to thrive syndrome.
- Necrotizing enterocolitis.
- Hypermetabolic states, e.g. severe burns and trauma with paralytic ileus.
- Gastrointestinal fistulas.
- Inflammatory bowel disease.
- Cardiac cachexia.
- Chemotherapy and bone marrow transplant.
- Chronic idiopathic intestinal pseudo-obstruction.

Parenteral nutrition is much more difficult to administer than other intravenous infusions such as dextrose saline. The nutrient solutions are a rich growth medium for micro-organisms, so special preparation facilities are required. The nutrient solutions are also hypertonic – except fat – which means that special techniques are required to maintain venous access.

GENERAL PRINCIPLES OF TPN

(1) Parenteral feeding requires considerable clinical, pharmaceutical and nursing skills as well as special laboratory facilities for biochemical

monitoring using small blood samples. Children who may require prolonged TPN should be cared for by specialized centres where all the necessary facilities are available.

(2) TPN has no advantages over enteral feeding when the gut is functioning. Intravenous feeding is expensive, may be associated with numerous complications [4,5,6] and it is difficult to provide an energy density greater than 1 kcal/ml.

(3) Parenteral feeding is not an emergency procedure. Dehydration, acidosis and other gross electrolyte disturbances should be corrected before TPN commences.

(4) Daily requirements for all nutrients vary according to age and growth rate. Nutritional aims should allow for basal metabolic requirements and the level of physical activity as well as for growth and development. Adjustments should also be made to compensate for previous deficiencies and estimated further losses. Intravenous feeding should always be prescribed individually to meet the needs of each child.

(5) Nutrient requirements for children vary qualitatively as well as quantitatively. Some products have been developed specifically for paediatric use. Where there is a choice, these products are more likely to provide optimal nutritional support and may be associated with fewer metabolic complications than products designed for adult use.

(6) TPN must be built up gradually to allow metabolic adaptation to the infusion of nutrients. During this time, the solution should remain balanced in fluid provision and in energy to nitrogen ratio. With the exception of trace elements, the solution should be nutritionally complete within 3–5 days for effective support.

(7) There is usually little clinical or nutritional justification for prescribing TPN for less than five days.

(8) The complete exclusion of luminal nutrients during TPN is associated with marked atrophic changes in gastrointestinal and pancreatic function. Enteral feeding should begin as soon as possible even if tolerance is limited and the quantity of feed taken is nutritionally insignificant. This is likely to reverse villous atrophy, protect against bacterial colonization and may reduce the risk of cholestasis and long term TPN-induced liver disease.

(9) Maintenance of oral feeding is also important. Severely limited oral intake in infancy may result in delayed oral motor skills, which will affect weaning and speech development. Oral stimulation should be continued by any available methods. The skills of a speech therapist are useful in the management of these children.

(10) Once TPN is established, the time required for the delivery of parenteral infusions may be reduced to between 12–16 hours, depending on the child's age. This allows more freedom for normal play activities and may encourage oral feeding. TPN should always be withdrawn gradually over a few days, to avoid the risk of hypoglycaemia.

NUTRITION TEAMS

A multidisciplinary team approach is the best way of providing consistently safe, appropriate and effective nutritional support.

Members will vary, according to the functions of the nutrition team. Clearly the dietitian has an important role. The following members are also essential for effective parenteral nutrition support:

- a consulatant who oversees patient care
- a surgical registrar who may be solely responsible for the insertion of IV feeding lines and together with a medical registrar, will prescribe all the TPN
- a senior pharmacist who organises production of the intravenous solutions and advises on their content
- an intravenous therapy sister who liaises with the nursing staff to ensure that all procedures related to TPN are performed correctly
- and a senior biochemist who may advise on monitoring procedures and can assist in the interpretation of results.

THE ROLE OF THE DIETITIAN

Patient selection

Paediatric dietitians usually organise the provision of specialized enteral feeds in hospital. Thus the dietitian working with the nutrition team should be able to provide a detailed feeding history of children being referred for TPN. This will enable the team to decide if all enteral feeding options have been given an adequate trial before a child is accepted for parenteral feeding.

Assessing patients' nutritional requirements

Nutritional status should be monitored regularly (see page 3). Nutritional aims should be recorded and reviewed according to the child's progress. Actual nutritional intake (TPN received rather than TPN prescribed, as well as any enteral intake) should be calculated at least weekly, on a three-day intake basis.

Weaning from parenteral to enteral nutrition

An appropriate product should be selected to make best use of existing gut function and to eventually meet the child's nutritional requirements. The most appropriate route and method of administration should be chosen (see page 27). The strength and speed at which enteral feeding may be introduced should then be decided.

Finally, once enteral feeding is successfully established and provides at least 25% of the child's requirements, a corresponding reduction can be made to the TPN solution. Similarly when enteral feeding achieves 50% of his needs, the TPN will be reduced to provide 50% of his needs. Parenteral nutrition should not stop until at least 75% of requirements is provided by the enteral route.

A good account of transitional feeding has previously been published [7].

All children receiving TPN should be seen by the entire team at least weekly, when progress and nutritional adequacy of the TPN can be assessed, alterations to the treatment may be suggested and readiness for enteral feeding can be discussed. Some members of the team will also review patients daily themselves or in consultation with colleagues. For children with severe eating difficulties the advice of a speech therapist and a clinical psychologist may also be helpful.

The development of a team concentrates the involvement and expertise of caring for children on parenteral nutrition. It also limits the number of professionals involved in procedures such as catheter insertion and the prescription of TPN so methods may be standardized and the efficacy of particular practices can be monitored.

In centres where nutrition teams have been established, reported benefits include a reduction in mechanical line problems, reduced sepsis, fewer metabolic complications, shorter courses of parenteral feeding (due to faster transition to appropriate enteral formulas) and savings on the cost of providing parenteral nutrition [8].

NUTRIENT REQUIREMENTS AND SOLUTIONS

There is no comprehensive guide to the nutritional requirements of infants and children receiving TPN. Nutrient intakes vary at different centres and recommendations tend to be based on clinical experience. A number of centres have described their practices in detail [1,2,9,10,11]. Other reports provide a useful guide to the subject [3,12,13].

Fluid

Basal daily fluid requirements and other factors affecting fluid needs are described in detail elsewhere [13]. Age, size, fluid balance, the environment and underlying disease are all factors which alter fluid requirements [11,13]. For example, neonatal surgery, renal, cardiac and respiratory diseases may all limit available fluid volume; high losses due to diarrhoea, high output fistulas and fever may increase fluid needs.

The fluid allowance should always be determined first. Available fluid volume may influence choice of nutrient solutions as well as the route of administration. Children who are severely fluid restricted will only receive adequate nutrition if lipid and concentrated dextrose solutions are infused via a central venous catheter.

Normal fluid requirements [13]

Infants up to 10 kg:
    0–6 months   150 ml/kg/day
    6–12 months   110 ml/kg/day
the volume may be increased by 10 ml/kg/day until the required energy intake is achieved (maximum 200 ml/kg/day if tolerated).

Children over 10 kg:
>   11–20 kg: 1000 ml plus 50 ml/kg for each kg above 10 kg
>   21–30 kg: 1500 ml plus 20 ml/kg for each kg above 20 kg
>   31–50 kg: 100 ml/hour (2.4 litres/day)
>   >50 kg: 125 ml/hour (3.0 litres/day).

MACRONUTRIENT REQUIREMENTS

Energy

Most infants and children will achieve their expected growth rate if the energy intakes in Table 4.1 are provided. An energy:nitrogen ratio of approximately 250:1 is required to promote positive nitrogen balance.

Energy requirements may vary by up to 15% in illness [1]. A steady weight gain of 100–150 g per week is likely to indicate that the prescription is adequate.

Certain conditions are likely to increase energy needs. These include fever, sepsis, burns, trauma, major surgery and long term growth failure [1]. It is difficult to estimate additional energy requirements for children with these conditions. Intakes of 150% of the recommended intake may be needed following long term growth failure or severe burns [12]. However, patients rarely need such high intravenous energy prescriptions.

One study [14] found that actual energy and protein

Table 4.1 Estimated average requirements (EAR) for energy and protein

Age	Mean weight (a) kg	Energy intake (b) kcal/kg/day	Protein intake (c) g/kg/day	Nitrogen intake (d) g/kg/day
0–3 months	5.0	115	2.9	0.46
4–12 months	8.3	95	2.4	0.38
1–3 years	12.1	95	2.4	0.38
4–6 years	18.0	85	2.1	0.34
7–10 years	26.7	66	1.7	0.26
11–14 years	40.0	47	1.2	0.19
15–18 years	60.0	41	1.0	0.16

(a) Adapted from Annex 1 (Table 1.2) (DRVs)
(b) Derived from [34] (WHO)
(c) Based on 10% energy intake from protein
(d) Nitrogen intake (g) = $\dfrac{\text{protein intake (g)}}{6.25}$

requirements in children with acute non-lymphocytic leukaemia were significantly less than estimated requirements. Physical activity was thought to be reduced by the illness and their confinement to a laminar air flow unit. Clearly, reduced physical activity may offset the expected increase in energy requirements of very sick children.

Energy sources

Glucose and fat should both be used as non-protein energy sources. Although the use of intravenous fat emulsions has been associated with certain complications [15], such as acute allergic reaction, altered immune function and fat overload syndrome, the use of glucose as the sole energy source is no longer recommended. The latter caused problems such as hyperglycaemia, fluid retention, fatty infiltration of the liver [16], excessive carbon dioxide production [18] and essential fatty acid deficiency. In addition, the use of a balanced glucose-lipid regimen has been shown to reduce whole body protein turnover and produce higher net protein synthesis rates when compared to glucose alone [18].

Carbohydrate

The most important source of non-protein energy in parenteral nutrition is dextrose (D-glucose). Solutions which contain 5%, 10% and 50% glucose are mixed to provide any desired concentration. The energy content and approximate osmolality of various glucose concentrations is shown in Table 4.2. Glucose is an essential fuel in infants and is the most important substrate for brain cell metabolism. A continuous supply is essential for normal neurological function. Dextrose solutions have a high osmolality so most centres use 10% dextrose on the first day of TPN. The concentration of dextrose may then be increased daily as required, in a slow, stepwise manner, in

Table 4.2 Intravenous carbohydrate solutions

Solution	Energy kcal/l	Osmolality mOsm/kg
5% Dextrose	200	277
10% Dextrose	400	555
20% Dextrose	800	1110
50% Dextrose	2000	2775

1–2% increments if a central line is used. (Peripheral infusions do not usually contain more than 10% dextrose due to the increased risk of thrombophlebitis). A gradual increase in dextrose concentration allows time for an increase in the rate of endogenous insulin production which reduces the risk of glycosuria and osmotic diuresis [19].

The amount of glucose that can be directly oxidized to meet a child's energy needs is limited. Reports have suggested that infusion rates should not exceed 7 mg/kg/minute initially [20], but can be increased to 12–14 mg/kg/minute after 5–7 days feeding [1]. Total glucose intake should not exceed 18 g/kg/day [21].

Higher infusion rates result in conversion of carbohydrate to fatty acids. This process consumes up to 15% of available glucose energy [22]. As a guide, energy from carbohydrate should not exceed 60% of non-protein energy.

Fat

Intravenous fat preparations provide a concentrated source of energy in an isotonic solution. If the fluid intake is not restricted, the use of a fat emulsion will provide sufficient energy for growth via a peripheral vein. This avoids the complications associated with central venous access [23] and may prolong the life of peripheral lines in infants [24].

When fluid volume is limited, maximum energy intake can be achieved via a central venous catheter, by using up to 20% dextrose solutions along with intravenous fat. Lipid emulsions should normally contribute 30–40% of non-protein energy and should not exceed 50% of total energy.

A range of products which are similar in composition are available in the UK. All contain soybean oil with added glycerol and phospholipids and each product is available in 10% and 20% emulsions. These provide 1.1 and 2 kcal/ml respectively and are shown in Table 4.3.

The recommended intake of fat is 0.5–4.0 g/kg/day, providing serum lipids remain in the acceptable range. Clearance of lipids from the plasma is limited by the rate of activity of lipoprotein lipase. Hyperlipidaemia (>1.8 mg plasma triglycerides per litre) will result if the enzyme is saturated by excessive doses of fat or by rapid infusion. Maximum fat tolerance will be achieved by gradually increasing the volume of lipid emulsion by 1 g/kg/day over 4–5 days and by main-

taining a slow, steady rate of infusion over a 20 hour period so that all the administered fat should have cleared the circulation before the next infusion begins.

Serum lipids should be monitored regularly as the volume of fat increases and should always be taken four hours after the infusion is completed. (Peak levels of triglyceride and free fatty acids normally occur at the end of an infusion, returning to fasting levels 2–4 hours later [6]). Thereafter weekly monitoring is sufficient. It may also be useful to test baseline serum lipids prior to starting TPN. Children with failure to thrive frequently have raised triglyceride levels which return to normal when sufficient energy is provided.

A reduced dose of fat (0.5–2.0 g/kg/day) is usually recommended for children with hyperbilirubinaemia, sepsis, impaired immune function, blood coagulopathies, chronic liver failure and for very low birth-weight infants.

These products also provide a rich source of essential fatty acids, stores of which are limited in young infants. Biochemical evidence of deficiency has been noted after receiving fat-free TPN for only two days [24], yet essential fatty acid deficiency can be avoided by giving only 2–4% total energy as lipid emulsion. For example:

- 2.5 ml/kg/day of Intralipid 20% will provide 0.5 g fat/kg and 5% total energy for an infant
  i.e.
  2.4% total energy from n6 linoleic acid
  (Reference Nutrient Intake 1%)
  0.4% total energy from n3 linolenic acid
  (Reference Nutrient Intake 0.2%).

Therefore, even when fat tolerance is impaired, essential fatty acid deficiency can be avoided in most children.

The topical application of sunflower oil to prevent essential fatty acid deficiency remains controversial [26,27].

A 20% fat emulsion is usually used in infants and children since it contains half the amount of phospholipids per gram of fat compared to a 10% solution. Phospholipids are known to inhibit the activity of lipoprotein lipase.

Carnitine

Carnitine is not included in the parenteral solutions currently available. Compared with orally fed infants

Table 4.3 Intravenous fat emulsions–composition per litre

		Intralipid	
		Intralipid 20%	Intralipid 10%
Soybean oil	(g)	200	100
Phospholipid	(g)	12	12
Glycerol	(g)	22.5	22.5
Osmolality	(mOsm/kg)	350	300
kJ/kcal		8400/2000	4600/1095
		Lipofundin S	
		Lipofundin S 20%	Lipfundin S 10%
Soybean oil	(g)	200	100
Phospholipid	(g)	15	7.5
Glycerol	(g)	25	25
Osmolality	(mOsm/kg)	340	380
kJ/kcal		8520/2035	4470/1068
		Lipofundin MCT/LCT	
		Lipofundin MCT/LCT 20%	Lipofundin MCT/LCT 10%
Soybean oil	(g)	100	50
Medium chain triglycerides	(g)	100	50
Phospholipid	(g)	12	12
Glycerol	(g)	25	25
Osmolality	(mOsm/kg)	390	330
kJ/kcal		7990/1908	4430/1058
		Ivelip	
		Ivelip 20%	Ivelip 10%
Soybean oil	(g)	200	100
Phospholipid	(g)	12	12
Glycerol	(g)	25	25
Osmolality	(mOsm/kg)	360	310
kJ/kcal		8400/2000	4600/1095
		Soyacal	
		Soyacal 20%	Soyacal 10%
Soybean oil	(g)	200	100
Phospholipid	(g)	12	12
Glycerol	(g)	22.1	22.1
Osmolality	(mOsm/kg)	322	285
kJ/kcal		8400/2000	4600/1095

of similar gestational age, infants receiving carnitine-free TPN have lower plasma carnitine levels and lower levels of urinary carnitine excretion [28]. Children receiving long term TPN also have markedly reduced levels of plasma carnitine [29].

Carnitine supplementation may enhance keto-genesis and fat clearance and may improve nitrogen balance and weight gain in previously carnitine deficient infants [30,31]. However some studies have demonstrated no adverse effects on triglyceride and free fatty acid metabolism where blood and plasma concentrations of carnitine were much lower than expected [29]. They have also shown no significant improvement in the metabolism of fat emulsions accompanied by a carnitine supplement [32].

Protein

Crystalline l-amino acid solutions are used as the nitrogen source for parenteral nutrition. The amino acid composition of these products is modelled on a protein source of high biological value. The products listed in Table 4.4 have resulted in improved nitrogen utilization and reduced hyperammonaemia compared to the earlier protein hydrolysates.

The protein intakes suggested in Table 4.1 will be adequate for most children's needs. Nitrogen balance studies provide the best method of quantifying nitrogen requirements in sick children.

The ideal amino acid profile for parenteral feeding solutions in infants and children remains unclear [33]. Requirements for specific amino acids vary with age [34]; however in addition to the eight amino acids which are considered essential in adults, histidine, tyrosine, cystine and taurine are also required during infancy. Proline and alanine may also be 'semi-essential' [10].

A solution which contains insufficient quantities of essential amino acids will inhibit protein synthesis and may limit growth. Alternatively a solution which contains excessive amounts of an amino acid, such as glycine or phenylalanine, may result in hyperamino-acidaemia and even metabolic complications, leading to coma and brain damage. Plasma aminograms should therefore be checked regularly.

Most nitrogen sources have been designed for adult use. Of these Vamin (Kabi Pharmacia) has been considered the most appropriate solution for use in children (see Table 4.4). However Vamin has a high phenylalanine content and some centres have reported hyperphenylalaninaemia in neonates [8]. Vamin 9 contains 9.4 g nitrogen per litre. The dose is gradually increased over 3–5 days, from 15 ml/kg/day up to 40 ml/kg/day (0.38 gN/kg/day) [10,35].

Recently two products have become available for use in infants [36,37]. Vaminolact (Kabi Pharmacia) is based on the amino acid composition of breast milk and Primene (Clintec Nutrition Ltd) is based on the amino acid profile of cord blood. Thus, unlike other products available in the UK, these solutions contain taurine, which is essential for retinal development and normal bile acid metabolism [38,39]. Vaminolact contains 9.3 g nitrogen per litre and may be increased daily in a stepwise manner from 15 ml/kg/day to 40 ml/kg/day (0.37 gN/kg/day). Primene contains 15 g nitrogen per litre, so a smaller dose of up to 25 ml/kg/day (0.38 gN/kg/day) will cover most infants' requirements. Primene may be useful therefore when a moderate fluid restriction is indicated.

MICRONUTRIENT REQUIREMENTS

The exact intravenous requirements for micronutrients remains unclear [40]. Electrolyte requirements vary with age, clinical condition and blood biochemistry. The need for electrolytes is discussed in detail elsewhere [12,13]. Individual electrolyte solutions are usually added, to provide the exact requirements of each child. Increased amounts of calcium, phosphorous, magnesium, iron, copper, zinc, sodium and potassium are needed during growth so requirements are considered greatest in the first year of life [9].

Specific guidelines have been produced [41], based on previous reports [42,43] and currently available research. These guidelines for micronutrient intakes appear to maintain blood levels within acceptable

Table 4.4 Amino acid solutions for use in infants and children

| | Nitrogen g/l | Non-protein energy kcal/l | Electrolytes mmol/l | | | | | |
			K+	Mg2+	Na+	Cl−	Ca2+	Acetate−
Vamin 9	9.4	–	20	1.5	50	55	2.5	–
Vamin 9 Glucose	9.4	400	20	1.5	50	55	2.5	–
Vaminolact	9.3	–	–	–	–	–	–	–
Primene	15.0	–	–	–	–	15.6	–	25

Table 4.5 Guidelines for micronutrient requirements per day in term infants and children

Micronutrient		Recommended Intake
Sodium	(mmol/kg/day)	2–5
Potassium	(mmol/kg/day)	2–3
Chloride	(mmol/kg/day)	2–5
A	(μg)	500
D	(μg)	4.0
E	(mg)	2.8
K	(μg)	80.0
C	(mg)	25.0
B1	(mg)	0.35
B2	(mg)	0.15
B6	(mg)	0.18
Niacin	(mg)	6.8
B12	(μg)	0.3
Biotin	(μg)	6.0
Pantothenate	(mg)	2.0
Folate	(μg)	56.0
Iron		*

Copper	μg/kg/day	20	{300}
Selenium	μg/kg/day	2.0	{30}
Chromium	μg/kg/day	0.2	{5.0}
Manganese	μg/kg/day	1.0	{50.0}
Molybdenum	μg/kg/day	0.25	{5.0}
Iodide	μg/kg/day	1.0	{1.0}

		Infants	Children >1 year
Calcium	mg/l	500–600	200–400
Phosphorus	mg/l	400–450	150–300
Magnesium	mg/l	50–70	20–40
Zinc	μg/kg/day	<3 mths: 250	
		>3 mths: 100	50 {5000}

Adapted from [43]

Key { } = Maximum total intake
*   See explanation in text

ranges for children and infants, both on short term and long term TPN [44,45,46]. A summary is provided in Table 4.5.

Vitamins

Intravenous requirements for vitamins are generally higher than recommended enteral intakes. Adsorption to plastic TPN bags and giving sets [47], along with biodegradation due to light exposure may drastically reduce the child's vitamin intake. Vitamin A is most affected by these problems. A study using radiolabelled

vitamins in parenteral nutrition showed that only 31% vitamin A, 64% vitamin E and 68% vitamin D were received by the patient [48].

MVC 9 + 4 Paediatric (Lymphomed) is the only combined water and fat soluble vitamin preparation designed for children. Alternatively, Solivito N (Kabi Pharmacia) and Vitlipid N Infant (Kabi Pharmacia) may be used together. The recommended intakes provided by these products are shown in Table 4.6.

Trace elements

Trace element deficiencies have been described in neonates receiving TPN [49] so supplements are essential in long term feeding [50,51]. Requirements for trace elements vary: high fluid losses result in greater losses of magnesium and zinc whereas obstructive jaundice reduces requirements for copper and manganese (which are normally excreted in bile). Serum levels of trace elements should be measured before the child starts TPN, and three monthly thereafter.

Trace element mixtures are usually avoided in the first week of life to avoid toxic accumulation. Many centres add trace elements only if the child is fed parenterally for longer than a month.

Three solutions are currently used in children. Their composition is given is Table 4.7.

Pedel (Kabi Pharmacia) is the only trace element solution designed for use in infants and young children. The recommended dose is 4 ml/kg/day up to a maximum of 40 ml. It does not contain selenium and is low in zinc, so these trace elements must be added individually if plasma levels are low, or if a child is on long term TPN. Pedel does contain iron in higher concentrations than the adult trace element solutions, but even this product may not meet a child's needs. Intravenous iron supplementation is controversial due to the risk of adverse effects. Excess iron may enhance the risk of gram-negative septicaemia. Iron also has powerful oxidative properties and may increase demand for antioxidants such as Vitamin E. Iron-dextran preparations are rarely added to the intravenous solution, due to poor solubility and risk of anaphylaxis so additional iron is usually given by 'top-up' blood transfusions when required. Some centres do add low doses to parenteral nutrition for children on long term TPN, which reduces the risks of complications. Suggested doses vary from 0.1–0.15 mg/kg/day iron dextran [1,13].

Addamel (Kabi Pharmacia) may be used when

Table 4.6 Intravenous multivitamin preparations recommended for paediatric use

Vitamins		Solivito N* 10 ml	Solivito N* 1 ml	Vitlipid N Infant** 10 ml	Vitlipid N Infant** 1 ml	Paediatric MVC 9+4# 5 ml	Paediatric MVC 9+4# 3.25 ml
Thiamin	mg	3.2	0.32	–	–	1.2	0.78
Riboflavin	mg	3.6	0.36	–	–	1.4	0.91
Nicotinamide	mg	40.0	4.0	–	–	17.0	11.05
Pyridoxine	mg	4.0	0.4	–	–	1.0	0.65
Pantothenic Acid	mg	15.0	1.5	–	–	5.0	3.25
Biotin	µg	60.0	6.0	–	–	20.0	13.00
Folic Acid	mg	0.4	0.04	–	–	0.14	0.09
Cyanocobalamin	µg	5.0	0.5	–	–	1.0	0.65
Ascorbic Acid	mg	100.0	10.0	–	–	80.0	52.00
Vitamin A	µg	–	–	690	69.0	700.0	455.00
Vitamin D	µg	–	–	10	1.0	10.0	6.50
Vitamin K	µg	–	–	200	20.0	200.0	130.00
Vitamin E	mg	–	–	6.4	0.64	7.0	4.55

* Solivito N (Kabi Pharmacia)
  Dose 1 ml/kg/day (Maximum 10 ml)
** Vitlipid N Infant (Kabi Pharmacia)
  Dose 1 ml/kg/day (Maximum 10 ml)
\# MVC 9+4 Paediatric (Lymphomed)
  Dose 1–3 kg: 3.25 ml/day
      >3 kg: 5 ml/day

Table 4.7 Intravenous trace element solutions

		Pedel* 40 ml	Pedel* 4 ml	Addamel** 10 ml	Addamel** 0.5 ml	Additrace# 10 ml	Additrace# 0.5 ml
Calcium	mmol	6.0	0.6	5.0	0.25	–	–
Magnesium	mmol	1.0	0.1	1.5	0.08	–	–
Iron	µmol	20.0	2.0	50.0	2.50	20.0	1.0
Zinc	µmol	6.0	0.6	20.0	1.0	100.0	5.0
Manganese	µmol	10.0	1.0	40.0	2.0	5.0	0.25
Copper	µmol	3.0	0.3	5.0	0.25	20.0	1.0
Fluoride	µmol	30.0	3.0	50.0	2.5	50.0	2.5
Iodine	µmol	0.4	0.04	1.0	0.05	1.0	0.05
Phosphate	µmol	3000.0	300.0	–	–	–	–
Chloride	mmol	14.0	1.4	13.3	0.67	–	–
Sorbitol	mg	12.0	1.2	3.0	0.15	3000.0	150.0
Chromium	µmol	–	–	–	–	0.2	0.01
Selenium	µmol	–	–	–	–	0.4	0.02
Molybedenum	µmol	–	–	–	–	0.2	0.01

* Pedel (Kabi Pharmacia)
  Dose 4 ml/kg/day (Maximum 40 ml)
** Addamel (Kabi Pharmacia)
  Dose 0.25–0.5 ml/kg/day (Maximum 10 ml)
\# Additrace (Kabi Pharmacia)
  Dose 0.25–0.5 ml/kg/day (Maximum 10 ml)

infants attain one year of age and outgrow Pedel. It is a more concentrated source of trace elements so less fluid is used to provide the required intake. The suggested dose is 0.25–0.5 ml/kg/day (maximum dose 10 ml/day). Addamel does not contain phosphate so this must be added separately.

Additrace (Kabi Pharmacia) may be used in older children from 5–6 years. This product contains selenium with higher concentrations of zinc and copper. The suggested dose is 0.25–0.5 ml/kg/day (maximum dose 10 ml/day). It does not contain calcium, magnesium or phosphate so these minerals must be added separately.

ADMINISTRATION OF TPN

A detailed account of the techniques of TPN administration is available elsewhere [19,52].

Vascular access

TPN may be infused via a peripheral or scalp vein, or via a central venous catheter. Each route has advantages along with the risk of complications [53,54,55].

Peripheral lines are rarely associated with septicaemia and may be useful in short term TPN (7–10 days) when the fluid intake is not restricted and venous access is good. One major disadvantage is the risk of thrombophlebitis which occurs due to fibrin formation around the line, caused by the hypertonic solutions used for feeding. Infiltration is also a common problem: the peripheral line may penetrate the surrounding tissues resulting in leaking of the infusion. The pool of escaping fluid from the peripheral line into the surrounding tissues is known as extravasation. If undetected, this may cause severe tissue necrosis and scarring. The drip site must therefore be inspected frequently and changed regularly. Drips must be resited quickly to avoid the risks of rebound hypoglycaemia and suboptimal nutritional intake.

Central venous catheters (Broviac/Hickman silastic catheters) allow the infusion of much more concentrated solutions, so less fluid volume is required. These catheters are introduced into the superior vena cava via the subclavian vein, burrowing under the skin to provide a point of exit for the catheter remote from the site of energy to the vein. Silicone catheters such as these have a lower sepsis rate and inhibit fibrin formation so are less likely to block. The catheters are

tunnelled a few inches under the skin and have a subcutaneous Dacron cuff which helps to hold them in place. A central line infusion is more likely to supply sufficient energy for growth than a peripheral one. In addition, it can remain in place for months and allows free arm movement, so it is more suitable for long term TPN. The major disadvantage of central venous access is catheter-related sepsis. The incidence of sepsis varies according to insertion techniques and methods of catheter care [54]. One recent study highlighted the importance of specially trained nursing staff in reducing the incidence of catheter-related sepsis [56]. Nursing practice is probably a major factor in sepsis rate.

Peripherally inserted fine silastic central venous catheters (peripheral long lines) are often used in neonates. These have the advantages of long term venous access with a relatively simple insertion technique [3], which is similar to the procedure for peripheral venous cannulation, compared to the surgical procedure for insertion of central venous catheters. Insertion can be performed at the bedside, using the anti-cubital or temporal veins. The catheter tip must be positioned in the superior vena cava or upper right atrium, so these operate as effectively as central lines [57]. One disadvantage is the risk of dislodgement if it is not sutured in place.

Only parenteral nutrition should be given from a single lumen catheter. Separate venous access is then required for blood, plasma and drugs. Double lumen catheters are usually inserted when intravenous drug therapy and TPN are both required.

DELIVERY METHODS

Parenteral nutrition can be provided by a variety of systems [19,52]. The method of choice for use in infants and children is the 'big bag' system in which amino acids and dextrose are mixed and delivered simultaneously over 24 hours. The fat emulsion is delivered from a separate container but mixes with the amino acid and dextrose solution as close as possible to the peripheral or central line.

This system allows optimal utilization of all nutrients. In addition it reduces the frequency of line disconnections, saves nursing time and may reduce sepsis rates [19].

Some adult centres use 'all in one' mixes (containing amino acids, dextrose and lipids). These are difficult to produce in a stable form for children, so are rarely

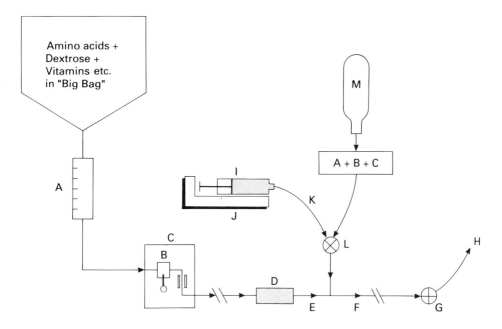

Key

A Burette administration set (used to monitor the volumetric accuracy of the pump)

B Cassette

C Volumetric pump

D Air-eliminating filter (0.2 μm) with an injection port below the filter

E Y-connector

F Fine bore extension tubing (allows freedom of movement)

G One way tap

H Short 25 cm extension tubing (permanently attached to the catheter and **G**)

I Syringe 60 ml, filled with fat emulsion

J Syringe pump

K Fine bore extension tubing

L One way tap

M Bottle of fat emulsion: alternative administration to **I** and **J** for older children, with larger volumes of fat

All connections are 'luer lock'

Note All apparatus **A** to **F** must be changed daily.

Adapted from [58]

Fig. 4.1 Equipment required for intravenous feeding

used in paediatrics. Another disadvantage of this system is that solutions containing lipids cannot be filtered.

Big bags require preparation in a pharmacy where special facilities and trained staff are available. Skill is required in compounding these solutions to ensure sterility and stability of the product, as well as optimal nutrient availability.

A TPN compounding room, containing a laminar air flow unit is used to transfer accurately measured quantities of sterile solutions into another sterile, sealed plastic bag. Although aseptic technique is used throughout the process, the number of additions to the bag should be kept to a minimum to reduce the risk of microbial contamination.

Specialist computer programs are used to ensure that the nutrient content of the bag is appropriate for the age, condition and biochemistry of each child. They can also be used to ensure nutrient stability and to avoid drug-nutrient interactions [19].

The parenteral solution is supplied premixed in a collapsible bag. An opaque plastic cover is used to protect vitamins in the big bag from photodegradation. When low rates of infusion are prescribed and the solution will remain in the burette for long periods, yellow, light protective sets (Avon Medicals Ltd) are also used [19].

EQUIPMENT

A constant flow rate should be maintained when infusing intravenous nutrients. Hyperglycaemia and fat overload syndrome will result if infusions are delivered too quickly. Alternatively the line may occlude and rebound hypoglycaemia may occur if the infusion slows down or stops. Various methods to control flow rate exist but only volumetric infusion pumps are sufficiently accurate for use in children. Examples include IMED 960 (Kabi Pharmacia) and IVAC 565 (IVAC). These machines pump measured volumes of solution through a cassette with a syringe mechanism so that the required volume is always delivered in the specified time.

Syringe pumps such as the MS2000 (Graseby Medical) are as accurate as volumetric pumps, but are more convenient to use when small volumes of solution are to be infused. These have a linear drive mechanism and can be set to deliver as little as 0.5 ml per hour.

The use of filters is recommended during intravenous infusion. Filters will remove any bacterial or fungal contamination and will prevent air embolism and entry of particulate matter. They must be inserted proximal to the point where lipid enters the line. Lipid emulsions cannot be filtered as the lipid molecules are generally larger than the filter pore size (0.2 μm).

A diagram showing all equipment required for TPN is shown in Fig. 4.1.

REFERENCES

1 Zlotkin SH, Stallings VA, Pencharz PB Total parenteral nutrition in children. *Paediatr Clin North Am*, 1985, **32**(2) 381–400.
2 Harries JT Intravenous feeding in infants. *Arch Dis Childh*, 1971, **46** 855–862.
3 Evans TJ, Cockburn F Parenteral feeding. In: McLaren DS, Burman D (eds.) *Textbook of Paediatric Nutrition*, 2nd edn. Edinburgh: Churchill Livingstone, 1990: 337–354.
4 Freund HR, Rimon B Sepsis during TPN. *J Parent Ent Nutr*, 1990, **14**(1) 39–41.
5 Pennington CR Parenteral nutrition: the management of complications. *Clin Nutr*, 1991, **10**(3) 133–137.
6 Drowgowski RA, Coran AG An analysis of factors contributing to the development of TPN – induced cholestasis. *J Parent Ent Nutr*, 1989, **13**(6) 586–589.
7 Braunshweig CL, Wesley JR, Mercer N Rationale and guidelines for parenteral and enteral transition feeding of the 3-to-30 kg child. *J Am Diet Assoc*, 1988, **88**(4) 479–482.
8 Puntis JWL, Booth IW The place of a nutritional care team in paediatric practice. *Inten Ther Clin Mon*, 1990, July/August 132–136.
9 Easton LB, Halata MS, Dweck HS Parenteral nutrition in the newborn: a practical guide. *Paediatr Clin North Am*, 1982, **29**(5) 1171–1190.
10 Candy DCA Parenteral nutrition in paediatric practice: a review. *J Hum Nutr*, 1980, **34** 287–296.
11 Cochran EB, Phelps SJ, Helms RA Parenteral nutrition in paediatric patients. *Clin Pharmacol*, 1988, **7** 351–366.
12 Kerner JA (ed.) *Manual of Pediatric Parenteral Nutrition.* New York: John Wiley, 1983.
13 Kerner JA Parenteral nutrition. In: Walker WA, Durie PA (eds.) *Paediatric Gastrointestinal Disease*, 1991, **41**(7) 1645–1675. BC Decker Inc, USA.
14 Merritt RJ *et al*. Calorie and protein requirements with acute non lymphocytic leukaemia. *J Parent Ent Nutr*, 1981, **4** 20–25.
15 Maynard ND Postoperative feeding. *Brit Med J*, 1991, **303**(26) 1007–1008.
16 Burke JF *et al*. Glucose requirements following burn injury. Parameters of optimal glucose infusion and possible hepatic and respiratory abnormalities following excessive glucose intake. *Ann Surg*, 1979, **190** 274–285.
17 Askanazi J *et al*. Respiratory changes induced by the large glucose loads of total parenteral nutrition. *J Am Med Assoc*, 1980, **243** 1444–1447.
18 Bresson JL *et al*. Protein metabolism kinetics and energy substrate utilisation in infants fed parenteral solutions with different glucose-fat ratios. *Am J Clin Nutr*, 1991, **54** 370–376.
19 Taylor C, Nunn T, Rangecroft L Parenteral nutrition for infants and children. In: Grant A, Todd E (eds.) *Enteral and Parenteral Nutrition*, 2nd edn. Oxford: Blackwell Scientific Publications, 1987.
20 Sauer P *et al*. Glucose oxidation in neonates, indirect calorimetry or stable isotopes? *Paediatr Res*, 1984, **18** 804 (Abstract 45).
21 Jones MO *et al*. The effect of glucose intake on substrate utilisation and energy expenditure in the surgical newborn infant. *Proc Nut Soc*, 1992, (Abstract 09).
22 Sauer P *et al*. Substrate utilisation of newborn infants fed intravenously with or without a fat emulsion. *Paediatr Res*, 1984, **18** 804 (Abstract 46).
23 Jakabowski D, Ziegler MD, Pereira G Complications of paediatric parenteral nutrition: central versus peripheral administration. *J Parent Ent Nutr*, 1979, **3** 29–32.
24 Phelps SJ, Cochrane EC, Kamper CA Peripheral venous line infiltration in infants receiving 10% dextrose, 10% dextrose/amino acids, 10% dextrose/amino acids/fat emulsion. *Paediatr Res*, 1987, **21** (Abstract 67A).
25 Friedman Z *et al*. Rapid onset of essential fatty acid deficiency in the newborn. *Paediatr*, 1976, **58** 640.
26 Press M, Hartop PJ, Protley C Correction of essential fatty acid deficiency in man by the cutaneous application of sunflower seed oil. *Lancet*, 1974, 597–599.

27 Hunt CE *et al*. Essential fatty acid deficiency in neonates: inability to reverse deficiency by topical application of essential fatty acid rich oil. *J Paediatr*, 1978, **92** 603–607.

28 Schiff D *et al*. Plasma carnitine levels during intravenous feeding of the neonate. *J Paediatr*, 1979, **95** 1043–1046.

29 Dahlstrom KA *et al*. Low blood and plasma carnitine levels in children receiving long term parenteral nutrition. *J Paed Gastr Nutr*, 1990, **11** 375–379.

30 Helms RA *et al*. Effect of intravenous L Carnitine on growth parameters and fat metabolism during parenteral nutrition in neonates. *J Parent Ent Nutr*, 1990, **14**(5) 448–53.

31 Christensen ML *et al*. Plasma carnitine concentration and lipid metabolism in infants receiving parenteral nutrition. *J Paediatr*, 1989, **115** 794–798.

32 Stahl GE, Spear ML, Hamosh M Intravenous administration of lipid emulsions to premature infants. *Clin Perinatol*, 1986, **13** 33.

33 Jackson AA Amino acids: essential and non essential. *Lancet*, 1983, May 7 1034–1036.

34 World Health Organization *Energy and Protein Requirements*. Report of a joint FAO/WHO/UNU Meeting. Geneva: WHO, 1985.

35 Puntis JWL *et al*. Egg and breast milk nitrogen sources compared. *Arch Dis Childh*, 1989, **64** 1472–1477.

36 Puntis JWL, Booth IW A clinical trial of two parenteral nutrition solutions in neonates. *Arch Dis Childh*, 1990, **65** 559–564.

37 McIntosh N, Mitchell V A clinical trial of two parenteral nutrition solutions in neonates. *Arch Dis Childh*, 1990, **65** 692–699.

38 Anon Taurine requirements in long term parenteral nutrition. *Nut Rev*, 1988, **46**(1) 15–16.

39 Cooper A *et al*. Taurine deficiency in severe hepatic dysfunction complicating TPN. *J Paed Surg*, 1984 **19**(4) 462–467.

40 Shenkin A Vitamin and essential trace element recommendations during intravenous nutrition: theory and practice. *Proc Nutr Soc*, 1986, **45** 383–390.

41 Greene HL *et al*. Guidelines for the use of vitamins, trace elements, calcium, magnesium and phosphorus in infants and children receiving total parenteral nutrition: report of the subcommittee on paediatric parenteral nutrient requirements from the committee on clinical practice issues of the American Society for Clinical Nutrition. *Am J Clin Nutr*, 1988, **48** 1324–1342.

42 American Medical Association Multivitamin preparations for parenteral use – a statement by the Nutrition Advisory Group. *J Parent Ent Nutr*, 1979, **3** 258–262.

43 American Medical Association Guidelines for essential trace element preparations for parenteral use – a statement by the Nutrition Advisory Group. *J Parent Ent Nutr*, 1979, **3** 263–267.

44 Greene HL *et al*. Evaluation of a paediatric multiple vitamin preparation for total parenteral nutrition in infants and children I. Blood levels of water soluble vitamins. *Paediatrics*, 1986, **77**(4) 530–538.

45 Greene HL *et al*. Evaluation of a paediatric multiple vitamin preparation for total parenteral nutrition II. Blood levels of vitamins A, D and E. *Paediatrics*, 1986, **77**(4) 539–547.

46 Marinier E *et al*. Blood levels of water soluble vitamins in paediatric patients on total parenteral nutrition using a multivitamin preparation. *J Parent Ent Nutr*, 1989, **13** 176–184.

47 Allwood MC Compatability and stability of TPN mixtures in big bags. *J Clin Hosp Pharm*, 1984, **9** 181–198.

48 Gillis J, Jones G, Pencharz P Delivery of vitamins A, D and E in parenteral nutrient solutions. *Parent Ent Nutr*, 1983, **7** 11–14.

49 Latimer JS, McClain CJ, Sharp HL Clinical zinc deficiency during zinc supplemented parenteral nutrition. *J Paediatr*, 1980, **97** 434–439.

50 Zlotkin SH, Buchanan BE Meeting zinc and copper intake requirements in the parenterally fed preterm and full term infant. *J Paediatr*, 1983, **103**(3) 441–446.

51 Pleban PA, Numerof BS, Wirth FH Trace element metabolism in the fetus and neonate. *Clin Endocrinol Metab*, 1985, **14**(3) 545–566.

52 Ball PA, Booth IW, Puntis JWL eds. *Administration of Parenteral Nutrition fluids. Paediatric Parenteral Nutrition*. Milton Keynes: KabiVitrum, 1988.

53 Synder CL, Saltzman DA, Leonard AS Central venous access in infants and small children: a new technique. *J Parent Ent Nutr*, 1990, **14**(6) 662–3.

54 Hansell D Intravenous nutrition: the central or peripheral route? *Int Ther Clin Mon*, 1989, **10**(6) 184–190.

55 Schmidt-Sommerfeld E, Snyder G, Rossi TM, Lebenthal E Catheter-related complications in 35 children and adolescents with gastrointestinal disease on home PN. *J Parent Ent Nutr*, 1990, **14**(2) 148–151.

56 Puntis JWLS *et al*. Staff training: a key factor in reducing intravascular catheter sepsis. *Arch Dis Childh*, 1990, **65** 335–337.

57 Puntis JWL Percutaneous insertion of silastic central venous feeding catheters. *Int Ther Clin Mon*, 1987, **8**(11) 7–10.

58 Grant A, Todd E *Enteral and Parenteral Nutrition* 2nd Edn. Oxford, Blackwell Scientific Publications.

Preterm and
Low Birthweight Nutrition

CHAPTER 5

Low Birthweight Infants

LOW BIRTHWEIGHT AND PREMATURITY

Low birthweight (LBW) infants are defined as weighing less than 2500 g at birth and those of very low birthweight (VLBW) less than 1500 g. Growth centile charts are available for low birthweight or preterm infants [1]. About one third of LBW infants show intrauterine growth retardation (IUGR) – i.e. weigh less than the 10th centile for postconceptional age – and are small for gestational age (SGA) or small for dates (SFD). About two thirds of LBW infants have a size which is appropriate for gestational age (AGA) – i.e. are between the 10th and 90th centiles – but are born before 37 weeks gestation and are considered to be 'preterm'.

The clinical management and nutritional requirements of the immature or preterm infant will be different from a mature IUGR infant born after 37 weeks. Preterm infants experience renal, hepatic, gastrointestinal and respiratory problems due to immaturity of organ systems. They are more likely to need assistance with breathing and are less likely to tolerate oral feeds. SGA infants have lower fat and glycogen stores, are more prone to hypocalcaemia and have greater difficulty in maintaining normal blood glucose levels than AGA infants of the same gestational age.

NUTRITIONAL REQUIREMENTS

The optimum growth rate for small infants has yet to be defined, but a weight increase of 15 g/kg/day has been suggested [1].

Although growth rates similar to those seen *in utero* might appear to be optimum, there are practical difficulties in achieving this and there may be some disadvantages in increasing growth velocity above that of a normal weight infant because of the extra stresses imposed by extrauterine life [2]. It is important to ensure that optimal nutrition is achieved as early as possible: there is now growing evidence that nutrient deprivation in early life has a considerable effect on long term outcome [3,4]. Since these infants have very little reserves of fat or glycogen they are extremely susceptible to even short periods without nutrition. Many of the nutritional recommendations for the LBW infant have been derived from those for normal term infants; relatively little is known about requirements for many nutrients.

The European Society for Paediatric Gastroenterology and Nutrition has compiled a report summarizing current knowledge [5]; the American Academy of Paediatrics has also reported on the subject [6] and a more recent review has been published [7]. Nutrient requirements for LBW infants are summarized in Table 5.1.

Fluid

Because of their relatively high losses LBW infants have a high fluid requirement; the theoretical minimum requirement is 130–160 ml/kg/day on an energy intake of 130 kcal/kg (543 kJ/kg). If volumes in excess of 220 ml per kg body weight are given orally or intravenously there is an increasing risk of patent ductus ateriosis, necrotizing enterocolitis and pulmonary oedema developing, particularly in the first two weeks of life [8]. In practice most LBW infants are on some degree of fluid restriction because of heart, respiratory or renal difficulties. Fluid intake can be reduced to 130 ml/kg/day, which should be regarded as the absolute minimum, providing extrarenal fluid loss is minimized and energy requirements can be met.

Table 5.1 Nutritional requirements of low birthweight infants

		per kg body weight per day
Fluid	(ml)	150–200
Energy	(kcal) (kJ)	130 (543)
Protein	(g)	3.0–4.0
Long chain	PUFA	nr
Sodium	(mmol)	3.5–5.0
Potassium	(mmol)	2.5
Chloride	(mmol)	3.1
Calcium	(mmol)	2.0–6.25
Phosphorus	(mmol)	1.4–3.1
Magnesium	(mmol)	0.4–0.65
Iron	(μmol)*	35–45 (max 270/day)
Copper	(μmol)	1.8–2.7
Zinc	(μmol)	21–23
Selenium	(μmol)	0.02–0.03
Manganese	(μmol)	0.05
Iodine	(μmol)	0.1
Chromium		nr**
Molybdenum		nr**
Vitamin A	(μg)	120–300
D	(μg)	10
E	(mg)	0.8–5.0
K	(μg)	5.0
C	(mg)	9.0
B1	(mg)	0.03–0.2
B2	(mg)	0.08–0.5
B6	(mg)	0.045–0.2
B12	(μg)	0.2–15.0
Niacin	(mg)	1.0–5.0
Folic acid	(μg)	0.08–50.0
Pantothenic acid	(mg)	0.4

Smaller infants (<1000 g) in general have requirements at the higher end of the range

* from 6–8 weeks
** no recommendations (nr)

Energy

The basal metabolic rate (BMR) rises from below normal to above that of term infants in the first few weeks of life. Growth retarded infants have a higher metabolic rate than those that are AGA. The high ratio of surface area to body weight, incomplete absorption, poor temperature control and stress contribute to the higher energy requirement that is necessary in order to achieve a high growth velocity. Small infants are nursed in a thermo-neutral environ-ment, with minimum handling, in order to reduce energy costs from stress or crying [9].

Requirements for energy are very variable and depend on the individual infant, postnatal age, degree of prematurity, diet, activity and amount of handling [5]. Most LBW infants require approximately 130 kcal (543 kJ)/kg/day, although if losses can be minimized and absorption is good, 100–110 (418–460) may be adequate. Intakes above 165 (690 kJ) kcal/kg/day may not result in better growth or may cause abnormally high fat deposition [10]. The energy:nitrogen ratio needs to be considered and is discussed in the fol-lowing section. Digestion of energy decreases in high energy formulas and such formulas have resulted in the formation of lactobezoars [11], so care should be taken when supplementing feeds.

Protein

The preterm infant has a low rate of protein gain to protein turnover and protein usage appears to be more efficient in the SGA infant [11]. Immaturity of the gastrointestinal tract and liver limit protein digestion, absorption and metabolism. Some amino acids such as cysteine, glycine and taurine, not considered to be necessary for older children, are essential for the LBW infant. High protein intakes overload the meta-bolic capabilities of the infant and cause high plasma levels of amino acids, hydrogen ions and ammonia and exacerbate metabolic acidosis [12]. Intakes of over 6 g/kg have been reported as causing long term neuro-logical impairment [13].

Protein and energy metabolism are interlinked and absorbed energy is the most important factor in deter-mining nitrogen retention; if energy intake is limited then the rate of protein synthesis will be low. The optimum protein:energy ratio for formulas appears to be 2.25–3.1 g/100 kcal (418 kJ) [14]. Care should be taken when supplementing feeds with energy that the protein:energy ratio does fall below this range.

Protein requirement in VLBW infants has been assessed at 3.0–4.5 g protein/kg/day; infants over 1000 g need approximately 3.0–4.0 g/day and moder-ately LBW infants 2.5–3.5 g/day, providing the energy intake is adequate.

Fat

Fat digestion is impaired compared to term infants and the preterm infant has a significantly reduced bile acid pool. Milk fat is resistant to pancreatic lipase but lingual lipase, which is stimulated by sucking, is thought to play an important part in digestion; tube feeding bypasses this enzyme. Breast milk itself contains a lipase which also aids fat digestion and which is destroyed by pasteurization.

The LBW infant has a high requirement for essential fatty acids; these requirements are met by human milk, but formulas should contain 500 mg/ 100 kcal (418 kJ) or 4.5% of the total energy as essential fatty acids [5]. There is now considerable evidence that the preterm infant lacks the desaturase enzymes necessary for the conversion of linoleic and alpha linolenic acids to long chain polyunsaturated fat (LCP) derivatives such as docosahexaenoic acid. Breast milk contains LCP but few formulas in the UK at this time contain LCP and there are no current recommendations for optimum levels in formulas. Differences in blood levels and phospholipid composition have been demonstrated between breast fed infants and those with no dietary source of long chain polyunsaturated fats [15,16]. Carnitine is also an essential nutrient for LBW infants [17]; it is adequate in breast milk but should be added to formulas.

Administration of some of the dietary fat as medium chain triglycerides may be advantageous in terms of greater digestibility, but formulas containing high levels of MCT have failed to demonstrate improvement in weight velocity compared to those containing smaller quantities [18].

Carbohydrate

Intestinal disaccharidases are present in the gut from about the 24th week of gestation, although levels of lactase are lower than in the term infant [19]. Glucose may be inadequately metabolized in the very premature infant, and intravenous and dietary carbohydrate may need to be limited. Minimum needs (oral plus IV) are 12–14 g/kg/day in order to prevent hypoglycaemia. Glucose polymers are well tolerated and may be used to increase the energy density of the diet if required [20].

Minerals and trace elements

For many micronutrients the exact requirements for LBW infants are not known. Where insufficient evidence exists, requirements are assumed to be similar to those of term infants and are based on mature breast milk. Nutrients discussed below are those where requirements are known to differ.

Sodium

In infants of less than 34 weeks gestation renal tubular function is poor and sodium supplements are necessary to maintain a plasma sodium of 130 mmol/l; because of increased urinary sodium losses and a high growth velocity sodium requirements are higher than those of the term infant. Infants weighing less than 1 kg may need in excess of 5 mmol/kg/day; those weighing 1.0–1.5 kg require 4–5 mmol/kg [21]. After 34 weeks or 1.5 kg, infants can usually cope on the sodium levels found in breast milk.

Iron

Although iron stores are low in preterm infants there seem to be few advantages in starting iron supplementation in the first 6–8 weeks or until regular blood transfusions have ceased, since iron will not be incorporated into body stores at this time.

Excess iron may be associated with increased risk of bacterial infection and with haemolysis if vitamin E intake is inadequate [22]. Homeostatic control of iron absorption is poor in preterm infants and there is a danger of overload if large oral supplements are given [23]. Iron added to breast milk appears to be more readily absorbed than that added to formulas [9]. Supplemental iron at a dose of 0.35–0.53 mmol [2– 3 mg] per kg body weight up to a maximum of 2.6 mmol [15 mg] daily should be given from 8 weeks and should continue until the end of the first year of life. Infants taking large quantities of supplemented formula may not require additional supplements for the whole of this time.

Copper and zinc

Copper deficiency has been reported in preterm infants [24]; preterm breast milk and formulas should provide sufficient copper but mature pooled bank milk may require supplementation.

Zinc accumulates in the fetus during the last trimester, so preterm infants have a high requirement. Zinc deficiency has been described, mainly in infants of less than 32 weeks fed on breast milk [25]. Preterm breast milk and formulas should provide adequate amounts, but plasma levels of trace elements should be monitored if there is any doubt.

Calcium, magnesium and phosphorus

The fetus acquires 80% of the normal term content of calcium, magnesium and phosphorus during the last trimester, with peak accretion rates at 34–36 weeks. Infants born before this time will be deficient in minerals. Preterm infants are prone to hypocalcaemia; late hypocalcaemia, occurring 3–15 days post delivery, is seen most often in winter and spring in infants with poor vitamin D status and a high phosphorus intake [26]. Osteopenia or rickets of prematurity is common and may lead to fractures, particularly in LBW infants who have a low intake of calcium and phosphorus [27].

Requirements for calcium and phosphorus are higher than for term infants and infants fed on human milk will require supplements, particularly of phosphorus. Loss of calcium and phosphate due to precipitation and settling of milks delivered by continuous infusion is likely. Mineral requirement depends on age; it has been suggested that infants under 1 kg require 210 mg calcium, 140 mg phosphorus and 10 mg magnesium/kg body weight, and infants weighing over 1.5 kg require 185, 123, and 8.5 mg respectively, although this is considered to be an overestimation by other groups [9].

The optimum calcium:phosphorus ratio for milks for LBW infants is not known precisely but it seems to be in the range 1.4–2.0 [5], although the optimum ratio is dependent on age, weight and calcium intake. It is important that excess phosphorus is not given as this impairs fat absorption and may lead to metabolic acidosis.

Vitamins

Vitamin A will need to be supplemented in infants fed largely on human milk, to provide 200–1000 µg/day but the low birthweight formulas probably contain adequate vitamin A. There are individual variations in sensitivity to and requirements for vitamin D. An intake of 20–40 µg/day should be provided from milk and supplements [5].

The requirement for vitamin E is affected by the amount of polyunsaturated fats and the amount of iron in the feed; both of these nutrients increase vitamin E requirement, but there is insufficient evidence available to recommend routine supplementation. Vitamin E is thought to be protective for a number of conditions in preterm infants – including bronchopulmonary dysplasia, retinopathy of prematurity and anaemia [28]. Excess vitamin E intake is associated with necrotizing enterocolitis [29]. A ratio of 0.9 mg alpha tocopherol per gram of fat is recommended in formulas [5].

An intramuscular dose of 1–1.5 mg vitamin K is advisable in the first few days of life in order to avoid haemorrhagic disease. Vitamin C, thiamin and folate levels may be low in heat-treated human milk and supplements are likely to be necessary; levels in preterm formulas should be adequate provided that energy needs are met from the formula.

NECROTIZING ENTEROCOLITIS

Necrotizing enterocolitis (NEC) is an inflammatory condition of the large bowel which occurs most commonly in first week of life, particularly in infants under 1.5 kg; it is only seen in infants who are receiving enteral feeds.

NEC may be due to hypoxic mucosal damage, bacterial infection or factors present in oral feeds; feed factors associated with NEC seem to be high volume feeding, hyperosmolar feeding (including oral drug solutions) and rapidly increasing fluid volume, though no factors have been shown conclusively to be associated with NEC [30]. Human milk protein, including pasteurized milk, seems to be protective [31].

Treatment for infants with suspected NEC is complete bowel rest and intravenous nutrition, although continuation of minimal enteral feeding (e.g. 0.5–1 ml/hour of mother's milk) may be useful since human milk contributes to gut maturation [32].

BRONCHOPULMONARY DYSPLASIA

Bronchpulmonary dysplasia (BPD) is a chronic respiratory disease seen mainly in LBW infants, resulting in respiratory failure and prolonged oxygen dependence. A number of nutritional factors have been associated with the incidence, or prevention, of BPD including antioxidant nutrients [33]. Infants with BPD exhibit growth failure which is directly related to the severity of the lung disease [34]. Poor growth is likely to persist into childhood [35]. They are usually fluid restricted [36] and have a high energy expenditure. However very high energy intakes may be undesirable as every 10 kcal/kg/day results in the production of 0.5 l of additional carbon dioxide which may not be excreted in infants with very poor respiratory function and which may contribute to metabolic acidosis.

MILKS FOR LOW BIRTHWEIGHT INFANTS

Human milk

The milk of mothers who deliver preterm has a different composition from that of mature human milk. It has a higher content of protein, sodium and iron although the energy content of mature and preterm milk appears to be similar. These differences are most marked during the first two weeks of preterm lactation; after this period the milk gradually changes and becomes similar in composition to term milk. Banked breast milk is often collected by the drip method and is lower in fat and energy than expressed milk. Table 5.2 lists the differences between mature (expressed) and preterm milk. For details of methods of handling and heat treatment of expressed breast milk see page 16.

Several studies show that LBW infants fed on human milk alone may be at a nutritional disadvantage:

they appear to have a reduced growth velocity [37], neurological development can be impaired [38] and they have a lower rate of protein accretion per gram of weight gain [39] when compared with infants fed a more energy-dense formula. It would appear from these and other studies that bank or human milk does not provide the optimum amount of a number of nutrients for LBW infants. Supplements of sodium, phosphorus, calcium, vitamins A, D, K and C are necessary. Additional energy, folate, thiamin, riboflavin, copper and zinc may be required, particularly in the smaller infant. However, the use of even small quantities of human milk significantly reduces the incidence of the bowel disease necrotizing enterocolitis [31]. Infants who received any human milk (from their own mother or from a donor) also had a higher intelligence quotient at age seven years [40], and it is likely that a number of factors in human milk are vital for the immature infant at this critical phase of development.

One method of increasing the nutrient content of human milk is to supplement it with additional protein and energy. This can be done by adding a small amount (5 g/100 ml) of a whey-based infant milk or a hydrolysed infant formula such as Prejomin (Table 6.13). Commercially produced enhancers for human milk are available. They provide extra protein, energy, minerals and micronutrients. Table 5.5 shows the composition of human milk supplemented with a breast milk fortifier.

Since the protein content of mature breast milk is low, additional energy should not be added without protein. The protein:energy ratio in human milk is 1.9 g:100 kcal; the recommendations for formulas is that the ratio should not fall below 2.25 g:100 kcal to allow for the less efficient use of non-human milk protein. If human milk is supplemented with energy, the ratio should not fall below 2 g protein:100 kcal.

Table 5.2 The composition of mature and preterm human milk

Nutrient		per 100 ml	
		Mature milk*	Preterm milk** (8–18 days)
Energy	(kcal)	69	71
Protein	(g)	1.3	1.8
Fat	(g)	4.1	4.2
Carbohydrate	(g)	7.2	5.6
Sodium	(mmol)	0.65	1.08
Calcium	(mmol)	0.85	1.45
Phosphorus	(mmol)	0.48	0.48
Iron	(μmol)	1.25	1.72
Zinc	(μmol)	4.59	6.93

* Holland *et al.* [50]
** Anderson *et al.* [51]

Standard formulas

The use of standard infant formulas containing 65–70 kcal/270–295 kJ per 100 ml has been shown to provide a less than optimal range of nutrients for the growth and development of LBW infants in the studies described above. In order to achieve their energy requirement, infants need to be fed very large quantities of milk, and this is often not achieved or desirable. If standard formulas are used they should be whey-dominant, since this type of milk has been

Table 5.3 Guidelines for composition of preterm formulas*

Nutrient		Recommendation per 100 kcal	per 100 ml (assuming 80 kcal/100 ml)	Comments
Energy	(kcal/kJ)	65–85/273–357		
Protein	(g)	2.25–3.1	1.8–2.5	Amino acid content should not be below that of breast milk
Fat	(g)	3.6–7.0	2.9–5.6	Not more than 40% MCT
Linoleic acid	(g)	0.5–1.4	0.4–1.1	Not more than 20% of total fatty acids
Linolenic acid	(mg)	55	44	No maximum recommended
Carbohydrate	(g)	7.0–14.0	5.6–11.2	Lactose not more than 8 g/100 ml; glucose sucrose, starch hydrolysates acceptable
Calcium	(mmol)	1.75–3.5	1.4–2.8	Ca:P ratio 1.4–2.0:1
Sodium	(mmol)	1.0–2.3	0.6–1.5	Intake not less than 1.3 mmol/kg
Iron	(µmol)	Approx 27	21	Intake should be 35–45 µmol/kg/day (max. 270 µmol total)
Zinc	(µmol)	8.4	6.7	No upper guide; no reason to exceed current levels of 17 µmol/100 kcal
Vitamin C	(mg)	7.0	5.6	No upper guide; no reason to exceed current levels of 40 mg/100 kcal
Folic acid	(µg)	60	48	No upper guide
Selenium Chromium Taurine Carnitine		No recommendation		

* ESPGAN [5]

associated with lower plasma aromatic amino acids and improved nitrogen retention and growth in some (though not all) studies [41,42].

Low birthweight formulas

A number of formulas designed for the low birthweight infant are available in the UK. They have a higher nutrient density than standard milks and contain all necessary vitamin, mineral and trace elements, although some infants may need an additional iron supplement.

Guidelines for the composition of these formulas have been published by the European Society for Paediatric Gastroenterology and Nutrition [5] and the American Academy of Pediatrics [6]. As yet there are no EC compositional guidelines. Table 5.3 sets out the ESPGAN recommendations and Table 5.4 gives

the composition of LBW milks available in the UK, all of which conform to the ESPGAN guidelines.

Other formulas

A small minority of infants will not be able to tolerate a cows' milk based formula; they should be treated according to their clinical symptoms and should receive a lactose-free or milk protein-free formula. Soya formulas are not recommended for LBW infants because of the possibility of altered calcium availability from these milks [6].

Summary

It appears that the most satisfactory regimen for LBW infants may be a combination of human milk to supply

Table 5.4 Low birthweight milks per 100 ml

Nutrient		Cow & Gate Nutriprem RTF	Cow & Gate Nutriprem 2*	Osterprem RTF	Premcare*	Prematil RTF	Prematil powder*	SMA Gold LBW RTF
Energy	(kcal)	80	74	80	72	70	70	82
Protein	(g)	2.2	1.8	2.0	1.85	2.0	2.0	2.0
Sodium	(mmol)	1.4	1.0	1.8	1.00	1.2	1.2	0.94
Calcium	(mmol)	2.7	2.0	2.0	1.75	1.75	1.75	1.92
Iron	(μmol)	16.10	19.68	0.70	11.70	1.79	1.25	11.98
Vitamin D (μg)		2.4	1.6	2.4	1.3	2.0	2.0	1.2

* powder form avialable for use outside hospitals

Table 5.5 Human milk fortifier

	Energy kcal	Protein g	Fat g	CHO g
4 sachets (3.84 g) human milk fortifier	14	0.7	–	2.7
100 ml expressed human milk	69	1.3	4.1	7.2
Totals	83	2.0	4.1	9.9

Human Milk Fortifiers:
   Mead Johnson Enfamil Human milk Fortifier (1 sachet/25 ml)
   Cow & Gate Nutriprem Breast milk Fortifier (1 sachet/50 ml)
   Milupa Eoprotin (3–4 g/100 ml)

approximately 50% of the energy requirements and a LBW formula supplying the remainder.

FEEDING LBW INFANTS

Pancreatic function is poor at birth – lipase, alpha amylase and trypsin secretion are lower than in the term infant. Lactase levels are low until about 35 weeks postconceptional age. The gut is able to tolerate nutrients by the 26th week of gestation, and partial enteral feeding may be possible from this time, although parenteral feeding is likely to be necessary for some weeks. In infants with a birthweight of over 1.5 kg enteral feeding can begin on day 1, providing there are no contraindications, and full enteral nutrition should be possible from day 10. Factors which may prevent (though not necessarily preclude) enteral feeding include perinatal asphyxia, mechanical ventilation, umbilical artery catheterization and sepsis [43].

It is important to initiate enteral feeding as soon as possible as it aids gut maturation and leads to earlier tolerance of full enteral feeding, and a lower incidence of hepatic dysfunction and bone disease [32]. Where enteral feeding is contraindicated, non-nutritive sucking accelerates maturation of sucking reflex and lingual lipase secretion [44].

Methods of feeding

A tube will be required for delivery of part or all nutrient requirements until at least 34 weeks of age, when the infant should be able to feed from the breast or bottle. Cup feeding of preterm infants has been advocated as an alternative to tube feeding for infants over 28 weeks [45].

Nasogastric tubes affect breathing and an orogastric tube may be preferable. Transpyloric feeding carries a lower risk of aspiration and it may be possible to achieve better volume tolerance initially. Although difficult to insert, a transpyloric tube may be preferable in the first few weeks of life.

Intermittent feeding results in greater hormone stimulation [46], but stomach capacity is small, gastric emptying is slow and oesophageal sphincter incompetence may cause reflux. Emptying is quicker on human milk and slower on high energy dense formula. Hourly or two hourly feeding will be needed until the infant reaches 1.5–1.8 kg.

For infants under 1.2 kg continuous feeding may be preferable [42] as it permits tolerance of high energy-density feeds and improved energy efficiency is likely [47]. With continuous feeds of breast or supplemented milk, fat tends to separate and adhere to containers, especially glass. Infusion systems for continuous feeding should be positioned so that they discharge milk in an upward direction to prevent separated fat remaining in the container at the end of the feeding period.

Progression of feeding

It is customary to continue a supplemented breast milk or LBW formula until the infant is 2.0 kg and growth velocity is normal; a standard infant formula or unsupplemented breast milk can be used from this time. With earlier discharge of preterm infants from hospital, there may be advantages in continuing a higher energy density formula in the community. Although small infants have been shown to consume very large volumes of milk [48], some infants may not be able to achieve an adequate energy intake [49]. Several powdered formulas designed for feeding the low birthweight infant in the community are currently available in the UK; their composition falls between low birthweight formulas for use in hospitals and a standard whey-dominant formula. Composition of these is given in Table 5.4. They are not prescribable and must be purchased from retail chemists.

Weaning the LBW infant

Factors to be taken into consideration when deciding on the time of weaning for a LBW infant are the degree of prematurity, the chronological age and the developmental level. It is suggested that weaning does not take place prior to 16 weeks post-delivery (as with a term infant), although it is unclear whether it is necessary to wait until the infant is 16 weeks corrected age, and not before the infant is 5.0 kg in weight. Parental pressure (usually because of the practical difficulties in maintaining a high milk intake) often result in solids being introduced at an earlier age. One formula used is to aim to introduce solids at the midpoint between 16 weeks chronological age and 16 weeks corrected age – e.g. if infant is 10 weeks preterm, 16 weeks corrected age is 26 weeks chronological age. In this case, weaning could be introduced at 21 weeks chronological age provided the infant is 5.0 kg by this time and appears to be able to eat from a spoon.

REFERENCES

1 Lubchenco LO *et al*. Intrauterine growth as estimated from live-born birth-weight data at 24 to 42 weeks gestation. *Paediatrics*, 1963, **32** 793–800.
2 Reichman B *et al*. Diet, fat accretion and growth in premature infants. *New Eng J Med*, 1981, **305** 1495–1500.
3 Lucas A *et al*. Early diet in preterm babies and developmental status in infancy. *Arch Dis Childh*, 1989, **64** 1570–1578.
4 Barker DJ *et al*. Weight in infancy and death from ischaemic heart disease. *Lancet*, 1989, **2** 577–580.
5 Committee on Nutrition of the Preterm Infant, European Society of Paediatric Gastroenterology and Nutrition. Nutrition and feeding of preterm infants. *Acta Paed Scand*, 1987, Suppl 336.
6 American Academy of Paediatrics Committee on Nutrition. Nutritional needs of low-birth-weight infants. *Pediatrics*, 1985, **75** 976–988.
7 Neu J, Valentine C, Meetze W Scientifically based strategies for nutrition of the high-risk low birthweight infant. *Europ J Pediatr*, 1990, **150** 2–13.
8 Bell EF *et al*. Effects of fluid administration on the development of patent ductus arteriosis and heart failure in premature infants. *New Eng J Med*, 1980, **302** 598–604.
9 Wharton BA *et al*. Nutrition and feeding of preterm infants. Oxford: Blackwell Scientific Publications, 1987.
10 Brooke OG Energy balance and metabolic rate in preterm infants fed with standard and high energy formulas. *Brit J Nutr*, 1980, **44** 13–23.
11 Roberts SB, Young VR Energy costs of fat and protein deposition in the human infant. *Am J Clin Nutr*, 1988, **48** 951–955.
12 Svenningsen NW, Lindroth M, Lindquist B Growth in relation to protein intake of low birthweight infants. *Early Hum Dev*, 1982, **6** 47–58.
13 Goldman HI *et al*. Clinical effects of two different levels of protein intake on low birth weight infants. *J Pediatr*, 1969, **74** 881–889.
14 Kayshup S *et al*. Growth, nutrient retention and metabolic response in low birthweight infants fed varying intakes of protein and energy. *J Paediatr*, 1988, **113** 713–721.
15 Koletzko B *et al*. Effects of dietary long-chain polyunsaturated fatty acids on the essential fatty acid status of premature infants. *Europ J Pediatr*, 1989, **148** 669–675.
16 Farquharson J *et al*. Infant cerebral cortex phospholipid fatty-acid composition and diet. *Lancet*, 1992, **340** 810–813.
17 Melegh B Carnitine supplementation in the premature. *Bio Neonate*, 1990, **58**(Suppl 1) 93–106.
18 Hamosh M *et al*. Fat absorption in premature infants: medium chain triglycerides and long chain triglycerides are absorbed from formula at similar rates. *J Pediatr Gastroenterol Nutr*, 1991, **13** 143–149.

19 Weaver LT, Laker MF, Nelson R Neonatal intestinal lactase activity. *Arch Dis Childh*, 1986, **61** 896–899.

20 Cicco R *et al*. Glucose polymer tolerance in premature infants. *Pediatr*, 1981, **67** 498–501.

21 Modi N Sodium intake and preterm babies. *Arch Dis Childh*, 1993, **69** 87–91.

22 Jansson J Medicinal iron and low birthweight infants. *Acta Paed Scand*, 1979, **68** 705–708.

23 Dauncey MJ *et al*. The effect of iron supplements and blood transfusion on iron absorption by low birthweight infants fed pasteurised human milk. *Paediatr Res*, 1978, **58** 889–904.

24 Blumenthal I, Lealman GT, Franklyn PP Fracture of the femur, fish odour and copper deficiency in a preterm infant. *Arch Dis Childh*, 1980, **55** 229–231.

25 Aggett PJ *et al*. Symptomatic zinc deficiency in a breast-fed preterm infant. *Arch Dis Childh*, 1980, **55** 547–550.

26 Itani O, Tsang RC Calcium, phosphorus and magnesium in the newborn: pathophysiology and management. In: Hay WR (ed.) *Neonatal Nutrition and Metabolism*. St Louis: Mosby-Year Book, 1991.

27 Halbert KE, Tsang RC Rickets in the newborn period and premature infants. In: Castells S, Finberg L (eds.) *Metabolic Bone Disease in Children*. New York: Marcel Dekker, 1990.

28 Ehrenkranz RA Vitamin E and the neonate. *Am J Dis Childh*, 1980, **134** 1157–1166.

29 Johnson L *et al*. Relationship of prolonged pharmacologic serum levels of vitamin E to incidence of sepsis and necrotising enterocolitis in infants with birth weight 1500 grams or less. *Paediatrics*, 1985, **75** 618–638.

30 Anderson DM, Kliegman RM The relationship of neonatal alimentation practices to the occurrence of endemic necrotising enterocolitis. *Am J Perinatol*, 1991, **8** 62–67.

31 Lucas A, Cole TJ Breast milk and necrotising enterocolitis. *Lancet*, 1990, **336** 1519–1521.

32 Gounaris A, Anatolitou F, Costalis C Minimal enteral feeding and gastrin levels in premature infants. *Acta Paediatr Scand*, 1990, **79** 226–227.

33 Rush MG, Hazinski TA Current therapy of bronchopulmonary dysplasia. *Clin Perinatol*, 1992, **19** 563–590.

34 Aerde JE Acute respiratory failure and bronchopulmonary dysplasia. In: Hay WW (ed.) *Neonatal Nutrition and Metabolism*. St Louis: Mosby-Year Book, 1991.

35 Sell E, Vaucher Y Growth and neurodevelopmental outcome of infants who had bronchopulmonary dysplasia. In: Merrit T, Northway W, Boynton B (eds.) *Bronchopulmonary Dysplasia*. Boston: Blackwell Scientific Publications, 1988.

36 Tammela OK, Lanning FP, Koivisto ME The relationship of fluid restriction during the 1st month of life to the occurrence and severity of bronchopulmonary dysplasia

in low birth weight infants: a 1-year radiological follow up. *Eur J Pediatr*, 1992, **151** 295–299.

37 Tyson TE, Lasky M, Miz CE Growth, metabolic response and development in very low birthweight infants fed banked human milk or enriched formula. *J Pediatr*, 1983, **103** 95–104.

38 Lucas A *et al*. Multicentre trial on feeding low birthweight infants: effects of diet on early growth. *Arch Dis Childh*, 1984, **59** 722–730.

39 Roberts SB, Lucas A The effects of two extremts of dietary intake on protein accretion in preterm infants. *Early Hum Dev*, 1985, **12** 301–307.

40 Lucas A, Morley R, Cole TJ Breast milk and subsequent intelligence quotient in children born preterm. *Lancet*, 1992, **339** 261–264.

41 Scott PH, Berger HM, Wharton BA Growth velocity and plasma amino acids in the newborn. *Paediatr Res*, 1985, **5** 446–450.

42 Cooke RJ *et al*. Effects of type of dietary protein on acid-base status, protein nutritional status, plasma levels of amino acids and nutrient balance in the very low birthweight infant. *J Pediatr*, 1992, **121** 444–451.

43 Robertson AF, Bhatia J Feeding premature infants. *Clin Paediatr*, 1993, **32** 36–44.

44 Miller MJ Non-nutritive sucking. In: Hay WW (ed.) *Neonatal Nutrition and Metabolism*. St Louis: Mosby-Year Book, 1991.

45 Musoke RN Breastfeeding promotion: feeding the low birth weight infant. *Int J Gynaecol Obstet*, 1990, **31**(Suppl 1) 57–59,

46 Aynsley Green A, Adrian T, Bloom S Feeding and development of enteroinsular hormone secretion in the preterm infant: effects of continuous gastric infusions of human milk compared with intermittent boluses. *Acta Paed Scand*, 1982, **71** 379–383.

47 Toce SS, Keenan WJ, Homan SM Enteral feeding in very low-birth-weight infants. *Am J Dis Childh*, 1987, **141** 439–444.

48 Lucas A, King F, Bishop NB Postdischarge formula consumption in infants born preterm. *Arch Dis Childh*, 1992, **67** 691–692.

49 Lucas A *et al*. Randomised trial of nutrition for preterm infants after discharge. *Arch Dis Childh*, 1992, **67** 324–327.

50 Holland B *et al*. *McCance & Widdowson's The Composition of Foods*, 5th edn. London: The Royal Society of Chemistry and Ministry of Agriculture, Fisheries & Food, 1991.

51 Anderson GH, Atkinson SA, Bryan MH Energy and macronutrient content of human milk during early lactation from mothers giving birth prematurely and at term. *Am J Clin Nutr*, 1981, **34** 258–265.

SECTION 4

Diseases of Organ Systems

CHAPTER 6

The Gastrointestinal Tract

GASTRO-OESOPHAGEAL REFLUX

Gastro-oesophageal reflux (GOR) is relatively common in infancy [1]. It describes a range of symptoms, from those infants who regularly posset some of their milk after every feed, to those who vomit more profusely. It excludes those with projectile vomiting where pyloric stenosis is the diagnosis. Posseting or vomiting will decrease with time, especially once solids are introduced to the diet. The mothers of infants who are thriving, despite vomiting, require reassurance that the problem will disappear eventually. The infant who fails to thrive, however, may require further investigation, particularly if thickened feeds and appropriate drug therapy have failed to stop or reduce vomiting. Surgery for fundoplication may be required.

The dietary management of infants with GOR is to thicken the infant's usual milk feeds. As a first step, however, the infant's usual milk intake should be checked to ensure that he is not simply being overfed. For the less severe vomiters, thickened feeds are very helpful. The choice of thickening agent is individual (Table 6.1). The thickness of the feed can be varied according to the infant's response but for the majority, the manufacturer's suggested concentration is sufficient. The thickening properties of some products may vary from time to time according to source materials used [2]. Neither Instant Carobel nor Nestargel add any nutritional value to the feed. Both products are prepared from carob bean gums containing complex non-digestible carbohydrates. They therefore pass through the gastrointestinal tract unchanged, and so mothers (who are already anxious about their infant) should be warned to expect a slight change in their infant's nappy to more bulky stools. In a very few infants diarrhoea may result. Cornflour or arrowroot can be used to thicken feeds, but careful cooking is required to break down the starch granules. Alternatively, Thixo-D, Thick and Easy and Vitaquick are modified food starches prepared from maize that do not require cooking, and can be mixed into feeds directly. These starch based thickeners will increase the energy content of the feed (4 kcal/g, 17 kJ/g of product).

For the breast fed infant, a gel of Instant Carobel or Nestargel can be made with water and given by teaspoon before and after a feed.

In addition to thickening feeds, advice should be given to widen the hole of the teat to allow the infant to suck comfortably. The infant should not be laid down immediately after a feed, but should be held in an upright position over the mother's shoulder or placed in a reclining seat or cradle. If juice or water is part of the infant's fluid intake, then this can be thickened too.

Once solids are introduced to the diet, the need for thickened feeds gradually decreases. The assumption of a more upright position as the baby learns to sit also helps to relieve the symptoms of GOR.

GOR is common in children with developmental delay where aspiration of stomach contents is a real risk [3]. Vomiting may not be problematic, but those with persistent GOR run the risk of developing oesophagitis. Barium studies may be difficult to perform in children with neurological handicap and thus oesophageal pH monitoring may be used as a method of assessment of the child. A continual 24 hour recording of pH levels will indicate the number of times reflux occurs, where reflux is indicated by a measurement of pH less than 4 [4].

Thickened feeds and drinks have a place in treatment but, for the tube fed patient, there may be difficulties in delivering the feed. Surgery for fundoplication is likely to be the route of correction in these

Table 6.1 Feed thickeners

Feed thickeners	% Concentration	Administration
Instant Carobel (Cow & Gate Nutricia)	0.3–1.5	Add directly to bottle before feeding
Nestargel (Nestlé)	0.5–1	Requires cooking prior to addition of milk powder
Thixo-D* (Cirrhus Associates)	1–3	Add directly to feed
Thick and Easy* (Fresenius)	1–3	Add directly to feed
Vitaquick* (Vitaflo)	1–3	Add directly to feed
Cornflour/Arrowroot*	2–4	Requires cooking prior to addition of milk powder

* The energy content of these products needs to be considered when being fed to infants and young children

Table 6.2 Oral rehydration solutions

	Na+	K+	Cl−	Glucose	Base
			Concentration mmol/100 ml		
Diocalm Junior (SmithKline Beecham)	6.0	2.0	5.0	11.1	1.0 citrate
Dioralyte (Rorer)	6.0	2.0	6.0	9.0	1.0 citrate
Electrolade (Nicholas)	5.0	2.0	4.0	11.1	3.0 HCO_3^-
Gluco-lyte (Cupal)	3.5	2.0	3.7	20	1.8 HCO_3^-
Rapolyte (Janssen)	6.0	2.0	5.0	11.1	1.0 citrate
Rehidrat (Searle)	5.0	2.0	5.0	9.1*	2.0 HCO_3^- 1.0 citrate

* also contains 9.4 mmol sucrose, 0.2 mmol fructose/100 ml

patients, and as malnutrition is a common problem, nutritional support may be required pre and post-operatively [5].

GASTROENTERITIS

On a world-wide scale, gastroenteritis is the main cause of death in childhood. Poverty and lack of hygiene and sanitation contribute to its spread. In the United Kingdom, gastroenteritis is still a significant cause of morbidity [6], especially in infants. The dietary management described below is that which might occur in the UK. The problems of gastroenteritis in developing countries are more complex and management is described elsewhere [7].

Gastroenteritis is the term used to describe acute infective diarrhoea. The infective agents are bacterial or viral in origin. The breast fed infant is less likely to develop gastroenteritis compared with the bottle fed infant [8]. The most important effect of gastroenteritis on the child is dehydration, which is particularly serious in the infant under six months. Dehydration leads to problems of electrolyte balance. In particularly severe gastroenteritis, intravenous fluid replacement will be required, but for others the correction of fluid and electrolyte loss by oral rehydration solutions (ORS) is the mainstay of treatment.

There are several oral rehydration solutions available (Table 6.2); most are powders to be reconstituted with water. Recommendations have been made for the composition of ORS [9]. The infant's usual milk feeds are stopped for 24 hours, in favour of ORS given at 200 ml/kg body weight. Thereafter, it is recommended that infants over six months of age should return to their usual full strength feed, whilst those under six months should be regraded to their usual feeds [10]. Controversy still exists on this latter point, and some advocate returning to full strength feeds straightaway [11]. If regrading is required, milk feeds should recommence at quarter strength, e.g. 30 ml formula milk with 90 ml ORS for a 120 ml bottle, and progress to half, three quarter and finally full strength. The strength of feed is usually changed each 24 hours, though an infant may be 'rapidly' regraded, the feed strength increasing every 12 hours. Breast fed infants should continue to be put to the breast with ORS offered after the feed to satisfy thirst.

Lactose intolerance following gastroenteritis is much less common than it once was. This lactose intolerance is largely secondary to mucosal damage caused by infection or cows' milk protein sensitization. The decreased sensitizing capacity of the protein in modern infant milk formulas has contributed to the decline in incidence of post-enteritis lactose intolerance [12]. The management of gastroenteritis is fully reviewed by Walker-Smith [11].

LACTOSE INTOLERANCE

A low lactose diet may be required for two reasons:

- primary lactase deficiency (congenital alactasia)
- secondary intolerance.

Table 6.3 Infant soya milks

Name	Manufacturer
InfaSoy*	Cow & Gate Nutricia Ltd
Isomil	Abbott Laboratories Ltd
OsterSoy*	Farley Health Products Ltd
ProSobee*	Mead Johnson Nutritionals
Wysoy*	SMA Nutrition

* Available also as Ready to Feed for hospital use

The basic principle of the diet is the same in both instances, but in congenital alactasia, avoidance of lactose is for life, whilst as a secondary consequence of, for example, gastroenteritis, diet is for a temporary period only.

Congenital alactasia

Congenital alactasia is extremely rare. The effect of the absence of the enzyme lactase, required to digest lactose, is apparent in the newborn infant as soon as milk feeds commence. Undigested lactose in the small bowel exerts an osmotic effect to produce watery diarrhoea, which is only relieved on the exclusion of lactose. Human milk and infant formulas contain lactose. As the nourishment of the infant depends upon such a milk, an alternative substitute is required to meet the infant's requirements. Galactomin 17 (a low lactose, casein based milk), soya formula (Table 6.3) or protein hydrolysate formula (Table 6.13, see later) is suitable and will meet the infant's full requirements without supplementation. Galactomin 17 and the soya milks listed in Table 6.3 are available on prescription in the UK for this condition. Solids are introduced at the usual time, and advice given on lactose free foods (see below). Regular follow-up is required to ensure an adequate diet at all times particularly in respect of calcium.

Secondary lactose intolerance

Secondary lactose intolerance can occur at any age as a complication of coeliac disease, gastroenteritis, cystic fibrosis, bowel surgery and any insult to the small bowel mucosa. Lactase is produced by mucosal cells in the brush border of the small bowel, and thus any insult to the mucosa will reduce lactase production resulting in watery diarrhoea, as the undigested lactose passes through the gut. The presence of reducing substances in the stool indicates lactose intolerance. As a secondary complaint, lactose intolerance will resolve with the management of the primary condition, and the need for diet is therefore temporary, anything from a couple of weeks to several months, and can never be predicted. It depends upon how unwell the child or infant was at presentation. Tolerance of lactose will be variable and of course, improve with time. Post-gastroenteritis, some children may be able to take milk-containing foods, but not cups of milk, whilst for others, milk-containing foods must also be avoided. As there is no possible way of determining the degree of tolerance it is usual to avoid lactose completely in the first instance, and then reintroduce lactose by trial at a later date.

Diet in infancy

The infant's usual milk feeds are altered to Galactomin 17, an infant soya formula, or protein hydrolysate feed. Milk free baby foods can be included at the appropriate time. Dried baby foods are more likely to contain milk. The choice of low lactose baby cereal or rusk is limited.

Diet for the older child

Foods permitted on a low lactose diet are noted in Table 6.4. Tins and packets of food are always potential sources of milk, so labels should be checked carefully. The British Dietetic Association publishes a list of manufactured foods free of milk, available to dietitians. Many supermarket chains and manufacturers will provide comprehensive lists of milk-free foods directly to the public; it is advisable for these lists to be checked by a dietitian.

The toddler and older child may be less compliant with a change of milk drink, but will usually take the substitute milk on cereals, in puddings or perhaps as a flavoured milk drink. If the milk drink is refused in any form, this presents a practical difficulty in varying the diet but is not of any nutritional consequence in the short term. However, a calcium supplement may be required if the child continues to refuse the milk substitute. Many cheeses contain only a trace of lactose and can be permitted in the diet [13] (Table 6.5). This, together with other foods, may negate the use of calcium supplements. Whilst liquid soya milks available from supermarkets are not suitable for the young

Table 6.4 Low lactose diet

Foods permitted	Foods not permitted
Galactomin 17, soya milk or hydrolysate	Milk, yoghurt, cheese (*except* those in Table 6.5)
Milk free baby cereal e.g. Milupa Baby Rice Flakes, Boots Baby Rice, Cow & Gate Pure Baby Rice, Farley's Original Rusk	
	Margarines containing whey powder
Meat, poultry, fish, eggs, some cheeses (Table 6.5)	Flavoured crisps and potato snacks
Butter, milk free margarine, oils	Tinned spaghetti in tomato sauce with added cheese, macaroni cheese
Vegetables, potato, fruits, nuts, plain crisps	
Rice, pastas	
Bread, crackers, crispbreads	Milk bread
Breakfast cereals e.g. cornflakes, Weetabix	Milk-containing baby rice, muesli, low sugar rusks
Juice, tea, coffee, fizzy drinks	
Boiled, pastille-type sweets, plain milk-free chocolate	Malted milk drinks
Jelly	Milk chocolate
Some tinned and packet foods will also be lactose free but should always be checked	Ice cream

NB Avoidance of the 'not permitted' foods and all cheeses, cream, butter, casein, caseinates, whey, hydrolysed whey, renders the diet free of cows' milk protein as well as lactase

Table 6.5 Cheeses containing trace of lactose only

Brie	Reduced-fat Cheddar
Camembert	Reduced-fat Cheshire
Edam	Soya cheese
Gouda	Vegetarian cheddar

infant due to their variable composition, their taste may be preferred by the older child and could be used from 2 years onwards. Some supermarket soya milks (e.g. Provamel, Unisoy Gold) are fortified with calcium. The calcium content of the child's diet should always be checked, however, and nutritional adequacy assessed.

Lactase enzyme in liquid or tablet form is available over the counter as the product Lactaid (Myplan Ltd). The enzyme is added to milk 24 hours before consumption to allow the enzyme to 'digest' the lactose. It is not a treatment generally advocated in paediatric practice, because there are other more easily obtained low lactose formulas available, which are preferable,

nutritionally, for the infant and young child on a restricted diet. Medicines, particularly powder and tablet forms should be checked to be lactose free; this sugar is often used as a filler and to sweeten medications.

Reintroduction of lactose

Lactose may be introduced to the diet again by accident. If no effect is noted the parents can experiment with expanding the child's diet. Other parents may be concerned at the suggestion of reintroducing lactose, remembering how unwell their child was previously. A staged reintroduction can be planned, beginning with foods known to contain small amounts of lactose and then progressing to, say, yoghurt and finally cows' milk itself. Recurrence of symptoms means a return to the lactose-free diet, but the parents should be reassured that this is something the child will eventually outgrow.

Reintroduction of lactose to the diet of the infant can be staged by introducing one part of normal infant formula to three parts of low lactose milk and gradually increasing to full strength, over four days.

SUCRASE-ISOMALTASE DEFICIENCY

Sucrase-isomaltase deficiency becomes apparent on the introduction of sucrose to the diet, and therefore is not normally detected until solids are introduced to the baby. Some babies may be intolerant of starch and glucose polymers. The symptoms of loose, watery stools may be intermittent according to sucrose consumption. Deficiency of the enzyme sucrase-isomaltase is a rare problem (the exact incidence is unknown) which requires permanent dietary restriction of sucrose for the relief of symptoms. It is thought to be inherited as an autosomal recessive trait [12] and thus dietary restriction is likely to be less severe in the heterozygote. An early diagnosis may be missed in some children due to the intermittent nature of the condition and even be attributed to 'maternal anxiety' [14]. Children will therefore present at any age. A jejunal biopsy that demonstrates absence or much reduced sucrase and isomaltase activity confirms the diagnosis. A sucrose tolerance test is less invasive, and may be the diagnostic tool. Failure to demonstrate a rise in blood sugars following an oral load of sucrose is indicative of malabsorption.

Treatment is to exclude sucrose from the diet with

Table 6.6 Low sucrose diet

Foods permitted
Milk, cream, cheese, plain yoghurt, low calorie yoghurts
Meat, poultry, fish, eggs
Butter, margarine, oils
Rice, pastas
Bread, cream crackers, Matzos, water biscuits, wholemeal crackers
Breakfast cereals*   – porridge, Puffed Wheat, Readybrek, Shreddies, Shredded Wheat
Potato, plain crisps
Vegetables†   – asparagus, aubergine, beansprouts, broccoli, cabbage, cauliflower, cucumber, endive, marrow, mushrooms, peppers, radish, spinach, swede, tomato, watercress
Fruits†   – avocado, blackberries, cranberries, currants, dates, cooking gooseberries, grapes, lime, canteloupe melon, olives, William pear, raisins, redcurrants, rhubarb, Sharon fruit, sultanas
Unsweetened grape juice, sugarless fizzy drinks and fruit squash, cocoa powder
Marmite, gelatine, sugarless jelly
Glucose, lactose, fructose, honey, saccharin, aspartame
Cakes and biscuits made with glucose

* Contain <1% sucrose
† Contain <0.1% sucrose

an almost immediate benefit. Glucose, fructose and lactose are tolerated, but isomalt must be avoided. Sucrose should be strictly limited in the first instance, but individual patients will tolerate varying amounts of sucrose as they get older and should be allowed to experiment with a wider range of foods of known sucrose content. Details of foods permitted are given in Table 6.6. Isomaltase is required to split the 1,6-glucosidic linkages of starch and, therefore, some authors suggest avoidance of starch also [15]. A temporary restriction of starch is usually only necessary in infancy. Undigested starch does not appear to exert an osmotic load on the gut.

Food composition tables enable the diet to be constructed, bearing in mind portion sizes and individual preferences, e.g. an exchange system of fruits may be appropriate. Ament *et al.* [16] suggested that their patients did not tolerate more than 2% sucrose in the

diet. A list of foods of known sucrose content for individual children can be drawn up. As sucrose tolerance will vary with age, and be variable between individuals, there can be no guidelines for the amount of sucrose allowed. Loose stools associated with the consumption of sucrose may be acceptable. However, if significant diarrhoea recurs, sucrose intake must be reduced as persistent malabsorptive diarrhoea can lead to growth failure.

Sucrose occurs in the normal diet mostly as an addition to other foods, but also occurs naturally in fruits and vegetables. Restriction of fruits and vegetables will naturally restrict vitamin C intake, and so a regular supplement should be given unless dietary assessment proves an adequate intake. Sucrose in foods such as biscuits, rusks, cakes, cereals will contribute to the child's energy intake, and may provide as much as 14–18% of their daily energy intake [17]. This lost energy source must be replaced, and glucose can be used instead of sucrose. Glucose is prescribable, under ACBS guidelines, for sucrase-isomaltase deficiency. Honey can also be used as a sweetener, containing less than 0.1% sucrose [18].

Compliance with the diet is most difficult for the later diagnosed child who has been used to sweets, chocolate, biscuits and cakes. As withdrawal of sucrose has such an immediate effect, compliance with the diet is reinforced, and indeed, some parents may notice a change in the child's temperament. Some parents who rely on 'convenience' foods to feed the family, will find the diet difficult to cope with, and need much support. An explanation of terminology on food labels is required to ensure that parents do not inadvertently give sucrose or isomalt. For example, 'sugar-free' sweets may contain isomalt and so be unsuitable, while 'low sugar' foods have a very variable sucrose content. Medicines, particularly syrups and cough mixtures should also be checked to be sugar free.

GLUCOSE-GALACTOSE MALABSORPTION

Glucose-galactose malabsorption presents in the immediate newborn period with profuse, watery diarrhoea, which can be fatal. It is a very rare inherited disorder (autosomal recessive) of glucose transport, and is thus an absorptive defect [12]. Normal levels of disaccharidases are present in the small bowel mucosa. Fructose is the only monosaccharide that is absorbed normally. The diet for treatment is very limiting, and avoids glucose, sucrose, lactose, galactose and starch. Dietary treatment is permanent, but the diet may be less restrictive with advancing years.

Breast feeding or infant milk feeding is abandoned and the baby is given Fructose Formula Galactomin 19 as his feed. This is a casein-based milk, with lactose removed and replaced with fructose. The presence of fructose increases the osmolality of the feed, when compared with normal infant formula, and therefore feeds should be introduced slowly starting with quarter strength. A modular feed, using either comminuted chicken meat or an amino acid base, is the only alternative but, at a practical level, is inconvenient for the mother to make when a readily available powder is obtainable. Fructose Formula Galactomin 19 is prescribable only for glucose-galactose malabsorption, and as a complete formula does not require supplementation. Parents should be shown how the feed mixes, particularly if a modular feed is used. Whilst Fructose Formula Galactomin 19 is manufactured as an infant milk, it remains as the older child's normal milk for drinks, puddings and cooking.

Weaning the infant with glucose-galactose malabsorption presents its difficulties as there are virtually no commercial baby foods suitable. Parents must therefore prepare much of their infant's foods, and the task of feeding their child must seem particularly daunting at this time. More frequent dietary counselling will be necessary at the time of weaning from an all milk diet to one of solids. Details of the diet are given in Table 6.7 and an example of a day's menu in Table 6.8.

As the child grows up, some carbohydrates other than fructose may be tolerated. The range of fruits and vegetables can be broadened, and small amounts of potato and cereal tried. Tolerance will vary between patients. Information is readily available [13,19,20] to scientifically construct the diet to suit individual patients, e.g. some older patients may tolerate strained Greek cows' milk yoghurt which contains 2% lactose, compared with 7.5% lactose of ordinary low fat yoghurt. Patients can be given lists of foods of known carbohydrate content to try, as appropriate to the individual.

Total energy intake must be assessed regularly, especially if the child reduces his Fructose Formula Galactomin 19 intake. Some carbohydrate in the diet is essential, and this is substantially provided in the diet by the special milk. Patients who do not comply with the diet risk failing to achieve their potential growth. Fructose can be added to sugar-free drinks to increase energy content of the diet and is prescribable for this condition.

Medicines should be checked to be carbohydrate free. If required, a special oral rehydration solution must be prepared using fructose, rather than glucose, as the base.

Table 6.7 Low glucose-galactose diet

Foods permitted
Fructose Formula Galactomin 19, comminuted chicken meat and fructose
Meat, poultry, offal, fish, eggs
Reduced-fat Cheddar and Cheshire cheese, Edam, Gouda
Butter, milk free margarine, oils
Fructose meringues
Vegetables* – asparagus, broccoli, cauliflower, courgette, cucumber, endive, leek, lettuce, marrow, mushrooms, spinach, turnip, watercress
Fruit* – avocado, lime, lemon, olives, rhubarb
Sugarless fizzy drinks and fruit squash, tea, coffee
Marmite[†], gelatin, sugarless jelly
Fructose, saccharin, aspartame
Home made mayonnaise

* Contain <1% glucose
† Contains 1.8 g starch per 100 g

Table 6.8 Day's menu for a young child requiring a low glucose-galactose diet

Breakfast	Fructose Formula Galactomin 19 Scrambled egg
Mid AM	Fructose Formula Galactomin 19
Lunch	Cold chicken with courgette and mushroom Fructose Formula Galactomin 19
Mid PM	Sugarless juice and Fructose meringue
Tea	Minced beef with turnip and broccoli Sugarless jelly Fructose Formula Galactomin 19

COELIAC DISEASE

Treatment for coeliac disease by gluten free diet is lifelong. The correct diagnosis that has excluded transient gluten intolerance is therefore essential and is clearly defined by the European Society for Paediatric Gastroenterology and Nutrition (ESPGAN) (1990) [21]. Guidelines require an initial jejunal biopsy with alleviation of symptoms on strict diet. The presence of circulating serum IgA gliadin, IgA antireticulin and IgA antiendomysium antibodies at diagnosis, and absence on a gluten free diet, further confirm the diagnosis. Measurement of salivary IgA antigliadin antibody may be another future tool of diagnosis [22]. It is important that the diet is assessed for gluten content prior to the first biopsy to confirm that the infant or child has actually been exposed to gluten. The amount of gluten that is likely to be present in the diet of children is given in Table 6.9.

Coeliac disease may be diagnosed at any age, but occurs most commonly in pre-school years. Over recent years, there has been a decline in the number of children presenting with coeliac disease. Why this should be so is unclear, but a combination of factors is likely, with some suggesting changes in infant feeding patterns as a likely cause [23]. The diagnosis of the condition may be preceded by a considerable period of ill-health and lethargy, so that a positive finding is often greeted with relief by the parents that something can be done to improve the health of their child. Relief is mixed with anxiety over the perceived deprivation of foods from the normal diet. A proper and thorough explanation of the gluten free diet is essential. This is just as important where there may already be another member of the family with the condition, who may not have received a dietetic update for a number of years. Compliance is undoubtedly related to how the parents and the child perceive the condition, thus stressing the need for sound positive dietetic support. As a lifelong condition, the gluten free diet becomes part of daily routine that the child grows up with and considers a normal part of him.

It is the gliadin fraction of gluten found in wheat and rye that is toxic to the intestinal mucosa in coeliac disease. All foods containing these cereals must therefore be avoided. Controversy still exists over the exclusion of oats and barley. It is the policy of the Coeliac Society to advise avoidance, but some centres would allow patients to include oats. The basic concept of the diet is simple, but this is not to underestimate the difficulties of avoiding gluten in a society where tins and packets of food constitute part of the weekly shopping trolley, and school meal cafeterias serve pizzas, pies and sausages. Difficulties arise where parents feel they are depriving their child of something. Parents should be encouraged to adopt a positive attitude to the very many foods that are suitable for the gluten free diet. Parents of a newly diagnosed child with coeliac disease can gain comfort and support from other parents who have a child established on a gluten free diet. Information about the Coeliac Society, and knowledge of a local branch of the Society should always be given. A video, 'The Coeliac Condition', produced by the Coeliac Society may be helpful, particularly for close relatives, friends and other carers of the child.

Gluten free diet

All formula milks available in the UK are gluten free. Many manufactured baby foods are gluten free and will indicate this on the label, with a flash or the gluten free symbol (Fig. 6.1).

Foods appropriate for the gluten free diet are detailed in Table 6.10. Wheat is the staple cereal of the UK, so gluten free varieties of bread, biscuits, flour and pasta are widely available. The main dis-

Table 6.9 Estimated wheat protein intake*

Age (years)	Wheat protein (g/day)
<1	Variable with weaning
1–3	5–10
3–6	7–12
6–9	10–15
>9	15–30

* From: Francis DEM *Diets for Sick Children* 4e. Oxford: Blackwell Scientific Publications, 1987

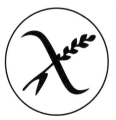

Fig. 6.1 Gluten-free symbol

Table 6.10 Gluten-free diet

Foods permitted	Foods not permitted
Milk, cheese, yoghurt, cream, butter, margarine	Sausages, battered fish, fish fingers, Scotch eggs, burgers
Meat, poultry, fish, eggs	
Vegetables, potato, fruits, nuts	Potato croquettes, some potato snacks
Rice, gluten-free pastas	Ordinary pastas, semolina, noodles
Gluten-free bread, cakes and biscuits	
Meringues	Ordinary bread, crispbreads, chapattis, biscuits, cakes
Some breakfast cereals e.g. Cornflakes, Rice Krispies	
Juice, tea, coffee, fizzy drinks	Wheat cereals e.g. Weetabix, muesli, Shreddies
Boiled sweets, some chocolates	
Cornflour, gluten-free flour, gluten-free baking powder	Ovaltine, Horlicks
	Liquorice; some chocolates e.g. Smarties
Check the Coeliac Society's *List of Gluten-Free Manufactured Foods* for all tinned, packet foods	Ordinary flour

Table 6.11 Manufacturers of gluten-free products

Manufacturers	Range of products
Farley Health Products Ltd	Farley biscuits
General Designs Ltd	Ener-G bread, pastas Pastariso pastas
Larkhall Natural Health Ltd	Trufree flours
Nutricia Dietary Products Ltd	Glutafin and Rite-Diet breads, mixes, pastas and biscuits
Procea Ltd	Tritamyl flours
Scientific Hospital Supplies Group UK Ltd	Juvela bread, biscuits
Ultrapharm Ltd	Aproten, Aglutella and Schar breads, biscuits, pastas, mixes

tributors of these products are detailed in Table 6.11. The World Health Organization *Codex Alimentarius* (1981) has proposed a standard for the amount of gluten that is permissible in gluten free products: the nitrogen content of the gluten-containing cereal should not exceed 0.05 g/100 g (0.3% protein), which is equivalent to about 100 mg gliadin per 100 g dry matter. Gluten free products based on wheat starch conform to this standard. However, studies giving patients with coeliac disease as little as 100 mg gliadin daily have induced jejunal injury [24]. There is some controversy as to whether gluten-containing 'gluten free' products are suitable for children who consume large quantities of these foods. Many gluten free products on the market are now made from cereals which are naturally free of gluten. Parents should be advised which products may be prescribed under ACBS guidelines. Compliance with the diet depends upon the use of gluten free foods e.g. bread, if the child is not to become hungry and therefore cheat on the diet. Parents must know how to obtain these gluten free foods (by prescription from their family practitioner), and it is useful to suggest that parents attend one particular pharmacist for their requirements, so that a continual supply of gluten free foods is assured for the regular customer.

Learning to bake with gluten free flour is not crucial nowadays as there are so many proprietary gluten free foods available. In addition to the prescribable basic gluten free foods, sweet, cream or chocolate covered biscuits, cakes and other foods may be purchased via mail order, pharmacists, or through outlets such as health food shops. A full list of those available can be obtained from the 'List of Gluten Free Manufactured Products' published annually by the Coeliac Society. This booklet should be made available to every newly diagnosed patient, and lists many proprietary foods.

The usual positive response to gluten free diet following diagnosis makes coeliac disease one of the rewarding conditions to treat in paediatric dietetics. Weight gain is dramatic, and the child regains lost ground, with a return to normal appetite. The child with undiagnosed coeliac disease may have had an excessive appetite due to malabsorption.

Until the bowel mucosa returns to normal, some children who may have suffered secondary lactose intolerance may require restriction of lactose for a short period. Some children may present with severe anaemia, and in most a low haemoglobin is usual. Iron supplements and vitamins are usually given, again until the bowel mucosa repairs and malabsorption is no longer a problem.

Coeliac disease is known to coexist with other diseases such as cystic fibrosis, Down's syndrome and diabetes mellitus.

Table 6.12 Food containing approximately 2 g wheat protein

1	Weetabix
20 g	Sugar Puffs
20 g	Shredded Wheat
2	rusks
3	cream crackers
2	digestive biscuits
100 g	spaghetti in tomato sauce
1	large medium slice bread

Gluten challenge

A gluten challenge, i.e. the introduction of a known amount of gluten into the diet again, may be required by some patients to absolutely confirm the requirement for lifelong gluten free diet. It is clear that not all patients will require a formal gluten challenge if criteria for diagnosing coeliac disease have been met. This is fully discussed elsewhere [21]. An important aspect of challenge is to ensure that sufficient gluten is given to constitute a challenge. The amount to be given is not clearly defined, but a minimum of 10 g wheat protein daily is recommended and parents can be instructed to give their child this amount by using foods listed in Table 6.12. Gluten powder has been used in doses of 20 g [25], but its incorporation into the diet is difficult and isolated gluten powder may not have the same physiological effect as gluten naturally found in food. Time taken to relapse on gluten is very variable.

CHRONIC DIARRHOEA

There are many reasons why diarrhoea may occur in infancy or childhood. It may be life threatening, particularly in the young infant who quickly becomes dehydrated. Routine investigations together with a clinical history may give a diagnosis fairly quickly and appropriate treatment is given. There are, however, infants who have chronic, sometimes profuse diarrhoea, for whom no immediate cause is found and for whom a trial of diet therapy may be required to move towards a diagnosis. Infants who fall into this category are those with severe protracted diarrhoea who, following a period of infective diarrhoea, may become temporarily sensitized to various dietary proteins.

Enteropathies have been ascribed to cows' milk protein, egg, soya, wheat, fish, chicken and rice [26–30]. Autoimmune enteropathy, congenital microvillous atrophy, acquired hypogammaglobulinaemia, familial protracted diarrhoea, together with food protein enteropathies are all situations where the following regimen may be tried.

Formulas based on hydrolysed protein are the first choice for the management of chronic malabsorption (Table 6.13, page 156). Soya milk formulas are not advised as they are based on a whole protein, which is potentially sensitizing; up to 30% of infants with cows' milk protein intolerance will be sensitized to soya protein [31]. In the absence of improvement on a protein hydrolysate feed the next logical step is a more elemental type of feed based on amino acids, e.g. Neocate. All of the feeds detailed in Table 6.13 are complete feeds, prescribable in the UK. The taste and smell of these special milks are often unpalatable to the infant so parents need support in using them and making them up. When introduced, solids should be free of potentially sensitizing proteins such as gluten, cows' milk, and eggs, as mentioned below.

Some infants will not respond to any of the above milks and require a more specialized feeding regimen. In practice, these infants are likely to be receiving intravenous nutrition at this stage and as the following regimen takes some days and even weeks to build up, then the infant's nutritional intake can be maintained. The regimen is based on the use of comminuted chicken meat and allows the manipulation of specific components and concentrations of ingredients in the feed. It is important that only one variable is altered at a time, e.g. an increase in volume of feed offered to the infant should not be made at the same time as increasing the concentration of carbohydrate in the feed. By changing one variable at a time it is easier to relate cause and effect. An alternative protein source to chicken meat is a complete amino acid mixture, Code 124, made by Scientific Hospital Supplies Group UK Ltd, which can be substituted in the regimen described below.

The use of comminuted chicken meat has been fully outlined [32] but more recent literature recommends less protein in the final feed than was originally advocated; 5 g of appropriate carbohydrate per 100 ml feed is usually added while the protein content is increased over a four day period. Once full strength protein in the feed (Table 6.14) has been achieved then fat emulsion and further carbohydrate can be introduced in increments of 1 g/100 ml feed per 24 hours, to achieve a normal to high energy feed. Fat and carbohydrate should not be introduced simultaneously. A glucose polymer is usually used as a

Table 6.13 Hydrolysate and elemental feeds for use in chronic malabsorption in infants

Analysis per 100 ml Dilution	Pepti-Junior Cow & Gate (13.1%)	Pregestimil Mead Johnson (14.8%)	Nutramigen Mead Johnson (15%)	Prejomin Milupa (15%)	Pepdite 0–2 SHS (15%)	MCT Pepdite 0–2 SHS (15%)	Alfare Nestlé (15%)	Neocate SHS (15%)
Protein (g) Source	2.0 Hydrolysed whey protein	1.9 Hydrolysed casein and amino acids	1.9 Hydrolysed casein and amino acids	2.0 Hydrolysed bovine collagen and hydrolysed soya	2.1 Hydrolysed beef and soya protein	2.1 Hydrolysed beef and soya protein	2.5 Hydrolysed whey protein	2.0 Free amino acids
Fat (g) Source	3.7 Maize Oil MCT oil	2.7 Maize Oil MCT oil Lecithin	2.7 Maize Oil	3.6 Vegetable (unspecified)	3.5 Refined peanut and coconut oil; refined pork fat	2.7 Refined vegetable oils MCT oil Sunflower oil	3.6 MCT oil Milk fat Corn oil Soya Lecithin	3.5 Safflower oil Soya and coconut oils
CHO (g) Lactose (g) Source	7.2 / 0.1 / Glucose syrup	9.1 / ND / Glucose syrup and modified cornflour	9.1 / ND / Glucose syrup and modified cornflour	8.6 / NIL / Maltodextrins and pre-digested corn plus potato starches	7.8 / NIL / Maltodextrin	8.8 / NIL / Maltodextrin	7.8 / 0.1 / Maltodextrin plus Potato Starch	8.1 / NIL / Maltodextrin
Energy (kJ)	276	276	276	314	288	276	301	292
Energy kcal	66	66	66	75	69	66	72	70
Osmolality (mOsmol/kg H_2O)	210	338	320	210–220	237	277	200	353
Renal solute load (mOsmol/l)	110	125	126	127	123	123	163	116

ND = not detectable

Table 6.14 Comminuted chicken meat feed*

Ingredients/100 ml		Full protein low energy	Full protein normal energy	Full protein high energy
Comminuted chicken meat	g	30	30	30
Glucose polymer	g	5.0	10	10
50% Fat emulsion	ml	nil	3	6
Mineral Mixture with water to 100 ml**	g	0.8	0.8	1.0
Fed at 200 ml/kg actual body weight				
Analysis per 100 ml				
Protein	g	2.25	2.25	2.25
Fat	g	1.0	2.5	4.0
CHO	g	5.0	10	10
Energy	kcal	37	69	83
	kJ	155	291	346
Sodium	mmol	1.5	1.5	1.9
Potassium	mmol	2.1	2.1	2.5

NB Complete vitamin supplement required

* Adapted from Cow & Gate Literature 1991
** Mineral Mixture should not exceed 1.5 g/kg body weight or 8 g daily

source of carbohydrate as it has a lower osmotic load than monosaccharide. Occasionally glucose polymer may not be digested if the gut is particularly badly damaged and glucose is used, thus increasing the osmotic load of the feed. There are some documented cases of a rare temporary intolerance to glucose when fructose can be used as the source of carbohydrate [12]. Fat is given as Calogen, but a mixture of long chain and medium chain fat can be given if there is a problem with the digestion and absorption of long chain triglycerides (LCT) alone. Medium chain fat (in the form of Liquigen) will further increase the osmotic load of the feed. There is some fat in the chicken meat which will provide essential fatty acids. The feed is not nutritionally complete and therefore it is essential that a complete mineral and vitamin supplement is given, e.g. Metabolic Mineral Mixture or Aminogran Mineral Mixture, and Ketovite tablets and liquid.

Whether established on a protein hydrolysate formula, amino acid formula, or a modular feed, solids must not be forgotten about. The introduction of solids will be dependent on the infant's clinical state. Solids should be free of cows milk, egg, gluten and any other proteins originally implicated at the outset of illness (Tables 6.4, 16.10 and 6.10). Disaccharides are usually avoided initially (Table 6.6). At some point the child will be challenged with the excluded foods, but often not until 6–12 months after the original illness to allow the child to demonstrate adequate growth. Dietary proteins should be introduced singly and at intervals to assess tolerance. A lactose challenge may be performed by gradually replacing the glucose polymer in a modular feed with lactose, or offering 7% lactose solution to drink. If this is tolerated then a change to an ordinary infant formula or cows' milk can be made (depending on the age of the child), having first challenged with 5 ml cows' milk-based formula or cows' milk to determine that cows' milk protein is tolerated. A regrade onto cows' milk or normal infant formula over a few days is usually recommended.

Older children with intractable diarrhoea may be given the hydrolysate and elemental feeds detailed in Table 6.15. The Pepdite feeds are suitable for children over two years of age. Adult hydrolysate and elemental feeds should be used with caution in the under fives, and are generally not suitable as a sole source of nutrition. The same exclusions of potentially harmful dietary proteins as described for infants should be observed.

CONGENITAL CHLORIDE DIARRHOEA

Congenital chloride diarrhoea, also known as familial chloride diarrhoea or chloridiarrhoea, is a rare chloride-losing form of diarrhoea. Most of the reported cases originate from Finland and treatment is described by Holmberg *et al.* [33]. Watery diarrhoea persists throughout life, and the treatment aim is to maintain adequate electrolyte balance by supplements of sodium and potassium chloride. There is no dietetic role in this condition.

TODDLER DIARRHOEA

Toddler diarrhoea, also known as chronic non-specific diarrhoea or irritable bowel syndrome of childhood, is the most common form of diarrhoea in childhood without failure to thrive [34]. It is sometimes known as

Table 6.15 Hydrolysate and elemental feeds for use in chronic malabsorption in children

Analysis per 100 ml	Pepdite 2+	MCT Pepdite 2+	Flexical	Peptamen	Elemental 028*
	SHS	SHS	Mead Johnson	Clintec	SHS
Dilution	20%	20%	22.7%	liquid	20%
Protein (g)	2.8	2.8	2.2	4.0	2.0
	Hydrolysed beef and soya		Casein hydrolysate	Whey hydrolysate	Amino acids
Fat (g)	3.5	3.6	3.4	3.9	1.3
	maize and coconut oil	coconut and sunflower oil	soy oil MCT oil	sunflower and MCT oil	arachis oil
CHO (g)	11.4	11.8	15.2	12.7	14.1
	Maltodextrin	Maltodextrin	Glucose syrup solids tapioca starch	Maltodextrin, starch	Maltodextrin
Energy kcal	85	88	96	100	72
kJ	357	369	401	420	301
Osmolality mOsm/kg	351	389	550	260	496

* Unflavoured
Orange flavoured 711 mOsm/kg
E028 Extra is a newer formulation of amino acid feed but is not yet prescribable

the 'peas and carrot syndrome', descriptive of the presence of recognizable foods in the stool. Occuring between 6 and 24 months of age, the diarrhoea resolves with time between the ages of 2 and 4 years. Throughout, the child continues to thrive and gain weight, but the practical problems of frequent clothes and nappy changes should not be underestimated. Toddler diarrhoea may follow a period of gastroenteritis, colic, previous constipation, and some have noted a high incidence of bowel dysfunction in parents of affected children [35]. Considerable reassurance to the mother that the child will thrive and outgrow the problem is required.

The cause of toddler diarrhoea has not been clearly elucidated, but some observations have led to attempts to treat it. The observation of raised plasma prostaglandins in affected children suggests the use of loperamide (and aspirin) as an inhibitor of prostaglandin synthesis [36]. Cohen *et al.* noted that the majority of children referred with toddler diarrhoea had low dietary fat intake, and proposed an increased fat intake to 4 g fat/kg body weight [37]. In 38 out of 44 patients whose fat intake was increased, symptoms resolved. Supplementation of the diet with polyunsaturated fat has also been shown to resolve toddler diarrhoea in some patients (Dodge, personal com-

munication). Others have suggested reducing fluid intake in children with toddler diarrhoea who appear to drink excessively [38].

CROHN'S DISEASE

Crohn's disease is a chronic inflammatory disorder that can affect any part of the gastrointestinal tract. Most commonly, the small intestine is involved.

The incidence of Crohn's disease in childhood has increased [39] over recent years although it is thought now that the incidence may have levelled off [40] in the UK. It is rare in children under nine years of age [41]. Exacerbations of Crohn's disease are unpredictable. Children present with abdominal pain, anorexia, diarrhoea and vomiting. Aggressive nutritional therapy is required to treat the striking feature in this condition of poor growth. Classically, the child or young adolescent feels miserable and has no appetite for food. Indeed, he may be a fussy eater even when the disease is in remission. Depression is not unknown. Reasons for poor growth now become clear. Continual pressure to eat from parental and professional sources may stress the child and contribute towards exacerbation of the condition.

Over recent years, the use of elemental diet in the management of Crohn's disease has become standard treatment in many centres. Elemental diet may be used for two reasons: to induce remission; and as a supplementary feed to improve overall nutrition.

The diet is provided by a special feed (Table 6.15). There is clear evidence that elemental diet will induce remission but why this should be so is not known. The use of elemental diet will either reduce or even remove the use of steroids for treatment, which is beneficial in terms of growth. In addition to having some effect on the gut mucosa, the elemental diet obviously feeds the child and improves his nutrition. Some children can take elemental diet orally, in small amounts, but usually a nasogastric tube is required to get in the amount needed to meet energy requirements.

To induce remission, the child will be given elemental diet only for a period up to six weeks (or longer), by nasogastric tube. The diet can also be given by gastrostromy if this is the preferred route. Elemental diets have a high osmolality and therefore should be introduced slowly from quarter strength up to full strength over a period of three to four days. Continual pump feeding will reduce the risk of diarrhoea, and it should be possible to give the child a break in feeding of 4–8 hours over a 24 hour period, depending upon the amount of diet to be administered and the child's tolerance. A large feed volume is needed to meet energy requirements, so it is important to limit any extra permitted oral fluids, as they may be taken in preference to the elemental diet. Milk should be banned, but a little diluted juice, jelly and boiled sweets could be allowed. This often helps the child to cope psychologically with the treatment.

As children with Crohn's disease are so often malnourished, it is appropriate to aim initially for 100% of the Estimated Average Requirement (EAR) for energy, particularly as in theory the diet is more completely absorbed than normal foods. For some children, this may mean concentrating the elemental diet a little more than is recommended by the manufacturers. Care should be taken to monitor electrolyte balance. If weight gain is poor, then an increase up to 150% of EAR for energy may be required.

After the initial period of elemental diet alone, there is less agreement as to the appropriate diet therapy. Original papers on the use of elemental diet in the treatment of Crohn's disease suggested the slow introduction of foods to the diet again to help identify any foods that might exacerbate symptoms [42]. Wheat and dairy products were identified as causing prob-

lems for some adults. Belli *et al.* [43] describe a complicated re-introduction of foods for which no rationale is given. Most patients will return to their normal diet after elemental diet. Some workers would never suggest a 'trial and error' introduction of foods, on the basis that nutritional intake could be further compromised [41]. A few patients may describe foods that they consider to provoke symptoms and it would seem sensible to avoid these whilst ensuring adequate energy in the diet. Some centres suggest a low residue diet before returning to a full normal diet again.

Whilst elemental diets are useful in inducing remission in Crohn's disease, they can also provide an intermittent [43] or continual form of dietary supplementation to promote growth. It is of interest to note that in one study [44] weight gain was so dramatic that patients considered themselves to be obese, such was the difference in their body image in achieving more normal weight and height for age. The level of supplementation requires assessment of the child's usual intake, and nutritional status, but a minimum of a third of EAR for energy (and probably more) should be given as an overnight feed.

The coping problems of such an unpredictable condition should not be underestimated. Tube feeding may alleviate some of the stress associated with eating in these patients, and every effort should be made to improve nutritional status.

INTESTINAL LYMPHANGIECTASIA

This is a rare problem of the small intestine where there is severe protein loss from the gut. It presents as failure to thrive most usually in the first two years of life [12]. The treatment is dietetic; by reducing dietary long chain fat intake the dilatation of the small intestinal lymphatics is reduced. The abnormality may be localized, in which case surgery is corrective, but this is not usual. It is thought that the disorder is lifelong, and strict diet is recommended at least up to and including pubertal years to optimize growth [45].

A high protein, very low long chain fat (5–10 g) diet is required. Protein loss into the gut is severe and as much as 5–10 g protein per kg body weight [15] should be provided in the diet initially. A special formula milk, e.g. Portagen, or drinks of skimmed milk with supplementary protein, e.g. Maxipro HBV, Protifar, may be used in children over one year of age. Protein intake should be reviewed regularly, together with serum albumin and total protein concentrations,

Table 6.16 Feeds based on medium chain triglycerides (MCT)

Feed	% total fat as MCT	% total fat as LCT
Infants		
Monogen (SHS)	93	7
MCT Pepdite 0–2 (SHS)	83	17
Caprilon (Cow & Gate)*	75	25
Pepti-Junior (Cow & Gate)	50	50
Alfare (Nestlé)	48	52
Pregestimil (Mead Johnson)	42	58
Children		
Portagen (Mead Johnson)	86	14
MCT Pepdite 2+ (SHS)	83	17

* Formerly MCT 1
  available 1994

as once treatment starts, protein loss from the gut should decrease.

Reducing fat so strictly limits energy intake and this is best replaced with some medium chain triglyceride (MCT) fat as Liquigen. This can easily be incorporated into a milkshake with skimmed milk and flavouring, but care must be taken in introducing MCT fat to the diet due to its osmotic effect on the gut. MCT oil can also be used in cooking, and if used for frying, parents must be warned that MCT oil cooks food at a slightly lower temperature compared with other cooking oils and may more readily burn. MCT oil is not a source of essential fatty acids (EFAs). The amount of EFAs provided by such a low fat diet must be assessed. A fat-soluble vitamin supplement is required e.g. 5 ml Ketovite liquid.

For the infant under one year an MCT-based formula is required (Table 6.16). Extra protein may need to be added to these feeds to meet protein requirements e.g. Maxipro HBV. Feeds should be commenced at quarter strength, and increased to full strength over four days or longer according to tolerance of MCT. Feeds containing less than 70–80% MCT may not be appropriate for treatment, and sometimes a modular feed may need to be constructed. If the infant/child fails to grow well on a theoretically adequate diet, a further decrease in LCT may be required to reduce lymphatic dilatation. In this situation a modular feed comprising protein powder, Liquigen,

glucose polymer, vitamins and minerals can be formulated to suit the individual requirement. A source of essential fatty acids must also be included. A minimal LCT diet is given on page 148.

COLITIS

Cows' milk induced colitis is uncommon, but can present in the infant with chronic diarrhoea containing blood. Removal of cows' milk from the diet produces a swift response, and the problem usually disappears with time, although the length of time is variable between patients. Hill and Milla [46] describe 13 infants where milk was successfully reintroduced between the ages of 18 months and 8 years. Breast fed infants are susceptible to maternal dietary protein secreted into breast milk [47,48].

Treatment is strict exclusion of cows' milk either in the diet of the breast feeding mother or the young infant. An infant soya milk as detailed in Table 6.3 may be appropriate as a milk substitute. It is known, however, that up to 30–40% of infants who react to cows' milk protein, will also react to soya protein [49] and, therefore, a hydrolysed protein formula (e.g. Nutramigen, Prejomin) may be more appropriate. Cows' milk must be strictly removed from the diet (Table 6.4). It is particularly important that parents are aware of the forms milk protein may take in manufactured foods e.g. casein, caseinates, whey, hydrolysed whey.

Follow-up of these patients is important to ensure a nutritionally adequate diet, particularly as other foods may cause gastrointestinal symptoms in some children [46].

CONSTIPATION

Constipation is common in childhood. It is seen particularly in the pre-school years, especially when toilet training is in progress. It results in misery for the child and may be compounded by parental anxiety. The causes of constipation are usually multifactorial and have been clearly described [50]. As bowel habit is so variable between individuals, 'normal' bowel habit is difficult to define and, thus, constipation. Weaver *et al.* [51] found in a study of normal one to four year olds that 85% passed a stool once to twice a day, and 95% of those studied passed a stool at least every other day or up to three times a day. Clayden [50] defines constipation as 'a delay in the passage of stools leading to distress in the child'. This covers a wide spectrum of problems from the mildly affected, where diet therapy is helpful, to problems of encopresis (the passage of normal stools in abnormal places) where diet therapy is not the main tool of management. Although Hirschsprung's disease is usually diagnosed in the infant under six months, a significant number are diagnosed later [52] and intractable constipation may be a presenting feature of Hirschsprung's disease in the older child (page 87).

Constipation does not usually occur in the breast fed infant where a normal bowel habit may range from a passage of stool after every feed to once every 10 days [53], so that reassurance to the mother of what is normal may be all that is required. Bottle fed infants may produce a harder stool. Total fluid intake should be checked and the number of scoops of baby milk powder added to each bottle as over-concentration reduces the amount of fluid available to the infant and can be a danger. Extra fluid as water or diluted fresh orange juice is helpful. Francis [53] suggests the addition of one teaspoon of brown sugar to a feed as a temporary measure, but it should be stressed to the mother that habitual use of sugar could lead to excessive energy intake and dental caries.

The constipated child is generally the toddler who drinks more than 600 ml (often up to 2 l) of milk a day, who does not eat much, and may be fussy about his food choice. A poor appetite may be described in as many as 47% of patients referred with constipation [54]. A change in dietary habits will help the mildly affected child in the long term, but medicinal help in the form of lactulose is required short term along with dietary advice. Eating habits in these circumstances are often chaotic and sometimes may be associated with failure to thrive. Dietary change does not occur overnight, especially for the milk drinkers who may still bottle feed, and requires perserverance by the parents.

The dietary aims are to encourage sensible eating habits:

- reducing milk intake to encourage the inclusion of other foods may be the first step for some children
- regular meals and snacks should be encouraged; eating between these times should be forbidden
- fluid is important and at least six cups a day or more for the older child is a guide to work from
- the non-starch polysaccharide (NSP) content of the diet should be increased.

Dietary histories of this group of children often show poor intake of NSP which may be a family trait. Therefore, a family approach to altering eating habits is indicated to help the child. The total NSP content of the diet can be raised simply by including wholegrain breakfast cereals and some wholemeal bread. Wholegrain pastas and rice can be included if enjoyed, but are often rejected by children. Fruits and vegetables should be encouraged, reminding parents to leave the skin on appropriate fruits, and to try some raw vegetables.

There is lack of information on the actual dietary intake of NSP in young children [55,56]. Excessive intake is cautioned because of the potential danger of a high phytate intake (derived from cereal NSP) interfering with calcium and mineral absorption. An enthusiastic use of cereal NSP foods in the toddler can also lead to failure to thrive [57] due to the child consuming insufficient energy because of the bulky nature of an NSP-rich diet. For these reasons additional bran is not normally recommended for the young child with constipation.

REFERENCES

1 Carre IJ Management of gastro-oesophageal reflux. *Arch Dis Childh*, 1985, **60** 71–75.
2 *Manufacturer's Literature*. Trowbridge, Wiltshire: Cow & Gate Ltd, 1990.
3 Sondheimer JM, Morris BA Gastroesophageal reflux among severely retarded children. *J Pediatr*, 1979, **94** 710–714.
4 Tappin DM, King C, Paton JY Lower oesophageal pH monitoring – a useful clinical tool. *Arch Dis Childh*, 1992, **67** 146–148.
5 Booth IW Silent gastro-oesophageal reflux: how much do we miss? *Arch Dis Childh*, 1992, **67** 1325–1327.
6 Conway SP, Phillips RR, Panday S Admission to hospital with gastroenteritis. *Arch Dis Childh*, 1990, **65** 579–584.
7 Jelliffe DB, Jelliffe EFP *Dietary Management of Young Children with Acute Diarrhoea*. Geneva: World Health Organization, 1989.
8 Howie PW *et al.* Protective effect of breast feeding against infection. *Br Med J*, 1989, **300** 11–16.
9 ESPGAN Recommendations for composition of oral rehydration solutions for children of Europe. *J Pediatr Gastroenterol Nutr*, 1992, **14** 113–115.
10 Wharton BA *et al.* Dietary management of gastroenteritis in Britain. *Br Med J*, 1988, **296** 450–452.
11 Walker-Smith JA Management of infantile gastroenteritis. *Arch Dis Childh*, 1990, **65** 917–918.
12 Walker-Smith JA *Diseases of the Small Intestine in Childhood*, 3rd edn. London: Butterworths, 1988.

13 Holland B, Unwin ID, Buss DH *Milk Products and Eggs*. Cambridge: Royal Society of Chemistry, 1989.

14 Milla PJ, Muller DPR *Harries' Paediatric Gastroenterology*. Edinburgh: Churchill Livingstone, 1988.

15 Bentley D, Lawson M *Clinical Nutrition in Paediatric Disorders*. London: Baillière Tindall, 1988.

16 Ament ME, Perera DR, Esher LJ Sucrase-isomaltase deficiency – a frequently misdiagnosed disease. *J Pediatr*, 1973, 83 721–727.

17 Department of Health *Dietary Sugars and Human Disease*. London: HMSO, 1989.

18 Ministry of Agriculture, Fisheries and Food. Unpublished data.

19 Holland B, Unwin ID, Buss DH *Vegetables, Herbs and Spices*. Cambridge: Royal Society of Chemistry, 1991.

20 Holland B, Unwin ID, Buss DH *Fruit and Nuts*. Cambridge: Royal Society of Chemistry, 1992.

21 ESPGAN Revised criteria for diagnosis of coeliac disease. *Arch Dis Childh*, 1990, 65 909–911.

22 Hakeem V *et al.* Salivary IgA antigliadin antibody as a marker for coeliac disease. *Arch Dis Childh*, 1992, 67 724–727.

23 Stevens FM *et al.* Decreasing incidence of coeliac disease. *Arch Dis Childh*, 1987, 62 465–468.

24 Ciclitira PJ *et al.* Clinical testing of gliadin fractions in coeliac patients. *Clin Sci*, 1984, 66 357–364.

25 Rolles CJ, Anderson CM, McNeish AS Confirming persistence of gluten intolerance in children diagnosed as having coeliac disease in infancy. *Arch Dish Childh* 1975, 50 259–263.

26 Hill DJ *et al.* A study of 100 infants and young children with cows' milk allergy. *Clin Rev Allergy*, 1984, 2 125–142.

27 Iynkaren N *et al.* Effect of soy protein on the small bowel mucosa of young infants recovering from acute gastroenteritis. *J Pediatr Gastroenterol Nutr*, 1988, 7 68–75.

28 Ament ME, Rubin CE Soy protein – another cause of the flat intestinal lesion. *Gastroenterology*, 1972, 67 227.

29 Eastham EJ *et al.* Antigenicity of infant formulae and the induction of systemic immunological tolerance by oral feeding: cows' milk versus soy milk. *J Ped Gastroenterol Nutr*, 1982, 1 23–28.

30 Vitoria JC *et al.* Enteropathy related to fish, rice and chicken. *Arch Dis Childh*, 1982, 57 44–48.

31 Milla PJ The clinical use of protein hydrolysates and soya formulae. *Eur J Clin Nutr*, 1991, 45(Suppl 1) 23–28.

32 Larcher VF *et al.* Protracted diarrhoea in infancy. *Arch Dis Childh*, 1977, 52 597–605.

33 Holmberg C *et al.* Congenital chloride diarrhoea. *Arch Dis Childh*, 1977, 52 255–267.

34 Walker-Smith J Toddler's diarrhoea. *Arch Dis Childh*, 1980, 55 329–330.

35 Davidson M, Wasserman R The irritable colon of childhood (chronic non-specific diarrhoea syndrome). *J Pediatr*, 1966, 69 1027–1038.

36 Dodge JA *et al.* Toddler diarrhoea and prostaglandins. *Arch Dis Childh*, 1981, 56 705–707.

37 Cohen SA *et al.* Chronic nonspecific diarrhoea: dietary relationships. *Pediatrics*, 1979, 64 402–407.

38 Greene HL, Gishan FK Excessive fluid intake as a cause of chronic diarrhoea in young children. *J Pediatr*, 1983, 102 836–840.

39 Barton JR, Gillon S, Fergusson A. Incidence of inflammatory bowel disease in Scottish children between 1968 and 1983. *Gut*, 1989, 30 618–622.

40 Booth IW Chronic inflammatory bowel disease. *Arch Dis Childh*, 1991, 66 742–744.

41 Griffiths AM Crohn's disease. In: David TJ (ed.) *Recent Advances in Paediatrics*. Edinburgh: Churchill Livingstone, 1992.

42 Workman EM *et al.* Diet in the management of Crohn's disease. *J Hum Nutr*, 1984, 38A 469–473.

43 Belli DC *et al.* Chronic intermittent elemental diet improves growth failure in children with Crohn's disease. *Gastroenterology*, 1988, 94 603–610.

44 Aiges H *et al.* Home nocturnal supplemental nasogastric feedings in growth-retarded adolescents with Crohn's disease. *Gastroenterology*, 1989, 97 905–910.

45 Tift WL, Lloyd JK Intestinal lymphangiectasia long-term results with MCT diet. *Arch Dis Childh*, 1975, 50 269–276.

46 Hill SM, Milla PJ Colitis caused by food allergy in infants. *Arch Dis Childh*, 1990, 65 132–140.

47 Pittschieler K Cows milk protein induced colitis in the breast-fed infant. *J Pediatr Gastroenterol Nutr*, 1990, 10 548–549.

48 Lake AM, Whitington PF, Hamilton SR Dietary protein induced colitis in breast-fed infants. *J Pediatr*, 1982, 101 906–910.

49 ESPGAN Diagnostic criteria for food allergy with predominantly intestinal symptoms. *J Pediatr Gastoenterol*, 1992, 14 108–112.

50 Clayden GS Constipation. In: David TJ (ed.) *Recent Advances in Paediatrics*. Edinburgh: Churchill Livingstone, 1991.

51 Weaver LT, Steiner H The bowel habit of young children. *Arch Dis Childh*, 1984, 59 649–652.

52 Doig C Childhood constipation and late presenting Hirschprung's. *J Roy Soc Med*, 1984, 77 3–5.

53 Frances DEM Nutrition for children. Oxford: Blackwell Scientific Publications, 1986.

54 Clayden GS Management of chronic constipation. *Arch Dis Childh*, 1992, 67 340–344.

55 British Dietetic Association *Children's Diets and Change*. Birmingham: BDA, 1987.

56 Department of Health, Report on Health and Social Subjects No 41. *Dietary Reference Values for Food Energy and Nutrients for the United Kingdom*. London: HMSO, 1991.

57 Clark B, Cockburn F Fat, fibre and the under-fives. *Nursing Times*, 1988, 84(3) 59–64.

FURTHER READING

Walker-Smith J *Diseases of the Small Intestine in Childhood*, 3rd edn. London: Butterworths, 1988.

Milla PJ, Muller DPR *Harries' Paediatric Gastroenterology*. Edinburgh: Churchill Livingstone, 1988.

Burke V, Gracey M *Paediatric Gastroenterology and Hepatology*, 3rd edn. Oxford: Blackwell Scientific Publications, 1992.

Clayden GS Constipation. In: David TJ (ed.) *Recent Advances in Paediatrics*. Edinburgh: Churchill Livingstone, 1991.

Milla PJ *Disorders of Gastrointestinal Motility in Childhood*. Chichester: John Wiley, 1988.

CHAPTER 7

Anatomical Abnormalities of the Gastrointestinal Tract

There are a number of congenital malformations requiring surgery in the neonatal period. These malformations affect the oesophagus, stomach, duodenum and the small and large intestines. The type of feed and the method by which it is given will be governed by the area of gut affected and the surgery performed to correct the defect.

OESOPHAGEAL ATRESIA AND TRACHEO-OESOPHAGEAL FISTULA

Oesophageal atresia occurs in about 1 in 3000 births [1]. The oesophagus ends blindly in a pouch so that there is no continuous route from the mouth to the stomach. This means that at birth the infant cannot swallow saliva and is seen to froth at the mouth. Aspiration of this saliva causes choking and cyanotic attacks. The obstruction usually occurs 8–10 cm from the gum margin. Approximately 85% of neonates with oesophageal atresia will also have a distal tracheo-oesophageal fistula (TOF) where the proximal end of the distal oesophagus is confluent with the trachea (Fig. 7.1). In this case any reflux of stomach contents will enter the trachea and, hence, the lungs. Oesophageal atresia is associated with other anomalies, cardiac malformations being the most common cause of death [2]. The overall survival rate is estimated at 85% [3].

Obviously, the infant cannot be fed via the enteral route until the lesion is corrected surgically and will, therefore, require parenteral nutrition initially. Treatment of oesophageal atresia, whether associated with TOF or not, is undertaken as soon as possible after birth. It involves the repair of the oesophagus by anastomosing the upper and lower ends, after closing any TOF if present, so that both the oesophagus and

trachea are separate and continuous. This is possible in about 90% of affected babies.

Feeding the baby with oesophageal atresia and TOF

When the proximal and distal ends of the oesophagus can be joined in one procedure, once the lesion has been repaired these infants can be feeding orally within 48–72 hours of birth, ideally being breast fed, or receiving expressed breast milk or infant formula. In Puntis and co-workers' study, 50% of infants undergoing a primary anastomosis were breast fed for a median period of three months [4]. Contrast studies prior to feeding will show whether the oesophagus is intact.

If it is technically impossible to join the upper and lower ends of the oesophagus, a staged procedure is required. The oesophagus is temporarily abandoned and a cervical oesophagostomy may be formed to allow the infant to swallow saliva. The oesophagus is left for 3–6 months before attempting to join the upper and lower ends. Although cervical oesophagostomy prevents growth in the upper pouch of the oesophagus, the lower pouch hypertrophies and shortens the distance between the two ends. Alternatively, the upper oesophagus is left intact with a double lumen Replogle tube *in situ* for 6–8 weeks, through which continuous low pressure suction can be applied to remove accumulating saliva; the upper pouch probably lengthens in this case and hypertrophies. A gastrostomy is formed to allow enteral feeding to proceed. If a TOF is present it must be disconnected and the defect in the trachea closed. Feeding these babies undergoing a staged repair presents more of a challenge.

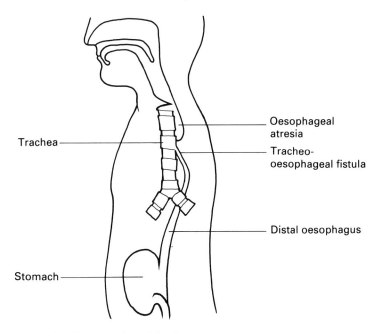

Fig. 7.1 Oesophageal atresia and tracheo-oesophageal fistula

The gastrostomy feed will be either expressed breast milk (EBM) or infant formula and should be given at the same volume and frequency as the infant would receive orally. In order for the baby to experience normal oral behaviour, sham feeding should begin as soon as possible. To allow for normal development and coordination, the sham feed should be of the same volume as the gastrostomy feed, and the feed should be of the same duration and frequency so that the baby learns to associate sucking with hunger and satiety. It is also important that a similar taste is offered in the sham feed as that being put into the gastrostomy so that there is no refusal of feeds on the grounds of taste once the infant later has an intact gut. The sham feed seeps out of the oesophagostomy, along with saliva and is usually dealt with by wrapping a towel or other absorbent material around the baby's neck (Fig. 7.2). Puntis *et al.* report that 38% of babies with oesophagostomies were breast fed for a median duration of 2.5 months [4]. It is now more regular practice for mothers who wish to give their babies breast milk to express their milk so that this can be given via the gastrostomy; the baby would be given infant formula by mouth for the sham feed. There are, however, problems with sham feeding:

- it is difficult to co-ordinate holding the baby, feeding from a bottle, mopping up feed from the oesophagostomy whilst giving a gastrostomy feed. This event may defeat nursing staff let alone the mother coping single handedly at home
- one third of babies with oesophageal atresia suffer from cardiovascular complications and may need ventilating, making sham feeding impossible
- the baby may tire quickly and not be able to suck for long enough to take the same volume orally as is going through the gastrostomy
- many babies have small stomachs and initially require small volumes of gastrostomy feed very frequently, e.g. 2 hourly, making it difficult to coordinate sham with gastrostomy feeding. However, this problem rapidly corrects itself if the feed volume is increased.

There may be no route for sham feeding if an oesphagostomy has not been formed as part of the initial corrective surgical procedure. Infants deprived of oral feedings for the first weeks to months of life can experience great difficulty in establishing sucking. This should not be a major problem if oral feeding is established within 2–3 months of life, but if oral

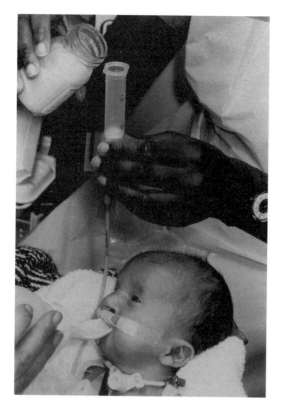

Fig. 7.2 Infant with tracheo-oesophageal fistula and cervical oesophagostomy receiving oral sham feeds whilst being fed via a gastrostomy tube. The infant also has a tracheostomy and cleft palate and takes oral feeds from a Rosti bottle

feeding is delayed any longer than this, it is associated with gagging and vomiting; the baby may avert its head at the very sight of the bottle or push out the teat with the tongue. Desensitization to this oral aversion is a long, slow process. It is important to remember that feeding is not just a process of providing nutrition; babies are very alert at feeding time and develop cognitive and motor abilities whilst feeding.

Babies with oesophageal atresia with or without TOF can grow well on breast milk and normal infant formulas if adequate volume of feed is taken. If there is a problem with weight gain, feeds can be concentrated and supplemented (page 7).

Weaning

In order to promote normal development, these babies should be weaned at the appropriate age though it has been observed that weaning in babies that have undergone a primary anastomosis is delayed to 6 months of age and the introduction of lumpy solids to 12 months of age [4]. Weaning solids should be sham fed if the oesophagus has not yet been joined up. There is controversy over what should go down the gastrostomy tube at this stage. A nutritionally adequate feed should be given in preference to weaning solids. In order to get strained weaning foods of the right consistency to go down the tube they have to be watered down, so diluting their energy and nutrient content. If this practice is continued in the long term, drastic failure to thrive results. In the study conducted by Spitz *et al.* of 148 children with oesophageal atresia, 27% of the patients were below the third centile for height and weight at 6 months and 5 years [3]. A contribution to this could well have been the practice of inappropriate solids being administered down gastrostomy tubes, as was common practice until very recently. If gagging is experienced when sham weaning solids are introduced, oral intake may be reduced to just tastes of food rather than giving large boluses in order to dispel the association between solid food and gagging. Both mother and child need to build up confidence about eating.

Feeding the older child

The attempt to join the oesophagus to the rest of the gastrointestinal tract may occur as early as 6 months of life, but may occur as late as 3–4 years in others. Until joined up, sham feeding of age appropriate foods should continue with nutritionally adequate feeds through the gastrostomy. Fortified baby milks may safely be used up to the age of one year or so, but will need to be replaced by a more nutritionally dense feed such as Paediasure or Nutrison Paediatric to maintain good growth in the older child (Table 3.3).

There are various methods of replacing the atretic oesophagus: gastric transposition involves pulling the stomach up into the chest and joining the end of the oesophagus to the fundus of the stomach; colonic interposition involves removing a piece of the colon and transplanting it between the oesophagus and the stomach. Oesophagostomies, if present, are closed at this time. Both procedures have their problems when feeding recommences. The advantage of the gastric transposition is that there is only one join in the gastrointestinal tract, but the stomach is now sited in a much smaller place in the thorax than it usually occupies in the abdomen. The volume of feed or meals that can be taken comfortably may be greatly reduced imposing a feeding regimen of little and often. The problem with colonic interposition is that two areas of the gut have undergone surgery and joining. The transplanted colon makes a rather 'baggy' oesophagus because of the nature of its musculature, and the repaired oesophagus may not have normal peristaltic function. The colon may suffer temporary dysfunction because of surgical trauma and malabsorption may ensue, necessitating a change to a predigested feed (Table 6.13). A third method of achieving oesophageal continuity is to perform a gastric tube oesophageal replacement procedure; a tube is formed from the greater curve of the stomach, using staples, which is then joined to the lower pouch of the oesophagus. The end result of surgery may be oesophageal continuity, but not necessarily normal oesophageal function.

Problems with oesophageal function following repair

Gastro-oesophageal reflux (GOR) is common following repair and may respond to medical management, e.g. thickening fluids (Table 6.1), positioning the baby appropriately after feeding or the administration of drugs such as metoclopromide and domperidone. These are dopamine antagonists which stimulate gastric emptying and small intestinal transit, and enhance the strength of oesophageal sphincter contraction. Cisapride, believed to stimulate gut motility by releasing acetylcholine in the gut wall, may also be used. H_2 receptor antagonists, cimetidine or ranitidine, may be administered. If GOR is severe and unresolved by these methods, surgical correction may be required by performing a Nissen fundoplication. This anti-reflux procedure involves mobilizing the fundus of the stomach and folding it behind the oesophagus, thus fashioning a loose wrap. Between 18% and 45% of children undergoing repair for oesophageal atresia have significant GOR leading to life threatening aspiration of feed and require such anti-reflux surgery [3,5]. Following unsuccessful medical management of GOR, 45% of the 31 babies described by Curci and Dibbins required Nissen fundoplication [5]. Together with children with neurological dysfunction, infants and children who have a repaired oesophageal atresia and TOF comprise the majority of patients needing such a procedure.

The change from receiving full nutrition from a gastrostomy feed to maintaining an adequate intake orally is slow and there is often a long period where the child needs supplementary gastrostomy feeds whilst learning to eat normally. Prior to being joined up, the child has not experienced the sensation of a bolus of food passing the entire length of the oesophagus. Although the child should have been exposed to sham feeding this method of feeding does not always lead to successful swallowing. Therefore, many children panic when offered any food other than in liquid form and the establishment of normal feeding has to proceed through stages of gradually altering the consistency of foods from purées to finely minced and mashed foods and then to the normal diet. After repair, whether the child has undergone a primary repair in the first few days of life or whether a staged procedure has been performed, a circular scar will form where the upper and lower segments of the oesophagus are sutured together. With perfect healing the scar will have the same diameter as the oesophagus and will grow with the child. However, if the gap between the upper and lower pouches is greater than 2 cm the two ends of the oesophagus have to be stretched to meet and this puts the repair under tension. This reduces the blood supply to the forming scar tissue, causing the tissue to shrink and form a stricture. Stricture occurs in about 20% of children and the normal passage of food is impeded. Bread, meat and poultry, apple and raw vegetables are the foods most often cited as getting stuck.

If there is reflux of stomach contents up into the oesophagus the acid will inflame the healing scar, which may also lead to stricture formation. Sometimes, the anastomosis joining the ends of the oesophagus leaks and this also causes a stricture to form. Anastomotic leaks occurred in 21% of infants receiving a primary repair in Spitz and co-workers' study [3]. Children with these problems will show difficulty in feeding and a reluctance to swallow. These strictures require repeated dilatations to soften the scar tissue and allow the easier passage of solid food. The oesophagus may also go into spasm at the site of the join and particulate foods like mince and peas get stuck.

The frightening experience of repeated choking leads to fraught mealtimes that both parents and children come to dread. One third of parents of babies with primary repair in Puntis *et al.*'s study reported problems with choking or coughing, 17% with vomiting and 20% with feed refusal at feeding times at least twice a day in the first year of life [4]. A similar frequency was seen in children after closure of oesophagostomy. The introduction of solids in these delayed repair children was significantly later than in both controls and children with primary repair, solid foods being introduced at 12 months and lumpy foods as late as 18 months. It is often easier to abandon the feeding of solids and go back to a completely liquid diet. If this is not supervized, the diet can quickly become very poor nutritionally. Children often become bored with food; if foods are liquidized to stop them getting stuck in the throat there is the danger that every meal will end up looking the same brown unappetizing mush. This can be improved by liquidizing the foods separately so that tastes and colours can be distinguished. Mealtimes can become very anti-social; choking and vomiting are common at meals and children may need hefty pats on the back or turning upside down to dislodge food that has stuck. Eating can be a very slow process for the child as foods have to be thoroughly chewed before swallowing can be attempted. Parents understandably feel inhibited about eating out of the home, which curtails the social experience of the child. It is often difficult for parents and carers to understand the problems with swallowing following repair of oesophageal atresia and force feeding the child may be a temptation. Adequate nutrition can usually be achieved with small frequent meals that are energy-dense, and the provision of fluids at mealtimes to help wash down the food. Such are the problems associated with eating that families need help, advice and encouragement from all professionals with appropriate experience, including dietitians, speech therapists and clinical psychologists as well as the medical and nursing professions. The Tracheo-Oesophageal Fistula Support Group (TOFS) is a self-help organization where carers of these children can share their experiences and offer advice.

Dysphagia may remain a problem for many years after repair, but improves with time. Half of the children in Puntis *et al.*'s study experienced feeding difficulties at the age of 7 years [4]. Chetcuti and co-workers interviewed 125 adults born with oesophageal atresia with or without TOF before 1969 to see how their congenital disease had affected their quality of life. Dysphagia and symptoms of gastro-oesophageal reflux was present in over half the adults, but most enjoyed a normal diet provided they drank fluids with their meals. Their social achievements and failures matched that of the rest of the population [6].

DUODENAL ATRESIA

Duodenal atresia is a common cause of congenital intestinal obstruction. Intestinal obstruction has an incidence of 1 in 1500. Duodenal atresia presents as significant vomiting after the first oral feed is given; the vomitus is usually bile-tinged as secreted bile cannot pass down the intestine. The obstruction is corrected by one of three surgical procedures: side-to-side duodenoduodenostomy, side-to-side duodenojejunostomy or diamond-shaped duodenoduodenostomy. The former procedure seems to be favourable in terms of allowing earlier feeding and discharge from hospital [7]. There are other anomalies associated with this atresia: Down's syndrome, oesophageal atresia, imperforate anus and cardiac malformations occur in over 50% of babies with duodenal atresia. Mortality is related to the severity of the associated anomalies. Mooney and co-workers report an improval in survival from 72% in 1973 to 100% in 1983 [8].

Total parenteral nutrition is used routinely to feed these babies in the first days of life. Once the amount of bile aspirate decreases (indicating that the lower gut is patent) and bowel sounds return, oral feeding can be commenced. The feeding problems following repair of duodenal atresia are usually associated with the motility of the duodenum. In utero, the duodenum proximal to the atresia is stretched because ingested material cannot get past the atretic area of gut. The musculature does not function properly once the obstruction is removed, resulting in a baggy proximal duodenum. The infant may feed normally, but milk will accumulate in the lax duodenum rather than continuing its passage down the gut. This can result in huge vomits, up to 200 ml at a time. Feeds need to be small and frequent to overcome this problem. A transanastomotic tube may be passed in the early days post-surgery to help in the delivery of feeds, though jejunal feeding tubes are associated with perforation and are easily dislodged. Mooney *et al.* found that transanastomotic tubes prolonged the time until oral feeding was tolerated by 10 days: babies without the tube tolerated oral feeds at 5.3 days; babies with the tube at 15.7 days [8]. Breast milk or normal infant formula should be used for feeding and, if administered correctly should provide adequate nutrition. If weight gain is poor the usual methods of feed fortification can be used. If GOR is present, feeds can be thickened and the baby should be positioned correctly after feeding. As the gut grows and matures with the infant, problems should resolve so that the older child will feed normally.

SHORT GUT SYNDROME

Small intestinal obstruction in the infant requires surgical resection to remove the obstruction and restore a continuous tract. Obstruction may be due to: small intestinal atresias (either jejunal or ileal); duplications; malrotation with or without volvulus. The removal of the obstruction and the surgical correction reduces the length of the bowel and thus its absorptive area. This will affect the absorption of water and nutrients and cause a diarrhoeal state. The degree of malabsorption will depend on how much of the small intestine is removed (or perhaps more importantly how much of the small intestine remains). Massive intestinal resection is defined as a resection of more than 30 cm [9], or alternatively where less than 75 cm of small intestine remains after surgery. Other conditions may also require resection of the small intestine (Table 7.1). The clinical effects of such surgery are known as the short gut syndrome. Survival of the infant will be determined by the remaining length of bowel; Wilmore reports a survival rate of 90% if more than 40 cm of small intestine remains after corrective surgery, 50% survival if 15–40 cm remains, and a remaining length of less than 15 cm to be incompatible with life [10].

Absorptive function of the small intestine

The site of the resection will determine how well the gut will function post-operatively. The absorptive functions of the jejunum and the ileum are given in Table 7.2. Resection of the jejunum does not usually cause any long term significant malabsorption because the ileum can adapt and is able to absorb carbohydrates, protein, fat, and the minerals and vitamins that are normally dealt with by the jejunum. Resection of the ileum has more profound results as the proximal jejunum cannot develop the mechanisms for absorbing vitamin B12 and bile acids. This may result in depletion of the bile acid pool and, hence, malabsorption of fat with resultant steatorrhoea; megaloblastic anaemia will be apparent once body stores of vitamin B12 are depleted. Massive resection of the jejunum and ileum will result in the malabsorption of all nutrients and water. Diarrhoea and electrolyte loss are the immediate

Table 7.1 Causes of small intestinal obstruction requiring resection in infants

Small intestinal atresia – jejunal or ileal
Malrotation with or without volvulus
Meconium ileus
Necrotizing enterocolitis
Intussusception
Duplication of intestine
Colonic aganglionosis
Inflammatory bowel disease
Long segment Hirschsprung's disease

Table 7.2 Absorptive functions of the jejunum and the ileum

Jejunum	Ileum
Glucose	Vitamin B12
Disaccharides	Bile salts
Protein	
Fat	
Calcium	
Magnesium	
Iron	
Water-soluble vitamins:	
thiamin	
riboflavin	
pyridoxine	
folic acid	
ascorbic acid	
Fat-soluble vitamins:	
vitamin A	
vitamin D	

consequences, followed by a dramatic growth failure. The presence or absence of the ileocaecal valve (ICV) after resection will have an effect on final outcome; if present it reduces gut transit time thereby minimizing fluid and electrolyte losses and maximizing absorption time. If this valve is removed, transit time is increased. A recent review by Galea *et al.* considers that if the ileocaecal valve is intact, infants with a remaining segment of small bowel of 20 cm are salvageable. However, if the ICV is removed, more than 30 cm of small intestine needs to remain to provide enough absorptive area for the infant to survive [11]. Loss of the ICV may also be related to bacterial colonization of the small bowel which will worsen the pre-existing diarrhoea.

Dietetic management

Whatever the cause of the primary lesion infants and children with the short gut syndrome need the same management: adequate nutrition within the confines of a gut that has lost the majority of its absorptive capacity. After resection the remaining gut will go into a state of ileus. Profuse watery diarrhoea will be present. Total parenteral nutrition (TPN) is required for at least 2–3 months following massive intestinal resection. Georgeson and Breaux have recently reviewed 52 neonates with short bowel syndrome and report a mean duration of some parenteral nutrition (not TPN) for a period of 16.6 months [12]. The duration of the parenteral nutrition was related to the presence or absence of the ICV: those with an intact ICV were fed parenterally for a mean duration of 7.2 months; those without an ICV required parenteral support for a mean of 21.6 months.

There are differing views as to when enteral feeding should be introduced: as soon as the ileus has resolved or after 1–2 months of gut rest [9,13]. Early introduction of enteral feeding will lessen the mucosal hypoplasia seen when enteral feeding is withheld. Continuous enteral feeding is much better tolerated than bolus feeds and should be commenced at very small volumes. A predigested formula, with the protein present as peptides, will be better absorbed than the amino acids found in elemental feeds. The digestion of long chain fat may present a problem because of bile salt deficiency and feeds with a significant proportion of the fat as medium chain triglycerides (MCT) may be advantageous. However, the osmotic effect of these shorter chain triglycerides in the gut may favour a mixture of LCT and MCT fat. Disaccharides should be avoided because of the reduced disaccharidase activity in the shortened gut. The better absorbed feeds will be Pregestimil, MCT Pepdite 0–2, Alfare and Pepti-Junior. Intolerance of glucose polymer may increase the diarrhoea associated with short gut in the early days and carbohydrate may have to be given in the form of monosaccharides. The comminuted chicken feed (Table 6.14) allows greater flexibility of feed design for the individual baby, and carbohydrate may best be given as a mixture of glucose and fructose. Any increase in steatorrhoea can be dealt with by the partial substitution of the LCT in Calogen with the MCT emulsion Liquigen. The osmotic effects of using monosaccharides and MCT in the feed may restrain their use. It is important to include some LCT in the feed as this form of fat is the most potent stimulus for mucosal adaptation, and also provides a source of essential fatty acids [13]. The 'chix' feed may be administered continuously by thickening the suspension with Nestargel at a concentration of 0.5%.

The process of enteral feed introduction is a very slow one. It is advisable to change only one constituent of the feed at a time, e.g. volume or concentration, so that any worsening diarrhoea can be more easily traced to the change in feed composition. Throughout this period adequate fluids and nutrition will be supplied by parenteral nutrition. Codeine may be given to help control the diarrhoea. The gastric hypersecretion which may follow resection can be controlled by the use of anticholinergic drugs [9]. Thus the inactivation of pancreatic enzymes in this potentially acidic environment is prevented. It is unusual, however, for acid hypersection to occur in children and is more common in adults.

The remaining ileum has the capacity to adapt after resection. Within a couple of months of resection hormonal changes and luminal nutrition cause significant changes in the lining of the ileum. There is mucosal hyperplasia so that the ileum has an increased number of cells that perform the normal digestive and absorptive function of the small bowel. Enteroglucagon is thought to be the major trophic hormone involved in this ileal adaptation [14]. As a result of this adaptation the gut is able, with time, to digest and absorb some of the more normal constituents of the diet.

Goulet *et al.* have shown that the time taken for adaptation to be completed is dependent on the length of the residual bowel [15]. In 31 infants with less than 40 cm of bowel adaptation was complete 27.3 months after resection. In the 51 infants who had 40 to 80 cm of remaining bowel, adaptation was completed at 14 months.

Some degree of malabsorption will, however, continue throughout the first year or two post-resection and a balance needs to be made between enteral and parenteral nutrition to prevent the child from failing to thrive and suffering from the conditions caused by the malabsorptive state, e.g. rickets (vitamin D, calcium and magnesium deficiency), neurological abnormalities (vitamin E deficiency). Serum levels of calcium, magnesium and the fat-soluble vitamins need to be checked regularly to see if further supplementation of these nutrients is necessary.

Although enteral nutrition is best absorbed by continuous feeding, the oral route must not be ignored.

Table 7.3 Weaning diet – milk, egg, gluten and disaccharide free

Breakfast	Milk-free baby rice mixed with milk substitute
Lunch	Purée chicken, meat, fish
	Potato, rice, gluten-free pasta
	Low sucrose vegetables e.g. cabbage, cauliflower, courgette, marrow, spring greens
Tea	Custard made with cornflour and milk substitute
	'Milk pudding' made with milk substitute and rice, sago or tapioca
	Sweeten with glucose

The infant needs oral stimulation and experience of feeding. Weaning should be started when the infant is old enough and well enough. Initially the diet should be free of disaccharides, and it is usual practice to avoid milk, egg and gluten. A typical weaning diet is given in Table 7.3. Diarrhoea will gradually decrease with time as the gut adapts, but it may take up to a year for the child to obtain adequate nutrition from the enteral route. Along with the weaning diet, the child should be tentatively tried with bolus oral feeds rather than receiving only continuous enteral feeds.

As the diarrhoea subsides, previously avoided foods can gradually be tried in the toddler's diet to assess tolerance. Gluten and egg may be introduced first; then disaccharides in the form of sucrose-containing vegetables and, later, fruit. Milk (and lactose) are tried last of all. Most children by this time will be able to tolerate a normal diet, though a degree of fat malabsorption may remain. Matsuo *et al.* reviewed eight children over a period of 2–19 years and found abnormal absorption of fat in those with a residual small intestine of less than 45 cm [16]. Ohkohchi *et al.* found similar results: nine infants were followed up for 1.5 to 14.6 years and severe steatorrhoea was noted in those with a bowel length of less than 50 cm [17].

There are some children in whom the adaptive process is less successful and they may become susceptible to abnormal water and electrolyte losses during intercurrent illness, especially a gastroenteritis. They may need intravenous fluids at these times to maintain fluid and electrolyte balance. Other children never achieve tolerance of a normal diet and need some degree of long term dietary modification to keep their malabsorptive diarrhoea in abeyance.

Infants requiring massive small intestinal resection have had improved survival rates with advances in surgical technique, TPN and dietetic management in the last 20 years. Dorney *et al.* quote survival rates before 1972 at 27%, rising to 69% after 1972 [18]. Weber *et al.* have looked at the survival rates and quality of life of 16 children with short bowel syndrome over a period of 2–10 years and found a 94% rate of survival [19]. They conclude that the advent of home parenteral and enteral nutritional support has not only improved survival, but allowed these children to enjoy a much improved psychosocial environment. These findings are echoed by Goulet *et al.* who quote an overall 90% survival rate in children with less than 40 cm of small bowel [15]. Survival has improved dramatically since the introduction of home TPN, with survival at 65% before 1980, and at 95% in those born after 1980 when home TPN became available.

Normal growth can be expected with proper nutritional management [15,16]. The long term problems that may be encountered include renal calculi, cholelithiasis and fractures [16]. Long term steatorrhoea may lead to low serum levels of vitamin D, total cholesterol and disruption of bile acid absorption. Nutritional supplements to offset this chronic fat malabsorption are probably necessary [17].

HIRSCHSPRUNG'S DISEASE

Hirschprung's disease describes a total absence of ganglion cells in the affected part of the large intestine. It has an incidence of 1 in 5000 infants [1]. Some 80–90% of cases present as complete intestinal obstruction, bilious vomiting and profound abdominal distension in the neonate, with a delayed passage of meconium. Surgery aims to clear the obstruction either by fashioning a colostomy as the initial procedure, followed by a pull-through procedure at a later date; alternatively a primary pull-through may be performed. Some children present later with intractable constipation alternating with diarrhoea which may be treated symptomatically with a high fibre diet. In long-segment Hirschsprung's disease there is small intestinal involvement; resection of aganglionic bowel will be necessary, leaving the infant with a shortened length of bowel. The dietary management is as described for short gut syndrome.

EXOMPHALOS AND GASTROSCHISIS

These conditions are not abnormalities of the gastro-intestinal tract, but are abdominal wall defects involving the exposure of the infant's intestine to the outside world. There is an incidence of 1 in 5000 to 10 000 births [1]. An exomphalos can be small or large and occurs when the lateral folds of the abdominal wall fail to meet *in utero*. Not only bowel, but also solid viscera like the liver are exposed, covered by a translucent membrane. Sometimes the bowel can be placed back inside the abdomen in one operation, but if it is a large exomphalos this is not possible. The exomphalos sac is covered with either a Prolene or Silastic prosthesis to protect it and the abdominal cavity is left to grow so that it will accomodate the bowel in stages.

In gastroschisis, a rupture of the umbilical cord *in utero* allows the intestine to escape outside the abdominal wall. Again the bowel is put back inside the abdomen in one go, if possible, or may need a staged procedure, tightening the prosthesic sac gradually [20]. Both Silastic and Prolene prostheses and primary fascial closure are considered acceptable procedures; the primary closure has the advantage of avoiding additional operations [21].

The pressure of the prosthetic sac or the closed abdominal wall forces the intestine back into the abdomen, but this continual pressure will upset its normal function and the gut may suffer a prolonged paralytic ileus. Most of these infants will need TPN for several weeks or months before bowel function returns and the use of TPN is of major importance in the survival of these infants [22]. Adam *et al.* found that delayed closure of the abdomen in exomphalos lead to more readily established enteral feeding [23]. However, Sauter *et al.* found no difference in the time taken to establish enteral feeding in babies with gastroschisis and exomphalos whether they underwent primary repair or a delayed procedure [21].

When bowel sounds return enteral feeding can be considered. Expressed breast milk or infant formula is usually tolerated if given as small frequent bolus feeds. Large boluses are not tolerated as the intestinal tract is under contant pressure and cannot accomodate a large amount of fluid at once. If the baby can be handled normally and does not need to be nursed flat, breast feeding is possible. If there is malabsorption, then a predigested feed is indicated.

Exomphalos and gastroschisis were fatal abnormalities prior to the 1970s. The advent of TPN and temporary prosthetic sacs, which allow delayed abdominal closure, has allowed the good survival rates seen today [20].

REFERENCES

1 Spitz L Surgical emergencies in the first few weeks of life. In: Milla PJ, Muller DPR (eds.) *Harries' Paediatric Gastroenterology*, 2nd edn. Edinburgh: Churchill Livingstone, 1988.
2 Chittmittrapap S *et al.* Oesophageal atresia and associated anomalies. *Arch Dis Childh*, 1989, **64** 364–368.
3 Spitz L *et al.* Esophageal atresia: five year experience with 148 cases. *J Pediatr Surg*, 1987, **22**(2) 103–108.
4 Puntis JWL *et al.* Growth and feeding problems after repair of oesophageal atresia. *Arch Dis Childh*, 1990, **65** 84–88.
5 Curci MR, Dibbins AW Problems associated with a Nissen fundoplication following tracheoesophageal fistula and esophageal atresia repair. *Arch Surg*, 1988, **123** 618–620.
6 Chetcuti P *et al.* Adults who survived repair of congenital oesophageal atresia and tracheo-oesophageal fistula. *Brit Med J*, 1988, **297** 344–346.
7 Weber TR *et al.* Duodenal atresia: a comparison of techniques of repair. *J Pediatr Surg*, 1986, **21**(12) 1133–1136.
8 Mooney D *et al.* Newborn duodenal atresia: an improving outlook. *Am J Surg*, 1987, **153**(4) 347–349.
9 Walker-Smith J Massive resection of the small intestine. In: *Diseases of the Small Intestine in Childhood*, 3rd edn. London: Butterworths, 1988.
10 Wilmore DW Factors correlating with a successful outcome following extensive intestinal resection in newborn infants. *J Pediatr*, 1972, **80** 88.
11 Galea MH *et al.* Short-bowel syndrome: a collective review. *J Pediatr Surg*, 1992, **27**(5) 592–596.
12 Georgeson KE, Breaux CW Jnr Outcome and intestinal adaptation in neonatal short-bowel syndrome. *J Pediatr Surg*, **27** 344–348.
13 Milla PJ The management of massive intestinal resection. *Maternal & Child Health*, 1986, **11**(2) 59–64.
14 Sager GR *et al.* The effect of altered luminal nutrition on cellular proliferation and plasma concentrations of enteroglucagon and gastrin after small bowel resection in the rat. *Br J Surg*, 1982, **69** 14–18.
15 Goulet OJ *et al.* Neonatal short bowel syndrome. *J Pediatr*, 1991, **119** 18–23.
16 Matsuo Y *et al.* Massive small bowel resection in neonates – is weaning from parenteral nutrition the final goal? *Surg Today*, 1992, **22**(1) 40–45.
17 Ohkohchi N *et al.* Evaluation of the nutritional condition and absorptive capacity of 9 infants with short bowel syndrome. *J Pediatr Gastroenterol Nutr*, 1986, **5**(2) 198–206.

18 Dorney SFA *et al*. Improved survival in very short small bowel of infancy with use of long-term parenteral nutrition. *J Pediatr*, 1985, **107** 521–525.

19 Weber TR *et al*. Short-bowel syndrome in children. Quality of life in an era of improved survival. *Arch Surg*, 1991, **126**(7) 841–846.

20 Randolph J Omphalocele and gastroschisis: different entities, similar therapeutic goals. *South Med J*, 1982, **75**(12) 1517–1519.

21 Sauter ER *et al*. Is primary repair of gastroschisis and omphalocele always the best operation? *Am Surg*, 1991, **57**(3) 142–144.

22 Hoffman P *et al*. Omphalocele and gastroschisis: problems in intensive treatment. *Zentralb Chir*, 1986, **111**(8) 448–456.

23 Adam AS *et al*. Evaluation of conservative therapy for exomphalos. *Surg Gynecol Obstet*, 1991, **172**(5) 395–396.

USEFUL ADDRESS

The Tracheo-Oesophageal Fistula Support Group (TOFS)
St George's Centre, 91 Victoria Road, Netherfield, Nottingham NG4 2NN.

CHAPTER 8

The Liver and Pancreas

THE LIVER

In order to understand the full implications of paediatric liver disorders, it is important to consider the metabolic functions that the liver performs. The liver is essential for glucose homeostasis. It stores glycogen and during fasting mobilizes glucose. Infants and children with liver disease commonly become hypoglycaemic due to impairment of this function. Reduced synthesis of plasma proteins (e.g. albumin and prothrombin) and amino acids also have profound clinical consequences.

Impaired lipid metabolism also has an effect on the nutritional status of an infant or child. Reduced bile salt production and bile flow can result in fat malabsorption and an associated decrease in absorption of fat-soluble vitamins. As liver disease progresses, treatment of the severe clinical symptoms and nutrient abnormalities becomes increasingly important (Fig. 8.1). The growth and development of children with chronic liver disease must always be given the greatest priority.

BILIARY ATRESIA

Extrahepatic biliary atresia (EHBA) is a rare disease with an incidence of 1 in 14 000 live births [1]. This diagnosis must be considered in infants with persistent neonatal jaundice lasting longer than 14 days. Symptoms include pale stools and dark urine, resulting from the progressive obstruction of the common bile duct and its branches. Commonly the baby will appear to thrive, yet, with nutritional assessment, it is evident that this is only achieved by the consumption of a greater than average volume of breast milk or infant formula – as much as 250–350 ml/kg body weight. As the disease progresses, the ability to

gain weight is reduced and failure to thrive may be the predominant reason for the infant being investigated [2].

The Kasai operation, hepatic portoenterostomy, clears jaundice in up to 90% of infants if performed in the first eight weeks of life [3]. Normal bile flow may then not be achieved for up to nine months even when successful bile drainage is noted [4]. Average survival for infants without the procedure is 11 months.

Infant feeding

The resultant intestinal deficiency of bile acids leads to reduced fat digestion and malabsorption of varying severity. Post Kasai infants require a specialized infant milk such as Pregestimil, Pepti-Junior, MCT Pepdite 0–2, Alfare or Caprilon, all of which have a fat source rich in medium chain triglycerides (MCT) and essential fatty acids (EFA) (Table 8.1) [5,6].

A volume of 150–180 ml/kg is prescribed for a full term baby. A gradual change from normal baby milk to the above formulas is recommended to avoid rejection on the grounds of palatability. Unfortunately, exclusively breast fed infants with biliary atresia have poor weight gain after Kasai procedures and a specialized formula is recommended. Breast feeding is continued as a source of comfort only. As with any other infant formula, the specialized formula should be continued until the infant is one year old.

An infant is usually discharged 10 days after the Kasai, having regained his preoperative weight. It is known that infants with biliary atresia need to consume a higher energy and protein intake than normal infants in order to thrive [7,8]. If weight gain is poor, energy supplementation of the specialized milk

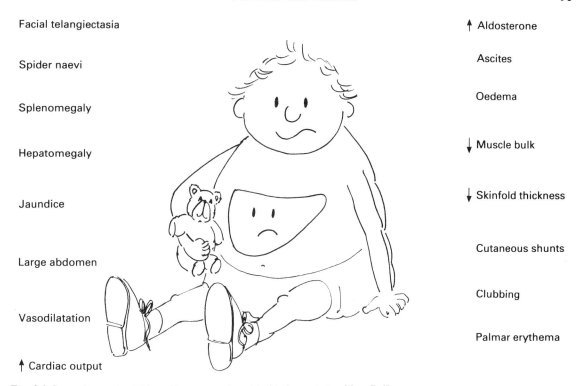

Facial telangiectasia

Spider naevi

Splenomegaly

Hepatomegaly

Jaundice

Large abdomen

Vasodilatation

↑ Cardiac output

↑ Aldosterone

Ascites

Oedema

↓ Muscle bulk

↓ Skinfold thickness

Cutaneous shunts

Clubbing

Palmar erythema

Fig. 8.1 Liver disease in children (figure reproduced by kind permission Nom Ball)

should be commenced immediately. Glucose polymer (maltodextrins) or a combination of glucose polymer and blended vegetable oils (Duocal powder) are equally suitable (Table 1.6).

Weaning

An infant with biliary atresia should be weaned on to solid food between 12 and 16 weeks ideally. Firstly, rice-based cereals mixed with the specialized milk should be offered. Home prepared liquidized food is as suitable as any of the manufactured baby foods.

Normal weaning advice should be given. If an infant has a chronic disease and has spent time in hospital, development can be adversely affected. The first foods offered may also affect food choice later in life [9]. Therefore, successful weaning is of great importance and varied taste and textures are essential for a baby with biliary atresia.

As solid foods are introduced, the infant may take less of the specialized milk and nutrition may become compromised. This is particularly evident when a beaker is used in place of the bottle; the smell and taste of these products are more noticeable and it is recommended that flavouring should be added to the milk to improve palatability. From six months, a baby can have the milk mixed with milk shake powders or syrups which improve taste and hence volume taken so that nutritional status is not affected.

Vitamin and mineral therapy

Vitamin and mineral status of infants and children with EHBA must be closely monitored. All newly diagnosed babies with biliary atresia are prescribed a multivitamin supplement (e.g. Ketovite 5 ml liquid and three tablets per day). Deficiencies of water-soluble vitamins have not been described in infants with biliary atresia [7]. Fat-soluble vitamin deficiencies are of great concern. They represent a constant potential risk and should be treated prophylactically [10]. Fat-soluble vitamin absorption may be further

Table 8.1 Specialized formula suitable for babies and infants with chronic liver disease

Formula	Energy kcal (kJ)	Major nutrients per 100 ml		
		Protein (g)	CHO (g)	Fat (g)
Pregestimil (Mead Johnson) (14.8%)	66 (280)	1.9 Casein hydrolysate (L-tyrosine, L-cystine, L-tryotophan)	9.1 Glucose syrup, modified corn starch	2.7 Corn oil, MCT oil (50%)
Pepti-Junior (Cow & Gate) (13.1%)	66 (280)	2.0 Whey hydrolysate	7.2 Glucose syrup (trace lactose)	3.7 Maize oil, MCT oil (50%)
MCT Pepdite 0–2 (Scientific Hospital Supplies) (15%)	66 (280)	2.1 Soya and meat protein hydrolysate and amino acids	8.9 Maltodextrin	2.7 Sunflower oil (monoglyceride) MCT oil (83%)
Caprilon (Cow & Gate) (12.7%) formerly MCT1 available 1994	64 (269)	1.5 Protein enriched whey powder	7.0 Maltodextrin, lactose	3.6 Maize oil, sunflower oil, MCT oil (75%)
Alfare (Nestlé) (10.5%)	65 (273)	2.2 Whey hydrolysate and amino acids and peptides	7.0 Maltodextrin and potato starch (trace lactose)	3.3 Corn oil, milk fats, MCT oil (48%), lecithin

Dilutions of formula powder for reconstitution with water are given as %

impaired by the use of cholestyramine (Questran) which is administered if a child remains jaundiced post-operatively. Cholestyramine is given as an anti-pruritic drug to bind bile acids and can therefore impair fatty acid transport. All supplementary vitamins should be given at least two hours apart from the administration of the cholestyramine in order to allow maximum absorption of the fat-soluble vitamins.

Vitamin K When a baby is diagnosed as having biliary atresia, vitamin K supplementation (Phyto-menadione, Konakion) is commenced using 1 mg of an intravenous preparation orally. This administration should be reviewed if the baby develops a normal prothrombin time, clears his jaundice (serum bilirubin <20 µmol/l) and appears to be improving clinically. Otherwise this supplement is continued long term and is gradually changed over from the intravenous preparation to 5 or 10 mg tablets given once or twice weekly.

Vitamin D The supplementation of vitamin D varies considerably between units specializing in paediatric

liver disease. Generally, all newly diagnosed babies with biliary atresia receive an intramuscular dose of 30 000–60 000 i.u. (750–1500 µg) vitamin D, depending on their weight, prior to discharge after the Kasai operation. This dose is then repeated at monthly intervals for a period of three months.

The synthetic alfacalcidol [1-alpha-(OH) vitamin D] and calcitriol [1,25(OH) vitamin D] forms are advocated. On each occasion that the baby is seen, the serum calcium, phosphate and alkaline phosphatase levels should be checked and he should be examined for evidence of rickets. An x-ray of the wrist may be taken to evaluate possible radiological change if rickets is apparent [11]. If a small baby develops rickets clinically and biochemically, it is usual to supplement with phosphate and occasionally calcium at a level of 1 mmol/kg/day. As well as rickets, children with chronic liver disease can develop osteoporosis and pathological fractures, the exact causes of which are unknown.

Vitamin E Vitamin E deficiency can cause progressive neuromuscular and neurological deterioration.

These abnormalities have been found in babies and children with a serum vitamin E level of 0.4 mg/l or more importantly a vitamin E/lipid ratio of 0.6 mg vitamin E/g of lipid or less. All babies are given a single intramuscular dose of 10 mg/kg vitamin E post Kasai. In the cholestatic baby, 15 mg of alpha-tocopherol acetate is continued orally and if further supplementation is required this can be increased to 200 mg/kg/day. If this does not correct the deficiency intramuscular injections of 10 mg/kg fortnightly is usual.

Minerals Iron deficiency is common in children with biliary atresia. Iron losses due to gastrointestinal bleeding or epistaxis are common. Nutritional intake of iron in babies is usually sufficient with the use of the complete specialized milk, yet chronically sick, older children with oesphageal varices and cirrhosis tend to have a reduced dietary intake. Iron is deposited in the diseased liver and spleen, and this may contribute to anaemia. Iron deficiency is treated with a therapeutic dose of oral iron.

Zinc deficiency is associated with chronic malabsorption and may contribute to the anorexia and poor growth of infants with biliary atresia [12]. It is difficult to determine this clinically as plasma zinc levels are not a good indication of total body zinc in patients with liver disease.

Retinol binding protein synthesis is zinc dependent, so deficiency can have an effect on vitamin A status [13]. In practice, zinc supplementation may be given orally at an acceptable level of 1 mg/kg/day.

Nutritional assessment

For an infant who receives little benefit from the Kasai operation, continual nutritional assessment and support is essential to prevent severe malnutrition and ensure optimum growth. Full nutritional assessment should be completed at each admission or clinic visit [14]. Measurement of weight and weight for height or length is not a good indicator of nutritional status. An increased body weight in infants with liver disease can be due to enlarged liver and spleen and fluid retention. Serial measurements of head circumference, abdominal girth, mid arm circumference, triceps and subscapular skinfolds as well as the weight and height or length of the individual are essential to assess status correctly [15–19]. If these parameters

are seen to fall, changes in medical management may be indicated, and immediate nutritional intervention is needed [20].

Feed supplementation

If the liver disease progresses, energy and protein supplements are used to give an average of 160 kcal/kg/day (672 kJ/kg/day) energy and 4.0 g/kg/day protein. This can be achieved in various ways. Powdered supplements can be added to the existing specialized formula, or a complete feed can be designed with various nutrient 'modules' for greater specificity (Table 8.2).

The source of protein for infants with compromised liver function is still being researched in the specialist centres throughout the world. Evidence appears to have renewed an interest in the role of branched chain amino acids (BCAA). It appears that the use of BCAA results in an improved nutritional status and this is reflected in greater muscle mass [21,22]. Products rich in BCAA such as Generaid powder are more widely used and new products are being developed all the time. Generaid Plus is the first complete milk rich in BCAA and MCT, currently recommended for children over the age of one year.

NUTRITIONAL SUPPORT FOR THE OLDER CHILD WITH LIVER DISEASE

After the first year of life, specialized infant milks are no longer considered the main form of treatment for children with liver disease. As the diet becomes more varied, the intake of these milks will decline. If weight gain is unsuccessful the special milk should be continued and, if refused orally, given via a nasogastric tube. Generaid Plus has been used orally and as a specialized nasogastric tube feed for children with liver disease from one year up to fifteen years of age (unreported trials are still continuing at Kings College Hospital, London).

If a child is in a stable nutritional state, ordinary diet and cows' milk can be taken. Young children with chronic liver disease may develop loose stools when cows' milk is first introduced into the diet because of its fat content, so the introduction should be gradual. Even if malabsorption is not displayed, these children

Table 8.2 Modular feed for a six month old infant with extra hepatic biliary atresia. Weight 6.0 kg; feed 180 ml/kg = 1080 ml

		Energy		Protein (g)	Fat (g)	CHO (g)	Sodium (mmol)	Potassium (mmol)
		(kcal)	(kJ)					
25 g	Maxipro (SHS)	98	410	20.0	1.5	1.2	1.4	3.0
129 g	Maxijul (SHS)	464	1936	–	–	122.7	2.7	0.1
25 ml	Calogen (SHS)	113	472	–	12.5	–	0.2	0.1
35 ml	Liquigen (SHS)	146	610	–	17.5	–	0.6	0.3
14 g	Paediatric (SHS)	42	179	–	–	10.5	<1.0	tr
	Seravit	–		–	–	1.0	–
0.2 ml	30% Sodium chloride (50 mmol in 10 ml)	–			–	–	–	10.0
5 ml	Potassium chloride (20 mmol in 10 ml)							
Sterile water up to a total of 1100 ml					(2.9%)	(12.2%)		
Total		863	3607	20.0	31.5	134.4	5.9	13.5
Feeding 1080 ml		847	3541	19.6	30.9	131.9	5.8	13.3
Per kg		141	590	3.2	5.2	21.9	1.0	2.2

may still require energy supplements in order to gain weight.

Children over the age of two may be given energy and protein supplements which provide 1 kcal/ml such as Ensure and Fresubin. More energy dense supplements (1.5 kcal/ml) can be given to children over the age of five (e.g. Fortisip, Ensure Plus, Fresubin high energy). The variety in flavours and the packaging of these products make them very appealing to children. New product developments in this field continue and may include a drink supplement which includes BCAA and MCT fat, and a confectionery bar of similar specification for use where there is the need for severe fluid restriction.

Healthy eating guidelines for a high fibre, low fat, low sugar diet are unsuitable for a child with chronic liver disease.

Infections

Ascending cholangitis causes progressive liver damage, and this complication is taken seriously. Clinical symptoms are fever without obvious cause and possible reappearance of jaundice and a reduction in stool pigment. Episodes of ascending cholangitis usually result in the infant or child being admitted to hospital for treatment with a minimum of five days intravenous antibiotics. Infections of this type can lead to a reduced oral intake of both milk and solids, and also a deterioration in liver function. For these reasons nutritional support is an essential part of the admission. Weight loss commonly occurs with infection, and feed supplementation will help to minimize this.

Ascites

Ascites can affect nutritional status greatly. It is important to ensure it is managed aggressively with the use of diuretics (e.g. spironolactone) and salt-poor albumin infusions if the serum albumin level is low. Treatment by fluid restriction alone can compromise nutritional status severely [23]. Imposed restrictions are commonly 80–100 ml/kg body weight. Feeds should be fully supplemented with energy and protein (Table 8.3). Energy-dense feeds of 1.6–2.0 kcal/ml (6.7–8.4 kJ/ml) are commonly used by giving up to 25% carbohydrate and 7% fat concentrations in the feed. These feeds are well tolerated by infants.

Solid food should continue and be energy supplemented where possible.

Table 8.3(a) Feed on fluid restriction with BCAA. For an eight month old child with extrahepatic biliary atresia. Weight 7.0 kg with ascites; estimated dry weight 6.5 kg. Fluid restriction 100 ml/kg = 650 ml

			Energy		Protein (g)	Fat (g)	CHO (g)	Sodium (mmol)	Potassium (mmol)
			(kcal)	(kJ)					
98 g	Pregestimil	(Mead Johnson)	448	1873	12.5	17.9	61.6	9.4	12.5
18 g	Generaid	(SHS)	70	293	14.6	0.9	<0.9	0.8	1.6
100 g	Duocal	(SHS)	470	1965	–	22.3	72.7	<0.2	<0.1
Sterile water up to a total of 650 ml						(6.3%)	(20.8%)		
Total			988	4131	27.1	41.1	135.2	10.4	14.3
Per kg			152	636	4.2	6.3	20.8	1.6	2.2

Table 8.3(b) Alternative feed

	Energy		Protein (g)	Fat (g)	CHO (g)	Sodium (mmol)	Potassium (mmol)
	(kcal)	(kJ)					
243 g Generaid plus sterile water up to a total of 650 ml	1089	4557	26.7	46.2 (7.1%)	150.7 (23.2%)	7.3	29.2
Total	1089	4552	26.7	46.2	150.7	7.3	29.2
Per kg	168	700	4.1	7.1	23.2	1.1	4.5

Nasogastric tube feeding

The presence of ascites, plus an enlarged liver and spleen, leads to a reduced tolerance of feed volume. Where feeds are not completed orally, nasogastric tube feeding should be commenced. Gastrostomy feeding is contraindicated in infants and children with liver disease, as the presence of ascites leads to an increased risk of peritonitis. However older children with cystic fibrosis and liver disease have been treated successfully with gastrostomy tubes.

The presence of oesophageal varices, due to portal hypertension in this group of patients, often deters doctors and dietitians from recommending the use of nasogastric tubes. A recent oesophageal bleed requiring endoscopic investigation and injection with a sclerosing agent would confirm this concern. However, fine bore polyurethane or silicone tubes are considered less erosive to the oesophagus and allow tube feeding to commence soon after a bleed.

It is preferable for nasogastric tube feeding to be administered overnight to allow normal daytime feeding behaviour to continue. If this is not practical, however, more frequent feeds should be offered orally then completed via the nasogastric tube as a bolus. Oral stimulation should continue with the use of a dummy (comforter) in infants.

Hypoglycaemia can be a life threatening symptom of impaired liver function and those caring for children with liver disease must be aware of this and taught how to recognize early signs. All feeding pumps must be fitted with an alarm system to indicate any disturbance in the delivery of feed. Parents should be fully trained in the operation of the feeding system [8,24], and must know how to give carbohydrate quickly in an emergency.

With this intensive feeding regimen, good nutritional status can be achieved. Parents also report improvement in the infant or child's wellbeing and quality of life. This will ultimately improve his chance of being considered for and receiving a successful liver transplant.

Oesophageal varices

Bleeding from varices can be chronic yet mild, causing anaemia only. However, long term this may require a blood transfusion. Severe bleeding can be stopped by the administration of intravenous vasopressin and somatostatin. A Sengstaken tube, a special endoscopic tube with balloons attached, is sometimes required. This can be inflated within the oesophagus to apply direct pressure on the bleeding areas. The infant or child will normally be sedated for this procedure. Enteral feeding is inappropriate at this stage; hydration and nutrition is maintained intravenously. Once stable, endoscopy is performed and if varices are located, they will be injected with a sclerosing agent (e.g. ethanolamine). This procedure will be repeated at intervals until the varices are controlled.

Clear fluids will be allowed 12–24 hours after endoscopy depending on the extent of injection. A soft diet is then maintained for approximately one week. Normal dietary intake can then continue. In practice, parents find the risk of a further bleed so stressful that children are discouraged from eating dry, 'sharp' foods such as toast, crisps, biscuits, chips. A 'shunt' procedure (porto-systemic) may be performed to divert blood from the portal vein back to the heart, thus relieving the portal pressure. This may induce hepatic encephalopathy however.

Hepatic encephalopathy

Current dietary managment of children with biliary atresia promotes a high protein intake, 4.0 g/kg/day – an average of two and a half times that of the reference nutrient intake (RNI) for protein [25]. It is important to monitor the infant or child closely because hepatic encephalopathy (HE) can develop as liver function deteriorates. This occurs in chronic disease after shunting procedures for portal hypertension, or acutely following a large gastrointestinal bleed. HE will develop rapidly in fulminant hepatic failure (see later).

Restriction of protein is an accepted method of treating HE. This can have a deleterious effect on the nutritonal status of the baby or child. Therefore it is essential for the degree of encephalopathy to be assessed to determine the level of dietary protein restriction. Serum ammonia levels have been used as a measure of encephalopathy. In practice, however, an infant can show no clinical signs with a raised serum ammonia level and, in general, protein restriction is not required until symptoms are detected. The most common signs noted are increased drowsiness and irritability.

The prescription of lactulose and neomycin or metronidazole (to remove ammonia-producing bacteria from the gut) is part of the clinical treatment for HE. In HE, the plasma amino acid profile shows an increase in the aromatic amino acids phenylalanine, tyrosine, tryptophan and also methionine. Branched chain amino acids are low [26].

For babies or children with severe HE (grade 4/5), it is essential for an energy source to be given either intravenously or nasogastrically to prevent catabolism [27]. This can be in the form of glucose or glucose and fat. Protein intake can recommence at 0.5 g/kg within 24 or 48 hours if the child is stable.

Daily assessment is essential and if improvement is seen the protein intake can be increased by 0.5 g/kg each day until a normal intake is achieved.

No clear benefit from the use of feeds rich in branch chain amino acids in the treatment of HE has been shown [28,29,30].

ORTHOTOPIC LIVER TRANSPLANTATION

The success of liver transplantation in infants and children has promoted a greater interest in nutrition [31] as a pre-operative factor that can have an impact on ultimate survival. Previously children with liver disease were transplanted only when they reached a weight of 10 kg. This was due to a shortage of organ donations for infants. With major advances in surgery such as the ability to reduce a donor organ in size and the use of live related donors, infants are now transplanted at any age or size. This highlights the need to provide optimum nutritional support throughout the period of care pre- and post-transplant [32,33]. Any child with chronic liver disease who is to be considered for liver transplantation will require a comprehensive assessment which will include full assessment of nutritional status. Serial anthropometric measurements are essential to provide information which will determine the requirements for and also response to any intensive therapy (i.e. overnight nasogastric tube feeding) undertaken pre-transplant.

Post-transplant, infants and children will be given total parenteral nutrition for the first few days, then gradually changed to enteral feeding [34,35]. The feeding regimen should be tailored to the individual [36]. In some cases, nasogastric tube feeding continues post-transplant until oral intake is fully established. The specialized MCT-based milks may still be used post-transplant in the infant, especially if chronic rejection is a problem and the infant exhibits loose stools (a side effect of prescribed immunosuppressive drugs).

A diet appropriate for age is advised when liver function has normalized. Good nutritional status is essential for a quick recovery. Liver transplantation, as any major surgery, will affect a child's feeding and general behaviour. An infant or child can become withdrawn and appear uncooperative. This is described as a 'post ITU syndrome'. The aim is always to encourage a child to enjoy all aspects of feeding whilst ensuring that optimum nutrition is achieved.

NEONATAL HEPATITIS

Nutritional management of babies with neonatal hepatitis is similar to that of biliary atresia. If the serum bilirubin levels and liver function tests return to normal after the baby is six months old and weight gain is sufficient, an ordinary infant milk can be introduced. In practice, the majority of babies still require a specialized formula and supplements.

ALPHA-1-ANTITRYPSIN DEFICIENCY

Approximately 17% of babies investigated for jaundice are diagnosed as having alpha-1-antitrypsin deficiency. This inherited disorder of the liver can be severe. Dietary treatment is the same as for biliary atresia.

INTRA-HEPATIC BILARY HYPOLASIA AND ALAGILLE'S SYNDROME

Biliary hypoplasia is an inherited condition in which the baby can fail to thrive and 20% of these babies will have been born small for dates. Cholestasis can be severe and pruritis is very distressing for the baby

[37]. Alagille's syndrome has an incidence of one in 100 000 live births. It is a collection of features including biliary hypoplasia, cardiovascular disease, skeletal, ocular and facial abnormalities and also renal disease. Chronic malabsorption is common. These children suffer from severe failure to thrive as well as severe pruritis and xanthelasma which affect quality of life to a great extent. The reasons for such marked failure to thrive is not fully known, although pancreatic insufficiency could be contributory [38,39].

The basis of dietary treatment is the same as for biliary atresia. The malabsorption can be helped by the use of enteric coated pancreatic supplements. The dosage must be assessed for the individual. With severe disease, the use of overnight nasogastric tube feeding is common. Any renal impairment must be considered in the dietary management.

HEPATITIS

Autoimmune or aquired hepatitis may be treated with steroids. Side effects include excess weight gain, fluid retention and impaired glucose tolerance. Appropriate dietary advice should be given accordingly. In severe cases medical treatment cannot control the disease and liver failure may result.

FULMINANT HEPATIC FAILURE

Fulminant hepatic failure is defined as the rapid onset of acute and severe liver impairment within eight weeks of the onset of symptoms [40]. Heparctic encephalopathy (HE) is common. The cause is unknown and prognosis is poor. Infants and children presenting with fulminant hepatic failure often require liver transplantation.

These children are usually ventilated, so intravenous nutritional support is often prescribed. If the child improves, an enteral feeding regimen will be prescribed according to the total fluid allowance and biochemical results.

THE PANCREAS

PANCREATITIS

Pancreatitis in childhood is rare. The cause can be a congenital pancreatic duct abnormality, drug therapy

(e.g. steroid therapy) or injury to the pancreatic parenchyma often brought on by trauma [41]. In many cases, the actual cause is unknown.

The most common cause of acute pancreatitis is

blunt abdominal trauma (e.g. non-accidental injury as a result of child abuse). Injury to the liver and pancreas in children frequently results from road traffic accidents (e.g. damage caused by seat belts), or sports injuries such as horse riding. Acute pancreatitis occurs secondary to this insult. Infection (viral, bacterial, fungal, or parasitic helminthic worm infestation), vasculitis, gallstones, imflammatory bowel disease and metabolic disease (e.g. Reye's syndrome) are all noted causes of acute pancreatitis.

Chronic pancreatitis is probably underrecognized as a cause of severe abdominal pain in children. It can be hereditary, caused by an abnormal pancreatic duct. Metabolic diseases are also associated with the chronic form of pancreatitis. These include cystic fibrosis, alpha-1-antitrypsin deficiency, and Wilson's disease. Pancreatic duct abnormalities are also associated with a choledochal cyst (dilatation of the biliary ducts).

Onset is commonly at the age of 10–12 years. Food avoidance, weight loss, growth retardation and even developmental delay can occur prior to the acute presenting symptoms of constant pain, nausea, vomiting and fever. Abnormal serum and urine amylase levels and standard liver function tests will confirm the diagnosis.

With an acute episode of pancreatitis, the child will have 'nil by mouth' and receive intravenous dextrose saline. Pain will be controlled. Hyperglycaemia and hypoglycaemia are a severe risk so blood sugar monitoring is essential. If symptoms persist total parenteral nutrition may be indicated. As amylase levels fall, indicating a return to normal pancreatic function, the child can start clear fluids and gradually return to a normal diet [41,42].

With chronic pancreatitis, fat malabsorption can be a problem. It is important to avoid the restriction of a low fat diet. In most cases, the child will benefit from the use of enteric coated pancreatic supplements (Creon, Pancrease, Nutrizym GR). These capsules should be taken with all meals and snacks. The dosage should be tailored to the individual child (Table 10.3). Energy supplements, such as glucose polymers in powder form (e.g. Maxijul, Polycal), or liquid form (e.g. Hycal, Polycal Liquid) may be prescribed to prevent weight loss.

SCHWACHMAN'S SYNDROME

Schwachman's syndrome is the second most frequently diagnosed cause of pancreatic insufficiency after cystic fibrosis. The disease is inherited and presents as exocrine pancreatic insufficiency, bone marrow and haematological abnormalities, with normal sweat electrolytes. Neutropenia is a common problem causing frequent infections which can compromise nutritional status [43].

The liver can also be affected in Schwachman's syndrome. Hepatomegaly is seen in two thirds of infants but less frequently in the older child. Liver function tests are elevated, yet the bilirubin level is normal. Malabsorption develops by 4–6 months of age. Failure to thrive and impaired growth soon become apparent.

Treatment

Treatment of malabsorption due to pancreatic insufficiency is with the administration of the enteric coated pancreatic enzymes (Creon, Pancrease, Nutrizym GR). Infants requiring pancreatic supplements are either given powdered enzyme (Pancrex) mixed with a small amount of milk, or the microspheres from the capsule of the enteric coated form mixed with fruit purée. If high doses of supplements are required, antacids and H_2 receptor antagonists (cimetidine or ranitidine) can also be prescribed.

Essential fatty acid deficiency is rare. Fat-soluble vitamin levels should be monitored regularly (page 116). A multivitamin preparation is recommended routinely and the use of intramuscular vitamin injections may be required.

Feeding behaviour problems are common in these children and should be tackled with the help of a speech therapist and psychologist. If failure to thrive is a problem, continual or overnight nasogastric tube feeding should be considered. Elemental or hydrolysatebased feeds are recommended in order to reduce the number of pancreatic supplements required.

NESIDIOBLASTOSIS

Nesidioblastosis, or organic hyperinsulinaemia, is the most common cause of severe hypoglycaemia in neonates and infants. It is an inherited condition shown histologically as an abnormality of all endocrine pancreatic cells, not just the beta cells which produce insulin.

The baby with nesidioblastosis will present with an increase in fatty tissue and hypoglycaemia soon after birth. An older child can present with behaviour changes or even convulsions. The child is commonly obese and generally tall for his age. The condition may go untreated due to the fact that the child has a mild form and has been fed frequently with no episodes of hypoglycaemia detected. Untreated hypoglycaemia can result in cerebral damage and permanent developmental delay.

Acutely, a central venous line is essential to ensure rapid correction of hypoglycaemia by intravenous glucose infusion. Temporary improvement can result from the administration of diazoxide. This inhibits insulin release, enhances the secretion of adrenaline from the adrenal medulla and stimulates glucose release from glycogen stores in the liver. Other medical treatments include glucagon and the somatostatin analogue octreotide. However in severe cases where medical treatment fails, subtotal (about 75%) or neartotal (95%) pancreatectomy is required [41]. The small piece of pancreas is left to protect the common bile duct. Secretion of enzyme and bicarbonate will be greatly reduced. Insulin injections are then required to treat the resulting diabetes mellitus.

Treatment

The aim of any dietary treatment is to prevent hypoglycaemia by giving frequent glucose-containing feeds orally or via a nasogastric tube [43]. However, as these infants require such large amounts of glucose to prevent hypoglycaemia (in the region of 12–15 mg glucose/kg body weight/minute may be required) much of which may need to be given initially as intravenous fluids via a central line, this will severely limit the volume of infant formula that can be taken. In order to improve nutrition, infant formula may be concentrated and then supplemented with additional carbohydrate so that the volume of intravenous fluids can be reduced. If the infant's blood glucose levels can be stabilized on diazoxide, then regular feeding with a normal infant formula can be resumed. Close blood glucose monitoring is essential. Fasting must be avoided. In the older child refused food must be replaced with carbohydrate containing drinks; if these are also refused glucose must be delivered by nasogastric tube. Intercurrent illness will often necessitate nasogastric feeding; intravenous glucose may be required. Parents and carers must be taught the signs of hypoglycaemia and how to deal with it.

If the infant or child cannot be stabilized on a regimen of diazoxide and frequent feeding then a partial pancreatectomy is performed. Post-operatively, insulin may need to be administered to control blood sugar levels, but some individuals can manage without insulin as the remaining pancreas adapts. Pancreatic enzyme supplements may be required if there is evidence of malabsorption once the child is taking a normal diet.

REFERENCES

1 Mowat AP *Liver Disorders in Childhood*, 2nd edn. London: Butterworths, 1987.
2 Weber A, Roy CC The malabsorption associated with chronic liver disease. *Am J Clin Nutr*, 1972, 23 604–613.
3 Mieli Vergani G *et al*. Late referral for biliary atresia – missed opportunities for effective surgery. *Lancet*, Feb 25, 421–423.
4 Ohi R *et al*. Progress in the treatment of biliary atresia. *World J Surg*, 1985, **9** 285–293.
5 Cohen MI, Gartner LM The use of medium chain triglycerides in the management of biliary atresia. *J Paed*, 1971, **79** 379–384.
6 Kaufman SS *et al*. Influence of Portagen and Pregestimil on essential fatty acid status in infantile liver disease. *Pediatrics*, 1992, **89**(1) 151–154.
7 Kaufmann SS *et al*. Nutritional support for the infant with extrahepatic biliary atresia. *J Paed*, 1987, **110** 679–686.
8 Charlton CPJ *et al*. Nutrition improved with intensive enteral feeding in children awaiting liver transplantation. Abstract in the proceedings of the first meeting of the Clinical Metabolism and Nutrition Support Group (of the Nutrition Society). Sheffield, UK, 1988.
9 Birch L The role of experience in children's food acceptance patterns. *J Am Diet Ass*, 1987, **87**(9), Supplement 36–40.
10 Ball CS, Mowat AP Liver disease – nutritional management. Nutrition and liver disease. In: *Clinical Nutrition of the Young Child*, vol 2. Nestlé Nutrition. New York: Vevey/Raven Press, 1992.
11 Daum F *et al*. 25-Hydroxycholecalciferol in the management of rickets associated with extrahepatic biliary atresia. *J Pediatr*, 1976, **88**(6) 1041–1043.
12 Suit S *et al*. Zinc status and its relations to growth retardation in children with biliary atresia. *J Pediatr Surg*, 1987, **2265** 401–405.
13 Morrison SA *et al*. Zinc deficiency: a cause for abnormal dark adaption in cirrhotics. *Am J Clin Nutr*, 1978, **31** 276.
14 Merrit RJ, Suskind RM Nutritional survey of hospitalized pediatric patients. *Am J Clin Nutr*, 1979, 32 1320–1325.
15 Sokol RJ, Stall C Anthropometric evaluation of children

with chronic liver disease. *Am J Clin Nutr*, 1990, **52** 203–208.

16 Tanner JM, Whitehouse RH Revised standards for tricep and subscapular skinfolds in British children. *Arch Dis Childh*, 1975, **50** 142–145.

17 Frisancho AR Triceps skinfold and upper arm muscle size norms for assessment of nutritional status. *Am J Clin Nutr*, 1974, **27** 1052–1058.

18 Frisancho AR New norms of upper limb fat and muscle areas for assessment of nutritional status. *Am J Clin Nutr*, 1981, **34** 2540–2545.

19 Sann L *et al*. Arm fat and muscle areas in infancy. *Arch Dis Childh*, 1988, **63** 256–260.

20 Chin SE *et al*. The nature of malnutrition in children with end stage liver disease awaiting orthotopic liver transplantation. *Am J Clin Nutr*, 1992, **56** 164–168.

21 Christie ML *et al*. Enriched branched chain amino acid formula versus a casein based supplement in the treatment of cirrhosis. *J Parenter Enter Nutr*, 1985, **9** 671–678.

22 Chin SE *et al*. Nutritional support in children with end stage liver disease: a randomized crossover trial of a branched-chain amino acid supplement. *Am J Clin Nutr*, 1992, **56** 158–163.

23 Smith J *et al*. Enteral hyperalimentation in under-nourished patients with cirrhosis and ascites. *Am J Clin Nutr*, 1982, **35** 56–72.

24 Holden CE *et al*. Nasogastric feeding at home: acceptability and safety. *Arch Dis Childh*, 1991, **66** 148–151.

25 Department of Health Report on Health and Social Subjects No 41. *Dietary Reference Values for Food Energy and Nutrients for the United Kingdom*. London: HMSO, 1991.

26 Rosen HM *et al*. Plasma amino acid patterns in hepatic encephalopathy of differing etiology. *Gastroenterology*, 1977, **72** 483–487.

27 Keohane PP *et al*. Enteral nutrition in malnourished patients with hepatic cirrhosis and acute encephalopathy. *J Parenter Enter Nutr*, 1983, **7** 346–350.

28 Swart GR, Frenkel M, Van den Berg JWO Minimum protein requirements in advanced liver disease; a metabolic ward study of the effects of oral branched-chain amino acids. In: Walser M, Williamson JR (eds.) *Metabolic and Clinical Implications of Branched-Chain Amino and Ketoacids*. North Holland, New York: Elsevier, 1981.

29 McCollough AJ, Mullen KD, Tavill AS Branched-chain amino acids in nutritional therapy in liver disease; dearth or surfeit. *Hepatology*, 1983, **3** 269–271.

30 Horst D *et al*. Comparison of dietary protein with an oral branched-chain enriched amino acid supplement in chronic portal systemic encephalopathy; a randomized controlled trial. *Hepatology*, 1984, **4**(2) 279–287.

31 Goulet OJ *et al*. Preoperative nutritional evaluation and support for liver transplantation in children. *Trans Proc*, 1987, **19** 3249–3255.

32 Stuart S *et al*. Preoperative evaluation, preparation and timing of orthotopic liver transplantation in the child. *Seminars in Liver Disease*, 1989, **9**(3) 176–183.

33 Hehir DJ *et al*. Nutrition in patients under going orthotopic liver transplantation. *J Parenter Enter Nutr*, 1985, **9** 695–700.

34 Byer SW *et al*. Liver transplantation therapy for children, Part I. *J Paed Gastr Nutr*, 1988, **7** 157–166.

35 Byer SW *et al*. Liver transplantation therapy for children, Part II. *J Paed Gastr Nutr*, 1988, **7** 797–815.

36 *Addenbrooke's Hospital Children's Liver Transplantation Protocol* (March 1990). Addenbrookes Hospital, Cambridge.

37 Singer JC *Alagille's Syndrome – Information for Patients and their Families*. Surrey: Children's Liver Disease Foundation, 1990.

38 Alagille D Management of paucity of interlobular bile ducts. *J Hepatol*, 1985, **1** 561.

39 Chong SKF *et al*. Exocrine pancreatic insufficiency in syndromic paucity of interlobular bile ducts. *J Pediatr Gast Nutr*, 1989, **9** 445–449.

40 Trey C, Davidson C *The Management of Fulminant Hepatic Failure*. New York: Grune & Stratton, 1970.

41 Davenport M, Howard ER Surgical treatment of pancreatic disease in childhood. In: Johnson CD, Imrie CW (eds.) *Pancreatic Disease – Progress and Prospects*. London: Springer-Verlag, 1991.

42 Aynsley-Green A Hypoglycaemia. In: Brook CGD (ed.) *Clinical Paediatric Endocrinology*. Oxford: Blackwell Scientific Publications, 1981.

43 Aynsley-Green A, Soltesz G Hypoglycaemia in infancy and childhood. *Current Reviews in Paediatrics*. Edinburgh: Churchill Livingstone, 1985.

USEFUL ADDRESS

Children's Liver Disease Foundation
138 Digbeth, Birmingham B5 6DR.

CHAPTER 9

Diabetes Mellitus

The parents of a child who is diagnosed as having a chronic disease (including a newly diagnosed diabetic child) are initially shocked and devastated. Parents can also feel a sense of guilt: they may feel that their child has developed diabetes because they have permitted him to eat sweets excessively; alternatively, if they have a family history of diabetes that they are responsible for their child's condition.

An effective, family-based dietary education programme which is going to result in the modification of a child's eating habits can only begin when parents are allowed to grieve and come to terms with the diagnosis of diabetes in their child. It is vital to develop a rapport with the family so that a high quality of consistent dietetic care can be provided. Frequent and short teaching sessions are preferable, with the entire family if appropriate. Unlike insulin, blood sugars and hypoglycaemia, food is familiar to all, so it may be beneficial to commence the diabetic instruction process with food and diet related topics before the nursing and medical staff begin detailed teaching.

THE DIABETIC DIET

Aims

- to meet the child's nutritional requirements

Children with diabetes have the same basic nutritional needs as their non-diabetic counterparts.

- to contribute towards optimising blood sugar levels, avoiding swings between hyper- and hypoglycaemia

The distribution of carbohydrate throughout the day is important and should balance the effects of the injected insulin. A pre-prandial blood glucose of 4–6 mmol/l is ideal.

- dietary modifications must ensure normal growth and development

Dietary energy should be sufficient for growth and allow for variable exercise patterns, but should not provoke obesity. Growth should be plotted at regular intervals using standard height and weight charts. Growth velocity charts are useful for anticipating the onset of obesity or stunting. Growth can be a useful indicator of diabetic control, as often poor physical development is a consequence of inadequate diabetic management. Obesity is less of a problem in diabetic children than in diabetic adults but, if children do gain weight disproportionately to their height, suitable dietetic advice should be given at a very early stage.

Particular care should be taken to monitor the weight of adolescent girls as this group is most prone to obesity [1].

- the diet should minimize the development of diabetic complications such as cardiovascular and microvascular disease

If insufficient carbohydrate is allowed then children will tend to compensate by eating more protein and fat, which is undesirable.

RECOMMENDATIONS

Two documents have published recommendations for people with diabetes.

The British Diabetic Association's 1980 document [2], updated in 1992 *Dietary Recommendations for People with Diabetes: An Update for the 1990s* [3], recommends that at least 50% of the dietary energy should be derived from carbohydrate, mainly fibre-rich polysaccharides.

More specifically '*Dietary Recommendations for*

Children and Adolescents with Diabetes' were made in 1989 by the British Diabetic Association [4]. These suggest that dietary carbohydrate should never be restricted below the usual family intake (40–45% energy). They also recognize that the energy distribution between carbohydrate, fat and protein will differ depending on age: breast fed infants will obtain approximately 55% energy from fat, 5% from protein and 40% from carbohydrate, whereas a five year old may derive 35% energy from fat, 15% from protein and 50% from carbohydrate. Traditional dietary regimens have emphasized only the carbohydrate component. Present day practice adopts a more holistic dietary approach.

An increase in carbohydrate, particularly from high fibre sources, and a reduction in fat is recommended. In addition the energy content of the diet should be tailored to the individual. This is of major importance in order to minimise the risk of chronic degenerative disease such as obesity and coronary heart disease.

Carbohydrate

The current recommendation for the diabetic child is that carbohydrate provides greater than 40% energy. The formula: 120 g carbohydrate + 10 g for every year of life reflects current thinking and provides a baseline of daily carbohydrate that should provide at least 40% energy from carbohydrate.

For example, a two year old boy will be prescribed 120 g + 20 g (140 g) carbohydrate daily. His estimated average energy requirement is 1190 kcal [5], hence a minimum of 47% energy should be derived from carbohydrate.

It should be noted however that the Dietary Reference Values for Food Energy [5] were not designed for the individual but for groups. Allowance should be made for the child's body weight and activity. A boy growing along the third centile for weight will weigh 14.4 kg, whilst a boy growing along the 97th centile will weigh 23.2 kg. Both are growing within normal limits, yet their weights vary by 8.8 kg. These two boys will require different energy and carbohydrate intakes.

Fibre (non-starch polysaccharide)

The British Diabetic Association recommends a fibre intake of 2 g/100 kcal/day [4], but admits that this will mean a large change for some children and their families, and that an intake of 1 g/100 kcal is a reasonable first step. Gradual changes in fibre intake are necessary to minimize colic, flatulence and abdominal distension. High intakes can impair the absorption of calcium, iron and zinc due to the high level of phytate in high fibre foods, although it can be argued that these foods themselves, being less refined, have a higher vitamin and mineral content than lower fibre foods.

High fibre foods are less energy-dense than refined carbohydrate ones, therefore the child's total energy intake may be compromised if the diet contains large quantities of fibre. However children can safely include a number of high fibre foods in their diet, e.g. wholemeal bread, high fibre breakfast cereals, baked beans and high fibre baked goods. A large proportion of children will eat at least one portion of fruit each day; many do not like vegetables, but will take them when included in soups and stews. Often raw vegetables will be taken in preference to those that are cooked.

High fibre pulses appear to be particularly beneficial for blood sugar control and many children will eat them in the form of baked beans, peas, sweetcorn, kidney beans or lentil soup.

Fat

Fat is necessary in children's diets to provide adequate energy, fat-soluble vitamins and essential fatty acids. However if an older child's fat intake is higher than 35% energy or rapid weight gain is a problem at any age, the following advice can be given to reduce dietary fat:

- take grilled and oven-baked foods in preference to fried foods
- cut off visible fat on meat
- take fish and poultry instead of red meat
- cut down on the quantity of crisps eaten to 2–3 bags per week (often a compromise of a maximum of one bag per day has to be conceded); use reduced fat crisp varieties
- take reduced-fat cheeses or varieties that are lower in fat (cottage cheese is not popular with children, so it seems more realistic to limit the amount of high fat cheese and encourage lower fat varieties such as Edam or half-fat hard cheese)
- Use semi-skimmed or skimmed milk, provided appetite is good and an adequate energy intake can

be maintained. A supplement of vitamins A and D should be considered for children under the age of 5 years who are taking a reduced fat milk.

Protein

Children with diabetes should have protein intakes not in excess of that taken by other children. In the diets of most children, protein provides 15% of dietary energy, although actual requirements are considerably lower than this [5].

Sugar

School children take 20–30% of their carbohydrate as added simple sugars. Replacing these with polysaccharides high in fibre in a diabetic child's diet results in a considerable increase in the bulk of food eaten. For this reason it is hard for diabetic children to increase the proportion of energy eaten as dietary carbohydrate if it is to come from high fibre sources.

It is now recognized that the use of sugar taken as part of a mixed meal does not have a detrimental effect on blood sugar control in well controlled insulin dependant diabetics who are not obese [6,7]. It is also recognized that the rate of absorption of carbohydrates depends on a great many factors, and the idea that sucrose always causes a rapid rise in blood sugar is perhaps too simplistic.

Rapidly absorbed carbohydrate such as a chocolate biscuit can be included in the dietary allowance at the end of a main meal, when the glycaemic response will be lower. The inclusion of a controlled amount of 'sugary' foods has a number of benefits:

- it makes the child feel that his diet is not too different from that of his peers
- it may increase dietary compliance
- it increases palatability and variety
- it discourages the use of diabetic products.

Sugar and exercise

Exercise has the effect of lowering blood glucose levels by increasing the non-insulin dependent uptake of glucose by the cells. Insulin doses can be reduced before periods of heavy exercise, but a child's energy expenditure is so variable from day to day and hour to hour that it is more practical in most instances to cover additional activity with extra carbohydrate. Extra carbohydrate given prior to exercise need not be in the form of simple sugars, although these are often favoured by the child. In prolonged strenuous exercise it will be necessary to 'top up' blood sugar during the exercise period, and this is most practically achieved by using rapidly absorbed simple sugars such as a glucose drink.

The amount of extra carbohydrate required to cover a period of exercise will depend on the activity, the time of day in relation to injections, usual diet and on the individual child. Only 10–20 g extra carbohydrate may be necessary before light exercise; 50–60 g may be required by an enthusiastic child before and during a football match. The child should be encouraged to take blood sugar readings before, during and after exercise initially, so that the amount of additional carbohydrate can be tailored to the individual.

It is particularly important to avoid hypoglycaemia during potentially hazardous activities such as swimming or skiing, where altered concentration or consciousness could have serious consequences.

Low sugar and diabetic products

Low calorie drinks are extremely valuable in the diet of a child with diabetes. Other low sugar products marketed for the general population can also be useful – for instance reduced-sugar jams, fruit canned in natural juice. Diabetic products however are not to be recommended for the child with diabetes. They are expensive, can be unpalatable and in addition may contain sorbitol. The child should be encouraged to regard the diet as one of 'sensible eating' and not one which relies on the need to eat different or 'special' foods.

Sweeteners

Sorbitol is a sweetener with a similar energy value to carbohydrate. It is poorly absorbed and can cause osmotic diarrhoea, particularly in children, who have a lower body mass than that of the adult, for whom the products are designed. Fructose has no advantage over sucrose in terms of taste as a sweetener and gives less satisfactory results in baking. Although it does not require insulin for its metabolism it has a glucose-sparing effect in the body and causes a rise in blood sugar if large quantities are taken.

Non-nutritive sweeteners can be useful in drinks and desserts and to sprinkle on breakfast cereals. However many people find that saccharin has a bitter aftertaste. Aspartame has a limited use because sweetening power is lost when subjected to prolonged heating. Acesulfame K is another non-nutritive sweetener that is currently not widely used, but may gain popularity in the future as it is heat resistant and without aftertaste.

PRESCRIBING THE DIET

A dietary assessment is essential on diagnosis, so that the child's normal intake and meal pattern can be ascertained. The carbohydrate or energy allowance and distribution can then be tailored to the home situation. Providing the child is not overweight, the usual energy intake prior to the onset of diabetic symptoms can be used as a basis for deciding the diet. Carbohydrate should provide 40–50% of energy and fat kept as low as practical, depending on the child's age.

It is important for children to take carbohydrate at regular intervals so that hypoglycaemia may be avoided and hyperglycaemia prevented. Meals should be consumed at least 30 minutes after an insulin injection (unless low blood sugar dictates otherwise) in order to optimize post-prandial blood sugar profiles. Amounts of carbohydrate in excess of 50–60 g given at an one time may also produce an inappropriately raised postprandial blood sugar. A meal pattern of three meals and three snacks each day is appropriate for most children, although very young children and adolescents may need more snacks. Carbohydrate should be distributed throughout the day taking account of the peak periods of insulin action. Fig. 9.1 shows commonly used insulins and their action times, Tables 9.1(a) and (b) show a typical day's diet with carbohydrate distributed according to insulin regimen.

Measured diet

It is important that the child and his carers have an understanding of the nutritional content of foods. At present the 10 g carbohydrate system (using handy measures) offers the best system for children, where a daily allowance of carbohydrate is given along with a

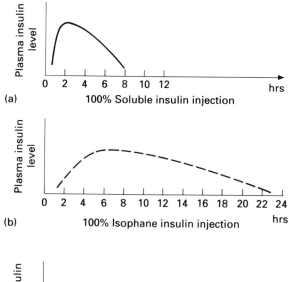

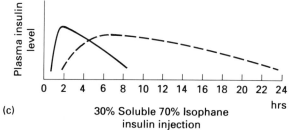

Fig. 9.1 (a) 100% Soluble insulin injection
(b) 100% Isophane insulin injection
(c) 30% Soluble 70% isophane insulin injection

suggested distribution of carbohydrate at each meal and snack time, although these may need revising when more is known about the glycaemic index of different foods or meals. A list of 10 g carbohydrate portions is given in Table 9.2; the British Diabetic Association also publish lists of 10 g carbohydrate exchanges. Examples of measured diets are given in Table 9.1; Table 9.1(b) gives an example of carbohydrate distribution for the prescribed insulin regimen shown in Fig. 9.2.

Unmeasured diet

Alternative methods of dietary advice which do not involve measuring or estimating the carbohydrate value of individual foods include the 'plate model' used by the Swedish Diabetic Association [7]. In this type of diet a meal or snack of approximately equal carbohy-

Table 9.1(a) A 3 year old girl is on a single daily injection of isophane insulin (Fig. 9.1b)

Insulin injection (7.00 AM)			gCHO
Breakfast (7.30 AM)	30 g	7 tablespoons porridge	10 g
		⅓ pint of milk	10 g
		½ large slice of wholemeal toast and polyunsaturated spread	10 g
Mid morning (10.30 AM)	10 g	1 banana	10 g
Lunch (12.30 PM)	40 g	1 plate of lentil soup	10 g
		1 large slice of wholemeal toast	20 g
		⅓ small tin of spaghetti	10 g
Mid afternoon snack (2.30 PM)	20 g	1 small box raisins	10 g
		1 digestive biscuit low calorie orange squash	10 g
Dinner (5.00 PM)	30 g	mince, carrots, 1 scoop of potato	10 g
		1 fruit yoghurt	20 g
Bedtime (7.00 PM)	20 g	1 glass of milk	10 g
		½ large slice of wholemeal bread and peanut butter as a sandwich	10 g

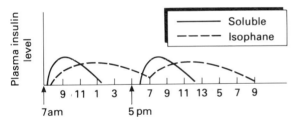

Fig. 9.2 Twice daily therapy of premixed 30% soluble 70% isophane insulin

Table 9.1(b) A 12 year old boy is on a BD regime of premixed 30% soluble and 70% isophane insulin and has a daily allowance of 240 g of carbohydrate (see Fig. 9.2)

Insulin injection (7.00 AM)			gCHO
Breakfast (7.30 AM)	40 g	2 Weetabix	20 g
		⅓ pint semi-skimmed milk	10 g
		½ large slice of wholemeal toast and polyunsaturated spread	10 g
Mid morning (10.00 AM – school break time)	30 g	Apple	10 g
		1 plain biscuit	10 g
		1 small box raisins	10 g
Lunch (12.30 PM)	50 g	2 wholemeal rolls with chicken and salad	40 g
		1 carton of diet fruit yoghurt Low calorie drink	10 g
Mid afternoon (2.30 PM – school break time)	20 g	Wholemeal scone and reduced sugar jam	20 g
(3.45 PM – after school)	10 g	1 packet crisps Low calorie drink	10 g
Insulin injection (5.00 PM)			
Dinner (5.30 PM)	50 g	Bowl of lentil soup	10 g
		Wholemeal pasta 135 g; bolognaise sauce; side salad	30 g
		1 scoop of ice cream Low calorie drink	10 g
Mid evening (7.30 PM)	20 g	1 glass semi-skimmed milk	10 g
		1 banana	10 g
Bedtime (9.00 PM)	20 g	1 large slice wholemeal toast with polyunsaturated spread Cup of tea	20 g

drate is given at regular intervals; the meal as a whole is assessed by eye and no attempt is made to quantify individual foods. The exact amount of carbohydrate is less important than the type, and the diet is high in fibre, which slows the absorption of carbohydrate from the gut. This method is widely used in the treatment of adult diabetes, but there is controversy over its use in childhood, particularly for very young children who may be erratic eaters and who may not accept or tolerate a high fibre diet [8]. A compromise may be to teach a measured diet initially on diagnosis, as many parents feel more secure using the 10 g

exchange system, then to move onto an unmeasured diet when appropriate.

Hypoglycaemia

Low blood sugars are likely to occur during or after exercise, if insufficient carbohydrate is eaten or if there is a long delay between injection and eating. A rebound hypoglycaemia can occur after a period of very high blood sugar levels.

Symptoms are similar to those seen in the adult and

Table 9.2 A brief list of 10 g carbohydrate exchanges

Bread
Wholemeal or white	=	½ large slice/1 small slice
Rolls, baps	=	½ roll

Breakfast cereals
All Bran, Branflakes	=	5 tablespoons
Cornflakes	=	5 tablespoons
Weetabix	=	1 biscuit
Porridge	=	7 tablespoons

Rice and pasta
Brown or white rice cooked	=	3 tablespoons
Spaghetti	=	10 long strands
Pasta e.g. macaroni	=	3 tablespoons
Spaghetti – tinned	=	⅓ small tin

Biscuits
Oatcakes	=	1 large
Crackers	=	2
Crispbread (wholewheat rye)	=	2
Digestive	=	1

Potatoes
Boiled	=	1 small
Mashed	=	1 scoop
Baked	=	1 medium
Chips	=	5 average sized
Crisps	=	1 small packet

Beans
Baked in tomato sauce	=	5 tablespoons
Dried uncooked	=	2 tablespoons

Fruit
Apple	=	1
Banana	=	1
Grapes	=	10
Orange	=	1
Pear	=	1

Milk
Semi-skimmed, whole, skimmed	=	1 glass (⅓ pint)
Natural/diet fruit yoghurt	=	1 carton
Fruit sweetened yoghurt	=	½ carton

Others
Jelly	=	3 tablespoons
Soup	=	1 ladle
Ice cream	=	1 scoop

NB All tablespoon measures are level

include pallor, sweatiness, irritability and fatigue. Children often find it difficult to describe their own symptoms, but might experience 'butterflies in the tummy', shaky legs or a buzzing in the head. 10–20 g

of rapidly absorbed carbohydrate should be sufficient to alleviate the symptoms of hypoglycaemia, but if the response is not adequate more can be administered after 10–15 minutes.

Hypostop is a rapidly absorbed glucose gel in a tube packaging which can be squeezed into the mouth if the child is not conscious or is uncooperative. Some centres advise that parents keep an emergency supply of glucagon injection to use at home if they are unable to resolve hypoglycaemic symptoms.

Glucose drinks like Lucozade and glucose tablets can be used to treat hypoglycaemia; jam, honey or syrup can also be useful. Ordinary sweets and sweet drinks should be used with caution as a routine treatment since children may fake hypoglycaemia in order to have these 'forbidden foods'. The suggestion of doing additional blood sugar testing at the time of a suspected hypoglycaemia is often enough to act as a deterrent. If hypoglycaemia occurs just prior to a meal then sufficient quick-acting carbohydrate should be given to alleviate symptoms and the meal or snack given soon after. If the next food is not due for an hour or more it is important to use a back-up of slower acting carbohydrate such as a digestive biscuit or piece of fruit in order to prevent blood levels dropping before the next meal. Regular episodes of hypoglycaemia indicate that the diet and insulin are out of balance and that the whole regimen needs assessing.

Illness

Children often do not wish to eat during periods of illness and infection. Blood sugars are likely to be high at these times, so it is important that insulin injections are continued. A change in the insulin regimen to several doses of a rapidly acting insulin may be advised, and the carbohydrate needs to be adjusted according to insulin dosage.

If the usual diet is refused it is not essential to completely replace all the carbohydrate, since blood sugars are likely to be high. A realistic aim is to give 70–80% of the normal intake. Small frequent doses of rapidly absorbed carbohydrate, preferably as a liquid, are often best tolerated. For example if the usual diet provides 180 g carbohydrate, distributed 40.10.40.20.40.30, then the aim would be to provide 35–40 g carbohydrate as hourly drinks between the usual breakfast and lunch times, 45–50 g between the usual lunch and evening meal and 50–55 g during the evening and night.

DIET THROUGHOUT CHILDHOOD

Regular and continued dietetic input is essential in order that the dietary advice is appropriate for the child's continuing and changing needs.

Babies

Adequate nutrition to promote growth is of major importance during the early months of life. Diabetic infants should have their carbohydrate allowance based on requirement for milk feeds, which are the principal source of nutrition. The feeding pattern of infants is one of frequent and regular feeds and this is ideal for the diabetic regimen. If at the time of diagnosis the infant is breast fed the mother should be encouraged to continue. However many mothers are anxious about hypoglycaemia if they are uncertain of the amount being consumed at each feed and will need reassurance. Whether breast or bottle fed, a baby's fluid requirement is 150–200 ml per kg per day; 150 ml breast or infant formula contains approximately 10 g carbohydrate. Providing growth and development is normal, the daily carbohydrate intake can be based on the baby's usual feeding pattern with the insulin dose adjusted accordingly. As with all infants, breast milk or infant formula should be the milk of choice until the child is 12 months old.

Weaning

Weaning can start at the usual time at around three to six months of age. Non carbohydrate foods may be used initially (e.g. 1–2 teaspoons puréed vegetables) as these will not alter the carbohydrate intake. This allows the baby to become accustomed to the different taste and texture of solids without any anxiety being generated by food refusal. Once the baby has become familiar with spoon feeding and the amount taken increased to 1–2 tablespoons, carbohydrate exchanges may be introduced. At first, 5 g carbohydrate exchanges are useful when only small quantities of food are being taken (e.g. half a rusk, 25 g potato, 5 g baby rice). The amount of mixed feeding will gradually increase and by the time the baby is one year old he will probably be having about 90 g carbohydrate as solids, the remainder of his carbohydrate intake coming from milk. Water and dilute low sugar squashes can be given as an additional drink.

Weaning is an anxious time for any parent and this anxiety is heightened if a dietary modification has to be observed. Tension about food must be relieved as a baby may refuse solids completely if his mother is fussing or worrying.

The Department of Health recommendations for vitamin supplements for infants and young children [9] also apply to the diabetic child. The first year of life is the period of most rapid growth. Dietary intake is constantly changing due to the child's progression through normal feeding and developmental milestones. It is essential that the dietitian is in frequent contact with the family to offer advice.

Hypoglycaemia is a real fear for parents and can be hard to recognize in babies. Advice should be given on how to recognize and treat symptoms. Extra milk, with or without additional sugar, Ribena or sweetened fruit juice may be used. Usually 10 g carbohydrate given as 150 ml baby milk or 75 ml baby milk plus one teaspoon sugar is usually sufficient to treat hypoglycaemia. It may be necessary to introduce a cereal-based weaning food (e.g. baby rice) earlier than three months of age if there is a problem with regular hypoglycaemia. Nocturnal hypoglycaemia is a concern of parents and milk and a cereal can be given before the baby settles for the night if he is no longer having night feeds and blood sugars are dropping overnight.

Toddlers

After one year of age the child can drink cows' milk and from two years semi-skimmed milk can be introduced as long as the child is taking a nutritionally adequate diet. Fully skimmed milk however contains too little fat (and hence energy) for the under fives and is not usually recommended. The introduction of skimmed milk over the age of five is a useful way to reduce the overall fat content of the diet. There is little fibre in the diets of children in their first year of life, but this can gradually increase from weaning. Some forms of fibre, such as Weetabix and baked beans, are popular with children; vegetable fibre and wholemeal bread need to be encouraged.

Small children do not understand the importance of their diet, so parents and health professionals must be flexible and compromise as much as is practical. Food strikes are common in children between two and four years of age. Most families manage to cope with the 'food refusal syndrome' without being manipulated, but the diabetic toddler poses a real problem: with hypoglycaemia always a possibility, food refusal can become a powerful weapon. Parents are torn between maintaining good glycaemic control with the accompanying risk of hypoglycaemia, and allowing the blood sugars to be a little raised. Advice should be given not to force feed and to rely on the child's falling blood sugar to cause hunger and a desire to eat. Some toddlers refuse breakfast after the insulin injection and Lucozade or another simple sugar may have to be given.

In addition to food strikes, some young diabetic children complain of incessant hunger. Measurements of height, weight and dietary intake should be done regularly to reassure parents that adequate nutrition is being maintained.

The British Diabetic Association Babysitting Notes (see Further reading) are useful at this stage.

Schoolchildren

While at school the teacher becomes one of the child's main carers and must know about diabetes, and in particular about hypoglycaemia. The BDA *School Pack* and *Coping with Diabetes at School* carry good explanations and should be given to each child's teacher.

Children with diabetes are advised to carry glucose tablets at all times and the teacher should be equipped with a glucose drink in case of hypoglycaemia.

Physical education teachers should be aware of the need for extra carbohydrate before exercise and to check that children are carrying extra carbohydrate during periods of prolonged exercise. Pockets may need to be sewn into shorts for this purpose. School lunches can present a problem: it is not always possible for children to go home and they may prefer to go to school lunch with their friends. Older children with a good grasp of their diet can choose their own meal and the cafeteria-style canteen allows a flexible choice of food. The organization and provision of diabetic meals can vary from area to area; it is not desirable for the diabetic child to have a 'special diet' away from his friends or at a different time from them. A normal main course should be suitable, with the dessert or pudding being replaced by fresh fruit or diet yoghurt. Discussion with the school cooks as well as teachers should help smooth problems. Advice can be given to parents about suitable packed lunches.

Children frequently eat sweets in the school playground and it is tempting for a child with diabetes to eat sweets also. Other less sweet snacks such as crisps, peanuts, raisins and chewing gum should be suggested as alternatives. The best attitude is to use positive reinforcement when the child is doing well, but if persistent cheating becomes a problem a 20 g carbohydrate 'sweet allowance' can be given on schooldays. These sweets should be allowed on condition that no other illicit foods are consumed during the day. If the sweet allowance is not effective and habitual 'bingeing' is causing a problem the services of a child psychologist may be needed: bingeing suggests underlying stress.

Adolescents

Adolescence is a period of rebellion and diabetic treatment is one more thing to rebel about. Snacking and eating out in the evening is common. Advice about alcohol and its hypoglycaemic effect will be necessary for some teenagers.

Adolescent girls have a tendency to become obese and appropriate advice is needed. Occasionally weight control can be achieved by simply cutting out crisps and fried foods. The amount of carbohydrate in the diet should only be reduced after very careful examination of the diet as a whole, as this may cause an increase in consumption of fat and protein. In order to get the message across, it is useful to point out the energy content of some of the carbohydrate portions – e.g. one packet of crisps provides 10 g carbohydrate and 150 kcal; one apple also contains 10 g carbohydrate but only 50 kcal.

Parties and eating out

Parties are highlights in a child's life and advice is required to ensure that children with diabetes can enjoy the party as much as everyone else. They can eat most of the party fare and it is important to ensure that sufficient carbohydrate is eaten to compensate for extra activity and excitement. The host can help by providing low calorie drinks for everyone.

Many of the fast food eating places publish the carbohydrate content of their foods. Children should be educated about their diet as soon as possible so that they are able to manage it independently, with support from parents as necessary. All children are different, but most children from the age of about eight should be actively encouraged to have a full understanding of their diet. Parents may need encouragement gradually to hand over responsibility of treatment to the child.

The incidence of diabetes is increasing in younger age groups and nutrition should provide normal growth and promote the avoidance of diabetic complications.

Parents may feel isolated and need much support and reassurance from the diabetic team. The British Diabetic Association has a role to play by producing useful publications (see Further reading), updates about food and organizing children's holiday camps and parent-child weekends. A local Parent's Group allows families in a similar situation to meet. Youngsters with diabetes should have a high quality life in which a suitably tailored diet is an essential part.

REFERENCES

1 Jackson R Growth and maturation of children with insulin dependent diabetes. *Pediatric Clinics N Am*, 1984, **31**(3) 545–567.
2 Report of the Nutrition Sub-committee of the Medical Advisory Committee of the British Diabetic Association. Dietary Recommendations for diabetics for the 1980s. *Hum Nutr: Appl Nutr*, 1982, **36A** 378–394.
3 Nutrition Subcommittee of the British Diabetic Association's Professional Advisory Committee. Dietary recommendations for people with diabetes: an update for the 1990s. *Diabetic Medicine*, 1992, **9**(2) 189–202.
4 Nutrition Subcommittee of the Professional Advisory Committee of the British Diabetic Association. Dietary recommendations for children and adolescents with diabetes. *Diabetic Medicine*, 1989, **6**(6) 537–547.
5 Department of Health Report on Health and Social Subjects No 41, *Dietary Reference Values for Food Energy and Nutrients for the United Kingdom*. London: HMSO, 1991.
6 Mann J What carbohydrate foods should diabetics eat? *Brit Med J*, 1984, **288** 1025–1026.
7 Slama G, Haardt M, Joseph P *et al*. Sucrose taken during mixed meal has no additional hyperglycaemic action over isocaloric amounts of starch in well controlled diabetics. *Lancet*, 1984, (12 July) 122–124.
8 Taitz LS, Wardley BL *Handbook of Child Nutrition*. Oxford: Oxford University Press, 1990.
9 Department of Health and Social Security Report on Health and Social Subjects No 32. *Present Day Practice in Infant Feeding, Third Report*. London: HMSO, 1988.

FURTHER READING

British Diabetic Association *Babysitting Notes*, BDA, 10 Queen Anne Street London W1M 0BP.
British Diabetic Association *School Pack*, London: BDA.
Coping with Diabetes at School, Ames Educational Services. Available from Ames Division, Miles Laboratories Ltd, PO Box 37, Stoke Court, Stoke Poges, Slough SL2 4LY.
British Diabetic Association Countdown, London: BDA.
Day J *The Diabetes Handbook – Insulin Dependent Diabetes*, Wellingborough: Thorsons, 1986.

CHAPTER 10

Cystic Fibrosis

Cystic fibrosis (CF) is the commonest recessively inherited genetic disease in caucasian populations, with an incidence of approximately 1 in 2500 live births [1]. The incidence in non-caucasians is lower, with estimates around 1 in 20 000 in black populations and 1 in 100 000 in oriental populations [2]. It is almost unknown in Japan, China and black Africa [3]. There is widespread dysfunction of exocrine glands which causes chronic pulmonary disease; pancreatic enzyme deficiency; intestinal obstruction in the neonate (distal intestinal obstruction syndrome); liver disease; infertility, especially in males; and abnormally high concentrations of electrolytes in sweat (Table 10.1). The CF gene was cloned in 1989 [4]. So far over 160 different mutations have been identified and, to some extent, this may account for the varying clinical features of the disease [5]. Before 1950, the majority of patients died in the first year of life. The average survival rates in the United Kingdom between 1977 and 1985 were 50% up to 20 years of age, and 25% up to 30 years [1]. Many CF centres in the United States of America, Canada and Australia report an 80% survival at 19 or 20 years. Patients with pancreatic insufficiency and steatorrhoea have a worse prognosis in terms of growth, pulmonary function and long term survival [6].

CLINICAL FEATURES

Most patients present with symptoms in the first year of life, but occasionally, if the disease is mild, it may be undiagnosed for many years.

Chronic respiratory disease

The lungs are normal at birth, but may become affected within a few weeks of life. Due to the ab-

normal secretions and resulting mucous there is obstruction in the small airways, with secondary infection which is progressive and destructive [3]. Common organisms cultured from the lung are *Staphyloccocus aureus*, *Haemophilus influenzae* and *Pseudomonas aeruginosa*; *P. cepacia* carries a relatively poor prognosis [7]. A major objective of respiratory management is to control infection and remove thickened bronchial secretions thereby maintaining respiratory function and delaying the rate of lung damage. This is achieved by:

- antibiotic therapy administered either intermittently, continuously or by aerosol
- regular chest physiotherapy
- use of bronchodilators, other anti-asthma treatment and oral steroids.

Gastrointestinal symptoms

CF is the most common cause of exocrine pancreatic insufficiency in childhood in Western countries. It is estimated that up to 90% of CF patients have obstruction of pancreatic ducts by viscid secretions, leading to a pancreatic insufficiency which will result in diarrhoea, steatorrhoea and failure to thrive. In the other 10% of patients, although enzyme secretion is diminished, it is still adequate for digestion and absorption of nutrients without the necessity for pancreatic enzyme supplementation [8]. Approximately 15% of babies present with a meconium ileus resulting from the blockage of the terminal ileum by highly proteinaceous meconium at birth [3]. 'Meconium ileus equivalent' or 'distal intestinal obstruction syndrome' (DIOS) may occur later in childhood or adult life.

Gastro-oesophageal reflux (GOR) has been frequently reported in CF. Although the reasons for this increased incidence are unknown, it has been sug-

Table 10.1 Clinical features of CF

Intestine	Meconium ileus
	Rectal prolapse
	Distal intestinal obstruction syndrome
	Steatorrhoea/diarrhoea
	Abdominal distention
	Failure to thrive/growth failure
	Intussusception
	Gastrointestinal reflux
Pancreas	Pancreatic failure
	Pancreatitis
	Glucose intolerance
	Diabetes mellitus
Liver	Hepatomegaly
	Cirrhosis
	Portal hypertension
Gallbladder	Cholecystitis
	Cholelithiasis
	Obstructive jaundice
Lungs	Repeated respiratory infections
	Asthma/wheezing
	Nasal polyps
	Bronchiectasis
	Hyperinflation
	Clubbing
	Haemoptysis
	Pneumothorax
	Cor pulmonale
	Growth failure/failure to thrive/weight loss
	Delayed puberty
Other	Salt depletion
	Sterility in males
	Arthritis
	Fat-soluble vitamin deficiency

gested that it may relate to a combination of increased transdiaphragmatic pressure due to the forced expiration of coughing and wheezing, and coughing raising the abdominal pressure intermittently [9]. Other gastrointestinal problems which may occur include acute pancreatitis, duodenal ulcer, coeliac disease, Crohn's disease and cows' milk protein enteropathy.

Effect on growth

CF is a well known cause of malnutrition and short stature. Patients have been reported to have poor weight for height, delayed puberty and the eventual size of those surviving to adulthood is commonly below average [10]. Bone age and onset of menarche may also be delayed [11]. Nutritional impairment is noted at birth with CF infants having an average birthweight of about 0.5 standard deviations lower than that of the normal population [12]. Growth patterns of 244 patients studied with CF show that 35% of females and 26% of males were on or below the third percentile for weight [13]. Berry and co-workers reported an average weight of one standard deviation below the mean in children aged between 3 and 8 years, with a relentless decline in weight to below the third percentile by 15 years of age [14]. However, near normal growth has been reported. In the Toronto clinic, in 1983, males conformed to a normal distribution on percentile charts for both height and weight and, although adolescent females were generally less than the 50th percentile for weight, their linear growth was normal [15].

Other clinical problems

Liver disease has a peak incidence during adolescence affecting more boys than girls and is associated with earlier death. Initially, liver disease may only be identified by abnormal liver function tests and ultrasound, but a few patients develop overt cirrhosis with portal hypertension and risk of bleeding oesophageal varices. Gallstones composed almost entirely of cholesterol may develop in older patients [3].

Glucose intolerance and diabetes mellitus is common in CF [16]. The incidence of diabetes mellitus was thought to be only 1–2% [17], but it may be higher than this, possibly 8–15% [18] with the incidence increasing with age. Koch has suggested that 2% of CF patients will develop diabetes between 10 and 15 years, 12% by 25 years and 17% over the age of 25 years [18]. The incidence of diabetes may be at least 40 to 200 times greater in CF than in the normal childhood and young adult populations. Pathological studies indicate that the number of islets of Langerhans and beta cells are decreased [19]. The diabetes in CF is non-ketotic and has a slow onset, but is usually insulin dependent [17]. Although the diabetes is generally considered mild, the development of diabetic complications has been described and is associated with a poor prognosis; Finkelstein *et al.* found that in a group of 448 CF patients 60% without overt clinical diabetes mellitus survived to the age of 30 years, whereas fewer than 25% with diabetes mellitus reached this age [20]. Other workers have found no difference in survival between diabetic and non-diabetic CF patients [21].

DIAGNOSIS

The sweat test remains the most reliable laboratory procedure to confirm the clinical diagnosis of CF [22]. Sweating is stimulated by pilocarpine iontophoresis to achieve an accurate collection of at least 100 mg sweat. Sweat sodium and chloride concentrations are below 40 mmol/l in normal children and lie between 80 and 125 mmol/l in almost all children with CF [23]. If sweat electrolyte results are slightly below the range expected for CF in a child suspected of having the disease, or in newborn infants, DNA testing may be helpful in confirming a diagnosis. Neonatal screening for CF is routinely performed in a number of centres using radioimmunoassay for trypsin [24]. A sweat test must be performed later to confirm the diagnosis. Antenatal diagnosis is possible in the first trimester of pregnancy by analysis of fetal DNA obtained from chorionic villus biopsy. In the small proportion of women where this test is unsuitable, a less specific assay of amniotic fluid microvillar enzymes can be carried out later in pregnancy.

NUTRITIONAL MANAGEMENT

There is evidence that improving a CF patient's nutritional status will improve a depressed immunological system, enhance growth, increase respiratory muscle strength, and possibly even improve survival [25]. Two CF clinic populations in Boston and Toronto were compared with respect to growth, pulmonary function and survival [26]. Although there was little difference between the two groups in pulmonary function, the Toronto males were taller, heavier and had a greater mean age of survival than the Boston males (30 years versus 21 years). The only difference in treatment policy was the high fat, high energy regimen offered by Toronto, and the low fat diet advocated by Boston. The better nutritional status of the Toronto patients, reflected in their superior growth, was concluded as being responsible for their improved survival.

Causes of malnutrition in CF

Malabsorption

Because pancreatic exocrine secretions in the CF patient contain less enzymes and bicarbonate, have a lower pH and are of a smaller volume, the physical properties of proteins and mucus within the lumen are affected. This results in obstruction to the small ducts and secondary damage to pancreatic digestive enzyme secretion causing malabsorption in 90% of patients. Other problems such as gastric hypersecretion, reduced duodenal bicarbonate concentration and pH, disorders of bile salt metabolism, disordered intestinal motility and permeability may all contribute to malabsorption. The severity of malabsorption is variable; there can be significant malabsorption of protein and fat-soluble vitamins despite adequate use of enzyme supplements [27] and up to 11% dietary energy may be lost in the stools [28]. Energy may also be lost in vomit following physiotherapy, or because of GOR. Up to 5% energy intake may be lost through the expectoration of sputum [10].

Increased energy expenditure

Resting Energy Expenditure (REE) of CF patients appears to be increased to about 110–130% of predicted values [29,30]. This excess in energy expenditure is attributed to increased work of breathing and the metabolic cost of chronic and pulmonary infection. An increase in REE does not necessarily imply an increase in total energy expenditure [31]; there may be a compensatory reduction in spontaneous physical activities [32].

Low energy intake

The results of dietary assessment surveys on CF patients are summarized in Table 10.2. Energy intakes seldom exceed the countries' estimated average requirement; no differences have been noted between males and females. Factors reducing appetite in CF include chronic respiratory infection, recurrent vomiting associated with coughing and psychological stress. Emphasis on weight gain and nutritional status may heighten parental anxiety about food which can result in undue pressure being exerted at meal and snack times. Media persuasion to eat a 'healthy' low fat, high fibre, low sugar diet, peer group pressure to follow the fashion and stay thin, and abandonment of animal

Table 10.2 Energy intake of CF patients on a normal diet

	MacDonald *et al.*, 1989 (UK)	Buchdahl *et al.*, 1989 (UK)	Thomson *et al.*, 1990 (UK)	Kalnins *et al.*, 1990 (Canada)	Lloyd-Still *et al.*, 1989 (USA)	Wootton *et al.*, 1990 (UK)
Number of patients studied	20	20	30	51	64	30
Age range (years)	6.6–16.6	5.3–17.3	(mean age = 11)	10–15	0.3–18	5.3–16.0
Energy intake of the respective RDI (%)	103	99	100	114	94.8	92
Range (%)	58–161	67–133	71–141	–	42–206	–
Mean daily fat intake (g)	101	73	–	–	–	76
Range (g)	38–148	36–133	–	–	–	–
% Fat energy	33.3	30	37.5	36.1	33.7	36

foods may all contribute to reduced food intake [33]. Inadequate energy intake will be influenced by poor use of dietary supplements, lack of financial resources, dislike of fatty foods, and the outdated recommendation for patients with CF to follow a low fat diet [27].

Aims of nutritional management

There are two main aims of nutritional management:

- to achieve optimal nutritional status
- to achieve normal growth and development.

Energy

Although it has been accepted that the energy requirements in CF should be increased, because of the heterogeneity of these patients it is impossible to give universal recommendations. Factors such as a child's age, sex, absorption, presence of respiratory infection, activity and nutritional status will affect energy requirements. Each individual's energy requirements will vary from time to time depending upon his clinical condition and activity levels. In reality the only practical method to gauge adequate nutrition is by closely monitoring weight gain and growth. Some children will grow normally by consuming no more than the estimated average energy requirement, whereas those with advanced pulmonary disease may need 50–60% more energy than normal. A useful guideline to follow is to assess the existing energy intake and increase this

value by a further 20–30% if weight gain or growth is poor.

To achieve a high energy intake, the first step is to maximize energy intake from ordinary foods. A good variety of energy rich foods should be encouraged such as full cream milk, cheese, meat, full cream yoghurt, milk puddings, cakes and biscuits. Extra butter or margarine can be added to bread, potatoes and vegetables. Frying foods or basting foods in oil will add additional energy. Extra milk or cream can be added to soups, cereal, desserts, mashed potatoes and used to top tinned or fresh fruit. Frequent snacks are as important as regular meals. However, it is necessary that parents establish a good routine for meals and snacks and do not allow children to substitute sweets and chocolate for savoury food at mealtime or else children will soon develop unsatisfactory eating habits which will be difficult to change in the future.

This type of dietary advice directly opposes current healthy eating recommendations and, not surprisingly, it is common to find opposition to it by parents, older patients, school teachers and even some health professionals, particularly dentists. An essential part of the dietitian's role is to ensure that all professionals connected with CF understand fully the rationale for this dietary treatment and that they give consistent and accurate advice about the diet.

Protein

Although exact protein requirements are unclear, it is generally accepted that the protein intake should be increased to compensate for excessive loss of nitrogen in the faeces and sputum [34]. Body protein stores are decreased with a low muscle mass and increased muscle catabolism [35]. In addition total body nitrogen is depressed in malnourished CF children [36]. It is recommended that 15% of the total energy intake should come from protein. Normally, the protein intakes of CF children are usually high, and do not warrant additional protein supplementation.

Fat

Fat is the most concentrated source of energy in the diet and the only source of essential fatty acids. It is now widely accepted that fat should be encouraged liberally and should provide 35–40% of the total energy intake. Prior to 1980, fat restriction was widely advocated for CF in order to reduce stearrhoea, increase protein absorption and improve the character of the stools. The Toronto CF clinic abandoned the low fat diet in the early 1970s which resulted in improved growth in their patients [37]. A comparison of high, moderate and low fat diets demonstrated that the children on higher fat diets had higher energy intakes and better growth [38]. The percentage fat malabsorption was not increased by a higher fat intake. Unrestricted fat intakes have lightened the treatment load for the parents and child. Although some children are positively enjoying the dietary freedom, others, even years after the liberalization of fat intake, take a more cautious stand and still choose to moderate their fat intake [39].

Carbohydrate

A high carbohydrate intake should be encouraged to provide 45–50% of the total energy intake. Starchy foods such as bread, potatoes and pasta as well as simple sugars should be encouraged, the latter providing a valuable energy source. Disaccharide intolerance may be a problem following surgery for meconium ileus. High fibre foods (non-starch polysaccharides) do not need to be restricted, but they do have a high satiety value which may be a problem if a child's appetite is poor.

Dietary supplements

Dietary supplements provide a useful source of energy when growth is inadequate or to compensate for poor nutrient intake during a respiratory infection. Unfortunately, their use is inconsistent both by health professionals and patients alike and it is not uncommon to find them discontinued by the patients themselves.

The range of prescribable dietary supplements has increased considerably in recent years. The cartoned fortified milkshakes such as Fresubin, Fortisip and Ensure Plus have proved popular with children. Care should be exercised when using some of the protein enriched supplements such as Fortimel as these are too high in protein to use as a routine supplement in young children. It is important to encourage children to take a variety of flavours to try and prevent boredom, although some children will only accept one specific flavour of one product and will refuse to try all others. Although the supplements taste better if served cold, the cartoned milkshakes are particularly useful for packed lunches. Good use should also be made of both home made and cartoned milkshakes which can be purchased in supermarkets. The latter are often presented in decorated cartons and are particularly attractive to young children. However they are expensive and are not usually fortified with vitamins and minerals.

Other useful energy supplements include the powdered glucose polymers, e.g. Maxijul, Polycal and Caloreen, and the concentrated glucose drinks, e.g. Hycal and Polycal Liquid. It is probably more convenient for parents to prepare a daily 15–20% glucose polymer solution with water and use this to dilute squash, rather than adding teaspoons of glucose polymer to individual drinks and puddings.

The quantity and timing of dietary supplements is important in childhood so as not to impair appetite and decrease nutrient intake from normal foods. Also, dietary supplements should not replace food at mealtimes. It is not uncommon to find young children taking large quantities of glucose polymer in drinks and then refusing most solid foods. Very concentrated glucose polymer solutions may also result in loose stools and diarrhoea which may lead parents to increase the pancreatic enzyme dosage inappropriately.

It is recommended that dietary supplements are given two to three times daily, either after meals or at bedtime. The quantity recommended is age dependent and the following is a useful guide of how much to give daily:

1–2 years	– 200 kcal (840 kJ)
3–5 years	– 400 kcal (1680 kJ)
6–11 years	– 600 kcal (2520 kJ)
over 12 years	– 800 kcal (3360 kJ)

If a patient has an acute infection or is currently being considered for enteral feeding these quantities can be exceeded.

Enteral feeding

Chronic malnutrition is common in adolescents and young adults with CF and it has been shown that up to 30% of patients are malnourished [40], despite the use of a high energy, high protein diet. As a result many CF centres are using overnight enteral feeding by the use of either nasogastric, gastrostomy or jejunostomy tubes. In a survey in the USA, enteral feeding was being practised in 73% of CF centres [41]. The following benefits have been observed from enteral feeding: increase in body fat, height, lean body mass and muscle mass; increased total body nitrogen; improved strength; and development of secondary sexual characteristics. Reduced weight loss during exacerbations of pulmonary infection has been noted and there is an increased sense of control over body weight and an improvement in body image [40,42].

Some workers have tried to issue guidelines on when enteral feeding should be started. These include failure to gain weight over a six month period, or the child being less than 80% ideal weight for height [43]. Other workers have suggested more exacting guidelines and have indicated that enteral feeding should begin if there is no weight gain over a three month period, or if the patient's weight/height ratio declines to less than 85% of ideal [42].

Short term overnight enteral feeding will usually produce immediate weight gain but, as soon as feeding is stopped, weight loss may quickly result [44,45,46]. However, intermittent overnight feeding for two weeks whilst in hospital to coincide with the administration of intravenous antibiotics every few months may be sufficient to improve and maintain nutritional status in some patients [47] and is worth consideration if a patient cannot have enteral feeds at home. Long term enteral feeding studies, where patients have been fed for up to three years, have demonstrated that patients have gained weight and grown satisfactorily; there is some evidence to suggest that pulmonary function may decline at a slower rate [48].

Many types of feed preparations have been used for enteral feeding in CF. These include elemental, semi-elemental and polymeric feeds. There is little published data comparing the efficacy of these feeds in CF. It has been hypothesized that elemental feeds have a good buffering effect and potentially act to buffer gastric contents at night [49] and are better absorbed in CF, but they are expensive and are lower in energy than polymeric feeds. It is also often stated that pancreatic enzymes are not needed with elemental feeds, but most elemental feeds contain some fat. Steatorrhoea is no greater using polymeric than elemental formulas provided pancreatic enzyme supplements are given [50].

The role of high fat feeds in CF is uncertain. Fitting's work has suggested that low carbohydrate, high fat feeds do not seem necessary for nutritional support in patients with chronic obstructive lung disease [51]. However, Kane and Hobbs have recently demonstrated that giving the high fat feed Pulmocare resulted in lower CO_2 production (VCO_2) and respiratory quotient in CF patients with moderate to severe pulmonary disease, than did feeding with a high carbohydrate feed [52].

In practice, most CF patients over 20 kg will tolerate an energy-dense polymeric feed providing at least 1.5 kcal/ml (6.3 kJ/ml). Initially the feed should supply at least 30% of the patient's estimated energy requirement. However, enteral feeding can significantly increase resting energy expenditure [53]. In addition, basal energy expenditure increases as pulmonary disease progresses [52], but voluntary oral intakes decrease with nocturnal feeding [53]. It is important, therefore, that the feed energy content is reviewed regularly and increased in order to sustain improvement in the nutritional status. Although enteral feeding does help to correct impaired nutrition, the weight/height ratio is rarely returned to normal and there may be a time lag of up to six months before there is an increase in linear growth velocity [13] if this improves at all.

For children weighing less than 20 kg, it is better to give an enteral polymeric paediatric feed, e.g. Nutrison Paediatric or Paediasure, providing 1 kcal/ml (4.2 kJ/ml). Commercial feeds that supply 1.5 kcal/ml (6.3 kJ/ml) usually have a higher protein profile and are unsuitable for the younger age groups. However, it may be necessary to increase the feed's energy density to 1.5 kcal/ml (6.3 kJ/ml) by additional glucose polymer and long chain fat emulsion such as Calogen. Patients are usually fed for a 10–12 hour period overnight, with a 1–2 hour break before their first physiotherapy in the morning. When feeding is first initiated, usually only 50% of the full strength feed is given on the first night and the volume is gradually increased to full volume over 3–4 nights. To aid compliance with older patients, it may be necessary to agree to them having one or two nights off the feed each week.

The method of pancreatic enzyme administration for tube feeds varies from centre to centre and no single method is better than another. In a USA survey in 68 CF centres, 82% gave pancreatic enzyme orally and the rest added powdered enzyme directly to the formula. 37% recommended that the enzymes were taken before starting the tube feed; 14% before and midway through the feed; 25% before and at completion of the feed; and 5% before, midway and after the feeding [41]. It is probably only necessary to give enzymes as enteric coated microspheres at the beginning of the feed and again before the patient goes to sleep. It does not seem necessary to waken a child in the middle of the night to administer extra pancreatic enzymes [53]. The dosage of pancreatic enzyme is arbitrary and can be estimated by using the amount of enzyme required for a normal meal and comparing its composition with that of the feed [43].

The route used for the feed will be influenced by the duration of feeding and by the preference of the patient, relatives and physician. Nasogastric, gastrostomy and jejunostomy feeds have all been used in CF and each method has merits and drawbacks (Table 3.4). Nasogastric feeding is used successfully in some CF centres in Britain, particularly in adult units [54]. However, gastrostomy feeding has become more popular in children, made easier by the development of the gastrostomy button (page 30). Jejunostomy feeding is rarely used in Britain for CF although it does carry less risk of aspiration [55]. Before tube feeding is commenced, the patient and family need to be fully educated.

Basic anthropometric measurements such as height and weight should be monitored at least monthly. Furthermore, as hyperglycaemia requiring insulin therapy has been reported in older patients receiving night time feeds, blood sugars should be monitored.

Occasionally, parenteral nutrition has been resorted to as a means of providing nutritional support in CF, but it has so far only been reported as being used in the short term and because of the high risk of complications and cost it should only be considered if a CF patient cannot tolerate a feed via the enteral route, e.g. post-operative management of patients who have had intestinal surgery.

Vitamin and mineral supplements

Fat-soluble vitamins

Deficiencies of vitamins A, D, E and K are well documented. Biochemical deficiency is not always accompanied by clinical effects, but it is reasonable to correct it when demonstrated.

Vitamin A

Vitamin A deficiency in CF is well documented and is associated with night blindness, xerophthalmia, bulging fontanelles and increased intracranial pressure. Serum levels of vitamin A and retinol binding protein tend to be low in CF. However, vitamin A supplemented CF patients are known to have a nearly 3.5 fold hepatic vitamin A reserve than normal controls. These observations suggest a defect in the mobilization of hepatic retinol or in its transportation from the liver into plasma or both [56]. Daily supplementation of up to 2400 μg (8000 i.u.) to 3000 μg (10 000 i.u.) is currently advised. Monitoring of blood levels ensures that adequate supplementation has been prescribed. However, if this is not possible, 2400–3000 μg/day usually restores the plasma levels to normal.

Vitamin D

Serum concentrations of major metabolites of vitamin D reported are variable, some authors detecting low values and others observing normal values. Rickets is rarely seen, but reduced cortical thickness and bone density, and bone demineralization have been documented [57,58]. A daily supplement of 20 μg/day (800 i.u.) is advisable.

Vitamin E

Blood levels of vitamin E are nearly always low unless supplements are given [11]. In older patients, undetectable serum concentrations of vitamin E have been noted in association with neurological syndromes [3]. Symptoms include progressive ophthalmoplegia, unsteadiness on walking, loss of reflexes, tremor and ataxia [57]. There may be some improvement following vitamin E supplementation. In addition, haematological abnormalities including anaemia may occur and may be reversed following vitamin E supplementation [59]. Almost all British CF centres give routine vitamin E supplementation and recommend

50 mg daily in infancy, 100 mg daily for children aged 1–10 years, and 200 mg daily for teenagers and adults.

Vitamin K

Deficiency of this vitamin has been noted in patients with liver disease and in young infants with CF, resulting in bleeding due to hypothrombinaemia, but clinical problems secondary to vitamin K deficiency are rare. Although it has been demonstrated that mean plasma vitamin K concentrations in CF patients was lower than in normal controls [60], the median value was similar and supplementation of vitamin K is only necessary if deficiency has been demonstrated.

Water-soluble vitamins

Routine supplementation is not necessary, although patients taking multivitamin supplements for their source of vitamin A and D will automatically receive additional supplements of some of the water-soluble vitamins. Theoretically patients on a high energy diet will need more thiamin as this is needed for energy metabolism.

Trace minerals

Iron   Serum iron levels are frequently low in CF patients [61], but iron supplementation is not routinely recommended.

Zinc   Although zinc deficiency has been reported in cystic fibrosis, plasma zinc levels appear to be low only in those with moderate to severe malnutrition. However, Safai-Kutti and co-workers recently reported low plasma zinc levels in well nourished patients and hypothesized that this was due to impaired zinc absorption rather than low dietary zinc intake [62]. Dietary intake of zinc should meet at least the dietary reference value. Routine zinc supplementation is not recommended unless deficiency has been demonstrated.

Selenium   Selenium is an essential co-factor for the enzyme glutathione peroxidase and is closely associated with vitamin E as part of the cellular antioxidant system. Several studies have demonstrated reduced levels of selenium in the blood in CF patients [63]. There is some controversy on actual glutathione peroxidase levels in CF; some

authors have reported this to be normal, whereas others have reported low plasma levels.

Selenium is potentially a toxic element if given in large quantities and routine selenium supplementation is not currently recommended. Further research is needed in this area.

Copper, calcium, magnesium   Plasma copper, calcium and magnesium have been reported as being normal in CF [64], although workers have demonstrated elevated copper levels in plasma and fingernail clippings.

Sodium   Normally there is no need to recommend a high consumption of salt, although salt depletion may occur in hot weather even in Britain and through physical exertion causing increased sweating. If the temperature is above 70°F (21°C), it may be good practice to recommend a salt supplement or to eat more salty foods. The amount given is arbitrary, but the following guideline may be useful.

0–1 year	2 mmols/kg of sodium in the form of sodium chloride solution (1 ml = 1 mmol of sodium)
1–5 years	2 × 300 mg sodium chloride tablets (10 mmol of sodium)
6–10 years	2 × 600 mg sodium chloride tablets (20 mmol of sodium)
11 years +	(3–4) × 600 mg sodium chloride tablets (30–40 mmol of sodium)

Anorexia may result from chronic salt depletion and contribute to poor growth. Significant hyponatraemia may be accompanied by vomiting. Hypoelectrolytaemia and metabolic alkalosis has been reported in infants [57].

INFANT FEEDING IN CYSTIC FIBROSIS

The nutritional requirements of CF infants have not been clearly identified but depend upon age, clinical and nutritional state at the time of diagnosis. Hypoproteinaemia and failure to thrive are classic early symptoms seen in cystic fibrosis infants [64,65]. However, even infants diagnosed early by neonatal screening have been shown to have nutritional deficits. Problems identified include reduced body mass, length, total body fat, total body potassium [66], hypoalbuminaemia and low level of tocopherol, linoleic acid [67], serum retinol, 25-hydroxyvitamin D [68], and zinc [69]. With pancreatic enzyme supplementation, appropriate diet therapy and vitamin supplementation, most CF infants should achieve normal nutritional status by the age of one year.

There is some evidence to suggest that asymptomatic infants diagnosed as having CF have a higher energy expenditure than normal [70,71], although most of these infants with pancreatic insufficiency will usually thrive on a normal energy intake, 100–120 kcal/kg (420–500 kJ/kg) in conjunction with pancreatic enzymes. If weight gain is inadequate or if meconium ileus has resulted in surgery and bowel resection, the energy requirement may be as high as 150–200 kcal/kg (625–840 kJ/kg).

Breast milk

Breast milk has enjoyed an upsurge in popularity in CF. Early reports concluded that CF infants should not be breast fed as it was associated with hypoproteinaemia, oedema and anaemia, though these infants were not receiving pancreatic enzyme supplements. In a recent CF survey from USA, breast milk or breast milk supplemented with protein hydrolysate milk was recommended by 77% of centres [72].

Breast milk has several theoretical advantages for CF infants. It is thought that breast milk lipase will help compensate for pancreatic lipase deficiency, will provide some immunological protection against infection and may be psychologically better for the mother. In addition, it has a high linoleic acid and taurine content [11]. Infants with CF have been shown to grow and gain weight adequately on breast milk with pancreatic enzyme supplementation [73,74]. One concern reported is the low sodium content of breast milk and the possibility of electrolyte depletion [75]. Urinary and serum electrolytes should be checked if a breast fed baby has poor weight gain.

The distress and anxiety associated with the diagnosis may lead to initial difficulties in establishing breast feeding; with encouragement and support from health professionals these will usually resolve. If, however, there is no weight gain over a two or three week period it may be necessary to consider supplementing the breast milk with extra energy or changing over to a formula milk. Supplementation of breast milk with protein hydrolysate is common practice in the USA [72,74].

Normal infant formula

Like breast milk, infants with CF have been shown to thrive satisfactorily on normal infant whey or casein based formula and pancreatic enzymes [73]. Normal formula milks are low in sodium and there has been one report of four CF infants who had a total of six episodes of electrolyte depletion between them when fed normal formula milk [75]. Energy supplemented formula is necessary when weight gain is inadequate on normal infant formula milk. Glucose polymers together with a long chain 50% fat emulsion, e.g. Calogen, are used [43]. The addition of 5 g glucose polymer and 3 ml of a 50% fat emulsion per 100 ml of normal infant formula provides approximately 100 kcal/100 ml (420 kJ/100 ml).

Protein hydrolysate formula

Protein hydrolysate formulas are favoured for CF infants in the USA. Farrel and co-workers compared 19 infants given a casein hydrolysate with 19 infants either breast fed or normal formula fed and demonstrated significantly better growth on the casein hydrolysate milk at twelve months of age [76]. Canciani and Mastella [77] demonstrated in 21 infants that fat and nitrogen absorption was better on a whey-based hydrolysate feed containing 49% medium chain triglycerides (MCT) than on normal infant formula. Infants were not given pancreatic enzymes on either feed.

Protein hydrolysate feeds are expensive and unpalatable and are probably unnecessary for the majority of CF infants. They may be beneficial following surgery for meconium ileus if infants develop a temporary disaccharide intolerance. Whey hydrolysates may be better tolerated than the casein hydrolysates currently available in Britain as they have a lower carbohydrate content. Pancreatic enzymes should still be given with protein hydrolysate formula, even if they contain a high proportion of their fat in the form of MCT.

Pancreatic enzymes: administration in infants

No pancreatic enzyme appears ideal to administer with infant formula milk or breast milk. It has been postulated that the uncoated powder preparations may be better as the infant's stomach secretes less acid and empties rapidly. The powdered enzyme remains active in the hypoacidic stomach, mixes with the feed and passes with it into the jejunum, thus acting early [78]. However, the powdered preparations have some disadvantages: they are unpleasant tasting; enzyme on the outside of a baby's mouth will not only cause local skin irritation but may irritate the mother's nipple in the breast fed infant. The powdered enzyme may be mixed with a little expressed breast milk or formula milk and given from a spoon. It should not be added to a bottle of formula milk as it will start digesting the milk. The powder may also get stuck in the hole in the teat. The powder may be mixed with water and syringed into the side of the baby's mouth.

In practice, the enteric coated granules (e.g. Creon, Pancrease and Nutrizym GR) appear more effective than the powdered enzyme for infants. The enteric coated granules can be mixed with a little expressed breast milk or formula and then given to a baby from a spoon or given on a wetted finger, but there is a tendency for these methods to cause choking. So far, the best method of administering these enzymes is to mix them with a small amount of fruit purée (which will hold the enzymes in a gel) and give them from a spoon at the beginning of the feed, but not all infants will accept them this way. A recommended starting dose is 0.5 capsule per 90–150 ml of feed or 0.5 capsule per breast feed.

Weaning

There is no need for early weaning in CF; any time between 3–6 months is recommended. Early weaning may significantly decrease the volume of infant formula taken so there is little benefit in this practice. Parents are encouraged to introduce home cooked or commercial weaning foods in the normal way. If the dried commercial baby foods are used, they can be made up with infant formula instead of water. From six months, adult yoghurt and milk puddings can be introduced, though cows' milk should not replace infant formula milk or breast milk for the first year of life. It is important that parents are encouraged to persist with trying to introduce more texture in the diet after the first six months. Often CF infants, like normal infants, will refuse to take lumpy/mashed weaning foods but will readily accept strained/puréed food. Parents will tend to stick with the strained consistencies as they feel that at least their infant is eating something. However, failure to introduce more texture and encourage chewing may lead to later feeding problems.

Toddlers and behaviour feeding problems

Behaviour feeding problems are common in young CF children. McCollum [79] noted that feeding problems were reported beyond the first year of life in 57% of a sample of 65 children with CF. Emphasis on weight gain may lead to the parents being excessively concerned about child health and food consumption. Mealtimes may become very tense and the child may exhibit strong negative behaviour by knocking the spoon away, turning the head away when offered food, spitting and vomiting. This can lead to the parents becoming even more anxious and eventually force feeding of the child may result. Mealtimes can become very unpleasant and painful resulting in even more determined food refusal behaviour and possible failure to thrive.

In severe behavioural feeding problems it may be necessary for referral to a psychologist. Behaviour management of food refusal in CF has been shown to be successful in a group of four young children [79]. In practical terms, the following strategies may be helpful to the dietitian in managing behaviour problems in the clinical setting [80]:

- set a time limit on feed times, perhaps 20 minutes
- initially offer foods which the child will readily accept and gradually increase the variety
- advise parents to reward the child for good feeding behaviour by positive verbal reinforcement or smiling; even small amounts of food consumed should receive praise and social attention
- advise parents to offer small, regular meals
- advise parents to take uneaten food away without comment and not to substitute uneaten food with sweets and chocolate
- advise parents not to discuss the child's feeding behaviour in front of others
- encourage parents to provide a pleasant unstressed eating environment
- advise parents to maintain a consistent approach to feeding during mealtimes
- encourage parents to allow their child to eat with other children e.g. at nursery or with neighbours' children, as children tend to eat more with their peers
- try and reassure parents that, if the CF child is well, there is no physiological cause for the food refusal.

PANCREATIC ENZYME SUPPLEMENTATION FOR THE OLDER CHILD

There are a large number of exogenous pancreatic enzymes available. They are based on animal pancreatic extracts and are presented in powder, tablet or capsule form. They all contain different proportions of lipase, amylase and protease (Table 10.3).

Originally, pancreatin was just available in powder form, Pancrex V and Cotazym. Although this reduced fat excretion it was not particularly effective even in high doses. Its inefficiency can be explained by peptic acid inactivation of the enzymes in the stomach and duodenum and partly by abnormalities of the micellar phase of fat absorption due to the low duodenal pH and reduced intraluminal bile acid [81]. In addition, pancreatin has been available for several years in the form of an enteric coated tablet, Pancrex V Forte. The coating is designed to dissolve when a pH of 6 is exceeded and so inactivation in the stomach is prevented. But it only works well when the postprandial intragastric and intraduodenal pH are re-

Table 10.3 Pancreatic enzyme preparations available in the UK

Product (Manufacturer)	Composition (per g of powder/ granules or per capsule/tablet) BP units		
	Lipase	Protease	Amylase
Powder			
Pancrex V (Paines & Byrne)	25 000	1400	30 000
Capsules			
Pancrex V '340 mg' (Paines & Byrne)	8 000	430	9 000
Pancrex V '125 mg' (Paines & Byrne)	2 950	160	3 000
Tablets			
Enteric-coated tablets			
Pancrex V (Paines & Byrne)	1 900	110	1 700
Pancrex V Forte (Paines & Byrne)	5 600	330	5 000
Enteric-coated microspheres			
Pancrease (Cilag)	5 000	350	3 000
Creon (Duphar)	8 000	210	9 000
Nutrizym GR (Merck)	10 000	650	10 000
Higher lipase enteric-coated microtablets			
Pancrease HL (Cilag)	25 000	1250	22 500
Creon 25 000 (Duphar)	25 000	1000	18 000
Nutrizym 22 (Merck)	22 000	1100	19 800

latively high [77]. There is little point in using enteric coated tablets or pancreatin powder in CF, although some centres still use the powder for infants.

In the early 1980s, enzymes in enteric coated microspheres were introduced onto the market (Creon, Nutrizym GR, Pancrease). The microspheres are either administered separately or in a gelatin capsule that dissolves in the stomach. Each capsule contains around one hundred individually coated 1–3 mm microspheres. The pancreatin in the released microspheres is protected from acid/pepsin digestion by a pH sensitive coat that does not dissolve until the pH exceeds 5.5 within the duodenum [82]. The greater surface area of the microspheres makes them disintegrate faster than enteric-coated tablets. Enteric coated microspheres should be able to achieve at least 90% fat absorption.

Studies demonstrate that the enteric coated microspheres are more effective than the conventional pancreatin powder and enteric coated capsules [82,83, 84,85] and there is little difference between the current enteric coated microspheres with respect to fat absorption and symptom scores when the same number of different capsules are used and patients consume a similar fat intake [86].

More recently, enteric coated microtablets of pancreatin containing higher doses of enzyme have been introduced on the market. These are Creon 25000, Pancrease HL and Nutrizym 22. So far there has only been one published study on the use of Pancrease HL capsules, but preliminary results from this study would indicate that it may be possible to reduce the number of pancreatic enzyme tablets taken by up to two thirds using the higher lipase preparations without adversely affecting fat absorption [87]. Further studies are awaited on the use of all three preparations.

The optimal dose of enteric coated microspheres varies for each patient and is usually more than recommended by the manufacturers [88]. The dose may vary from 1–2 to 12–15 capsules with meals. A useful starting dose is 2–3 capsules per meal (for children over one year) and the dose can be increased according to bowel frequency, stool consistency and abdominal discomfort. Although faecal fat estimations are useful in helping to determine the optimal enzyme dose, this investigation is not available at every centre. Without any objective measures of fat excretion, some patients and paediatricians may over estimate the dose of pancreatic enzymes needed, assuming that all abdominal symptoms are invariably due to pancreatic enzyme insufficiency [89].

Table 10.4 General guidelines for the use of pancreatic enzyme preparations

---

1 Give with every meal; during rather than all before or all after

2 Give extra enzymes (e.g. 1–2 capsules or tablets) with fatty or large snacks and milky drinks

3 Do not give enzymes with squash, lemonade, fruit or boiled and jelly sweets

4 Mix powdered enzyme either with a little soft food or jam or honey. Do not sprinkle over a complete meal

5 The enteric-coated microsphere capsules, e.g. Pancrease (Cilag), Creon (Duphar), Nutrizym GR (Merck) can be swallowed whole. Where swallowing is difficult the capsules may be opened and the contained microsphere taken with liquids or mixed with jam or honey. They should not be crushed or chewed

6 Do not mix granules with hot food

7 Increase the enzyme dose (e.g. by one capsule) if the stools are loose, fatty or more than twice daily

---

Pancreatic enzymes should be administered with all meals and snacks. Guidelines for using pancreatic enzymes are given in Table 10.4.

Adjunctive therapy to pancreatic enzymes

H_2 receptor antagonists such as cimetidine have been used as an adjunct to pancreatic enzymes. They aim to reduce both the volume and the acid concentration of gastric secretion [90] and thereby prevent acid/peptic inactivation of the enzymes. They may help increase efficiency of enteric coated enzymes [77] and are worth considering if patients have uncontrolled symptoms on large doses of pancreatic enzymes.

DIETARY MANAGEMENT OF DIABETES MELLITUS AND CF

No clear guidelines have been issued on ideal dietary management of diabetes for a patient with CF and little research has been conducted in this area. The traditional diabetic dietary recommendations, i.e. a high fibre, controlled unrefined carbohydrate (55% of the total energy intake), low fat (30% of the energy intake) and low sugar intake are difficult to apply to the child with CF.

The type of dietary control will depend upon the severity of the CF. In general terms, both hyperglycaemia and hypoglycaemia should be avoided and the blood sugar maintained between 4–10 mmol/l. Blood sugars should be monitored at least once daily. However, as malnutrition is still very common in CF, a more liberal dietary approach is possible. All diabetic CF patients require insulin.

Mild to moderate CF

- high energy intake
- 35–40% of energy intake from fat. Polyunsaturated and monounsaturated fats should be encouraged if possible. There is no evidence to state that the fat intake should be decreased in CF and diabetes
- 45–50% of the energy intake from carbohydrate, divided regularly throughout the day between meals and snacks
- if possible, at least 50% of the carbohydrate in the form of unrefined carbohydrate, particularly at bedtime
- whole protein milkshake supplements as needed
- nutritional status should be monitored closely.

Severe CF

- high energy intake
- 35–40% of the energy intake from any type of fat source
- 45–50% of the energy intake from carbohydrate, divided regularly into frequent small meals and snacks
- carbohydrate in any form, using simple sugars and dietary supplements, including glucose polymers and drinks if blood sugars are monitored carefully.

Poor diabetic control should be improved by alterations in insulin therapy rather than imposing dietary restrictions which may adversely affect nutritional status.

When treating CF with diabetes it may be necessary to involve the expertise of the diabetic team who need to fully understand and support the rationale for the different dietary approach.

REFERENCES

1 British Paediatric Association Working Party on Cystic Fibrosis Cystic fibrosis in the United Kingdom 1977–1985: an improving picture. *Brit Med J*, 1988, **297** 1599–1602.

2 Corey M *et al.* A comparison of survival, growth and pulmonary function in patients with cystic fibrosis in Boston and Toronto. *J Clin Epidemiol*, 1988, **41** 583–591.

3 Forstner G, Durie P Nutrition in cystic fibrosis. In: Grand RJ, Sutphen JL, Dietz WH (eds.) *Pediatric Nutrition. Theory and Practice*. Boston: Butterworths, 1987.

4 Brock DJH *et al.* Cystic fibrosis: the new genetics. *J Roy Soc Med*, 1991, **84**(Suppl) 2–9.

5 Tsui LC *et al.* Molecular genetics of cystic fibrosis. *Pediatr Pulmonol*, 1990, (Suppl 5) 58–59 (Abst).

6 Gaskin KJ *et al.* Improved respiratory prognosis in patients with cystic fibrosis with normal fat absorption. *J Pediatr*, 1982, **100** 857–862.

7 Simmonds EJ *et al.* Pseudomonas cepacia: a new pathogen in patients with cystic fibrosis referred to a large centre in the United Kingdom. *Arch Dis Childh*, 1990, **65** 874–877.

8 Sokol RJ The GI system and nutrition in cystic fibrosis. *Pediatr Pulmonol*, 1990, (Suppl 5) 81–83.

9 Cucchiara S *et al.* Mechanisms of gastro-oesophageal reflux in cystic fibrosis. *Arch Dis Childh*, 1991, **66** 617–622.

10 Wootton SA *et al.* Energy balance and growth in cystic fibrosis. *J Roy Soc Med*, 1991, **84**(Suppl 18) 22–27.

11 Dodge JA The nutritional state and nutrition. *Acta Paediatr Scand*, 1985, (Suppl 317) 31–37.

12 Goodchild MC Nutritional management of cystic fibrosis. *Digestion*, 1987, **37**(Suppl 1) 61–67.

13 Soutter VL *et al.* Chronic undernutrition/growth retardation in cystic fibrosis. *Clinics in Gastroenterol*, 1986, **15** 137–155.

14 Berry HK *et al.* Dietary supplement and nutrition in children with cystic fibrosis. *Am J Dis Childh*, 1975, **129** 165–171.

15 Corey ML *et al.* Improved prognosis in CF patients with normal fat absorption. *J Paediatr Gastroenterol Nutr*, 1983, 3(Suppl 1) 99–105.

16 Lanng S *et al.* Glucose tolerance in cystic fibrosis. *Arch Dis Childh*, 1991, **6** 612–616.

17 Knowles MR Diabetes and cystic fibrosis. New questions emerging from increased longevity. *J Pediatr*, 1988, **112** 415–416.

18 Koch C Diabetes mellitus in CF. The Danish experience. *Pediatr Pulmonol*, 1990, (Suppl 5; North American Fibrosis Conference) 108–109.

19 Krueger LJ *et al.* Cystic fibrosis and diabetes mellitus: interactive or idiopathic? *J Pediatr Gastroenter Nutr*, 1991, **13** 209–219.

20 Finkelstein SM *et al.* Diabetes mellitus associated with cystic fibrosis. *J Pediatr*, 1988, **112** 373–377.

21 Reisman J *et al.* Diabetes mellitus in patients with cystic fibrosis: effect on survival. *Pediatr*, 1990, **86** 374–377.

22 Simmonds E *et al.* Fractional measurements of sweat osmolality in patients with CF. *Arch Dis Childh*, 1989, **64** 1714–1720.

23 David TJ Cystic fibrosis. *Arch Dis Childh*, 1990, **65** 152–157.

24 Weller PH, West JV Neonatal screening – should we or shouldn't we? *J Roy Soc Med*, 1991, **84**(Suppl 18) 7–9.

25 Bently D, Lawson M *Clinical Nutrition in Paediatric Disorders*. London: Bailliere Tindall, 1988.

26 Corey M *et al.* A comparison of survival, growth and pulmonary function in patients with cystic fibrosis in Boston and Toronto. *J Clin Epidemiol*, 1988, **41** 583–591.

27 MacDonald A Cystic fibrosis. In: Thomas B (ed.) *Manual of Dietetic Practice*, 2nd edn. Oxford: Blackwell Scientific Publications, 1994.

28 Murphy JL *et al.* Energy content of stools in normal healthy controls and patients with cystic fibrosis. *Arch Dis Childh*, 1991, **66** 495–500.

29 Vaisman N *et al.* Energy expenditure of patients with cystic fibrosis. *J Pediatr*, 1987, **111** 496–500.

30 Buchdahl RM *et al.* Increased resting energy expenditure in cystic fibrosis. *J Appl Physiol*, 1988, **64** 1810–1816.

31 Shepherd RW *et al.* Increased energy expenditure in young children with cystic fibrosis. *Lancet*, 1988, **1** 1300–1303.

32 Spicker V, Roulet M, Schutz Y Assessment of total energy expenditure in free living patients with cystic fibrosis. *J Pediatr*, 1991, **118** 865–872.

33 Williams J, Handy DJ, Weller PH Improving oral energy intake in older children with cystic fibrosis. *J Hum Nutr Dietet*, 1989, **2** 279–285.

34 Beddoes V *et al.* Dietary management of cystic fibrosis. *Practitioner*, 1981, **225** 557–560.

35 Miller M *et al.* Altered protein, composition and muscle protein degradation in nutritionally growth-retarded children with cystic fibrosis. *Am J Clin Nutr*, 1982, **36** 492–499.

36 Baur LA *et al.* Nitrogen deposition in malnourished children with cystic fibrosis. *Am J Clin Nutr*, 1991, **53** 503–511.

37 Pencharz PB Energy intakes and low fat diets in children with cystic fibrosis. *J Pediatr Gastroenterol Nutr*, 1983, **2** 400–402.

38 MacDonald A *et al.* Low, moderate or high fat diets for cystic fibrosis. In: Lawson D (ed.) *Cystic Fibrosis: Horizons*. Chichester: John Wiley, 1984.

39 Daniels L, Davidson GP, Martin JA Comparison of the macronutrient intake of healthy controls and children with cystic fibrosis on low fat or nonrestricted fat diets. *J Pediatr Gastroenterol Nutr*, 1987, **6** 381–386.

40 Gaskin KJ *et al.* Nutritional status, growth and development in children undergoing intensive treatment for cystic fibrosis. *Acta Paediatr Scand*, 1990, **366**(Suppl) 106–110.

41 Thomas B, Blue B, Hemreid L Enteral feeding practices among CF centres. *Pediatr Pulmonol*, 1990, (Suppl 5) 267(A).

42 Ramsey BW *et al.* Nutritional assessment and manage-

ment in cystic fibrosis: a consensus report. *Am J Clin Nutrition*, 1992, **55** 108–116.

43 MacDonald A, Holden C, Harris G Nutritional strategies in cystic fibrosis: current issues. *J Roy Soc Med*, 1991, **84**(Suppl 18) 28–35.

44 Pencharz P *et al*. Energy needs and nutritional rehabilitation in undernourished adolescents and young adult patients with cystic fibrosis. *J Pediatr Gastroenterol Nutr*, 1984, **51**(Suppl 1) 5147–5153.

45 Moore MC *et al*. Enteral tube feeding as an adjunct therapy in malnourished patients with cystic fibrosis: a clinical study and literature review. *Am J Clin Nutr*, 1986, **44**(7) 33–41.

46 Daniels L *et al*. Supplemental nasogastric feeding in cystic fibrosis patients during treatment for acute exacerbations of chest disease. *Aust Paediatr J*, 1989, **25** 164–167.

47 Pierce A, Watson JBG, McKenna C The Irish experience with nocturnal supplementation in CF. *Pediatr Pulmonol*, 1990, (Suppl 5) 266(A).

48 Shepherd RW *et al*. Nutritional rehabilitation in cystic fibrosis. Controlled studies of effects of nutritional growth retardation, body protein turnover and cause of pulmonary disease. *J Pediatr*, 1986, **109** 788–794.

49 Levy L *et al*. Prognostic factors associated with patient survival during nutritional rehabilitation in malnourished children and adolescents with cystic fibrosis. *J Pediatr Gastroenterol Nutr*, 1986, **5** 97–102.

50 Kane RE, Hobbs PJ, Black P Comparison of low, medium and high carbohydrate formulas for night time enteral feeding in cystic fibrosis patients. *J Parent Ent Nutr*, 1990, **14** 47–52.

51 Fitting JW Nutritional support in chronic obstructive lung disease. *Thorax*, 1992, **47** 141–143.

52 Kane RE, Hobbs P Energy and respiratory metabolism in cystic fibrosis. The influence of carbohydrate content of nutritional supplements. *J Pediatr Gastroenterol Nutr*, 1991, **12** 217–223.

53 Taylor CJ, McIntyre S, Baxter PS Nutrition in cystic fibrosis. *Arch Dis Childh*, 1990, **65** 646–647.

54 Smith DL Teaching patients to insert a nasogastric tube. *Brit Med J*, 1991, **45** 139.

55 Boland MP *et al*. Permanent enteral feeding in cystic fibrosis: Advantages of a replacable jejunostomy tube. *J Pediatr Surg*, 1987, **22** 843–847.

56 Eid NS, Shoemaker LR, Samiec TD Vitamin A in cystic fibrosis. Case report and review of the literature. *J Pediatr Gastroenterol Nutr*, 1990, **10** 265–269.

57 Roy CC, Darling P, Weber AM A rational approach to meeting macro and micronutrient needs in cystic fibrosis. *J Pediatr Gastroenterol Nutr*, 1984, **3**(Suppl 1) S154–S162.

58 Hanly JG *et al*. Hypovitaminosis D and response to supplementation in older children with cystic fibrosis. *Q J Med*, 1985, **56** 377–385.

59 Kelleher J *et al*. The clinical effect of correction of vitamin E depletion in cystic fibrosis. *Internat J Vit Nutr Res*, 1987, **57** 253–259.

60 Choonara IA *et al*. Plasma vitamin K, concentration in cystic fibrosis. *Arch Dis Childh*, 1989, **64** 185–187.

61 Ehrhardt P, Miller MG, Littlewood JM Iron deficiency in cystic fibrosis. *Arch Dis Childh*, 1987, **62** 185–187.

62 Safai-Kutti S *et al*. Zinc therapy in children with cystic fibrosis. *Beitr Infusionsther*, 1991, **27** 104–114.

63 Richard MJ *et al*. Selenium and oxidant injury in patients with cystic fibrosis. In: Emerit I *et al*. (eds.) *Antioxidants in Therapy and Preventative Medicine*. New York: Plenum Press, 1990.

64 Kelleher J *et al*. Essential element nutritional status in cystic fibrosis. *Hum Nutr: Appl Nutr*, 1986, **40A** 79–84.

65 Bines JE, Israel EJ Hypoproteinaemia, anaemia and failure to thrive in an infant. *Gastroenterology*, 1991, **101** 848–856.

66 Greer R *et al*. Evaluation of growth and changes in body composition following neonatal diagnosis of cystic fibrosis. *J Pediatr Gastroenterol Nutr*, 1991, **13** 52–58.

67 Marcus MS *et al*. Nutritional status of infants with cystic fibrosis associated with early diagnosis and intervention. *Am J Clin Nutr*, 1991, **54** 578–585.

68 Sokol RJ *et al*. Fat soluble vitamin status during the first year of life in infants with cystic fibrosis identified by screening of newborns. *Am J Clin Nutr*, 1989, **50** 1064–1071.

69 Krebs N *et al*. Zinc status of infants with cystic fibrosis prior to therapy. *Pediatr Pulmunol*, 1990, (Suppl 5) 262A.

70 Davies PSW *et al*. Total energy expenditure in asymptomatic infants with cystic fibrosis. *Pediatr Pulmunol*, 1990, (Suppl 5) 260A.

71 Shepherd RW *et al*. Increased energy expenditure in young children with cystic fibrosis. *Lancet*, 1988, **i**, 1300–1303.

72 Luder E *et al*. Current recommendations for breastfeeding in cystic fibrosis centres. *AJDC*, 1990, **144** 1153–1156.

73 Halliday KE *et al*. Growth of human milk-fed and formula-fed infants with cystic fibrosis. *J Pediatr*, 1990, **118** 77–79.

74 Walker S Growth of breast fed versus formula fed infants with cystic fibrosis. *Pediatr Pulmonol*, 1990, (Suppl 5) 262A.

75 Laughlin JJ, Brady MS, Eigen H Changing feeding trends as a cause of electrolyte depletion in infants with cystic fibrosis. *Pediatrics*, 1981, **68** 203–207.

76 Farrell PM, Mischler EH, Sondel SA Predigested formula for infants with cystic fibrosis. *J Am Diet Assoc*, 1985, **87** 1353–1356.

77 Canciani M, Mastella G Absorption of a new semielemental diet in infants with cystic fibrosis. *J Pediatr Gastroenterol Nutr*, 1985, **4** 735–740.

78 The Consumers' Association Choosing and using a pancreatic enzyme supplement. *Drug and Therapeutics Bulletin*, 1992, **30** 37–40.

79 McCollum A, Gibson L Family adaptation to the child with cystic fibrosis. *J Pediatr*, 1970, **77** 57–78.

80 Singer LT *et al*. Behaviour assessment and management of food refusal in children with cystic fibrosis. *Developmental and Behaviur Pediatr*, 1991, **12** 115–120.

81 Carroccio A *et al*. Effectiveness of enteric-coated preparations on nutritional parameters in cystic fibrosis. *Digestion*, 1988, **41** 201–206.

82 Beverley DW *et al*. Comparison of four pancreatic extracts in cystic fibrosis. *Arch Dis Childh*, 1987, **62** 564–568.

83 Vyas H, Matthew DJ, Milla PJ A comparison of enteric coated microspheres with enteric coated tablet pancreatic enzyme preparations in cystic fibrosis. A controlled study. *Eur J Pediatr*, 1990, **149** 241–243.

84 Stead RJ *et al*. Enteric coated microspheres of pancreatin in the treatment of cystic fibrosis: comparison with a standard enteric coated preparation. *Thorax*, 1987, **42** 533–537.

85 Ansaldi-Balocco N, Santini B, Sarchi C Efficacy of pancreatic enzyme supplementation in children with cystic fibrosis: comparison of two preparations by random crossover study and a retrospective study of the same patients at two different ages. *J Pediatr Gastroenterol Nutr*, 1988, **7**(Suppl 1) 40–45.

86 Williams J *et al*. Two enteric coated microspheres in cystic fibrosis. *Arch Dis Childh*, 1990, **65** 594–597.

87 Morrison G *et al*. Pancreatic enzyme supplements in cystic fibrosis. *Lancet*, 1991, **338**(ii) 1596–1597.

88 Owen G *et al*. Pancreatic enzyme supplement dosage in cystic fibrosis. *Lancet*, 1991, **338** 1153.

89 Robinson PJ, Sly PD High dose pancreatic enzymes in cystic fibrosis. *Arch Dis Childh*, 1989, **64** 311–312.

90 Chalmers DM *et al*. The influence of long term cimetidine as an adjuvant to pancreatic enzyme therapy in cystic fibrosis. *Acta Paediatr Scand*, 1985, **74** 114–117.

USEFUL ADDRESS

The Cystic Fibrosis Trust
Alexander House, 5 Blyth Road, Bromley, Kent BR1 3RS.

CHAPTER 11

The Kidney

ACUTE RENAL FAILURE

Acute renal failure (ARF) can be described as a sudden decrease in renal function with retention of nitrogenous wastes and disturbance of water and electrolyte homeostasis. Oliguria (urine output <1 ml/kg body weight/hr in the young child) usually occurs simultaneously with the condition. However, occasional patients may have polyuria such as occurs with relief of urinary obstruction e.g. posterior urethral valves.

The causes of ARF in children are shown in Table 11.1 and are different from those in adult patients [1]. In newborns there are further considerations and causes [2].

The commonest cause of ARF in childhood in the United Kingdom is haemolytic uraemic syndrome (HUS). It typically follows a prodromal illness of diarrhoea which is often bloody [3]. Anorexia and vomiting often accompany and complicate the nutritional management, particularly in those occasional children who have had laparotomies for suspected appendicitis or colitis prior to the diagnosis of HUS.

Management of ARF

ARF requires close attention to fluid balance and monitoring of electrolytes and blood pressure. Some children may be conservatively managed, i.e. without dialysis. In such patients a greater need for fluid restriction can complicate the nutritional prescription whereas dialysis should allow the removal of fluid and uraemic toxins, thereby providing more 'nutritional space' and greater flexibility in nutritional regimens. Indications for dialysis include:

- hyperkalaemia
- fluid overload
- rapidly rising plasma urea and creatinine levels with oliguria
- metabolic abnormalities e.g. acidosis, hyperphosphataemia
- to create 'nutritional space'
- to remove specific poisons.

Dialysis and ARF

Peritoneal dialysis is the dialysis technique generally favoured for children [4] as it avoids the need for access to blood vessels and is a continuous 'gentler' form of dialysis. Haemodialysis or haemofiltration are implemented when peritoneal dialysis is complicated by leaks into the pleural cavity or because of abdominal surgery. Various types of haemofiltration are often used in intensive care areas to remove excess fluid.

Nutritional management of ARF

The paediatric dietitian should be involved at the onset as the dietary prescription may change with alterations in clinical management and stage of the illness [5]. Adequate nutrition will help prevent catabolism, control metabolic abnormalities and hopefully alleviate clinical symptoms and hasten recovery [6].

Dietary principles of ARF

The basic aims are an energy supplemented, reduced protein diet (Table 11.2). A potassium, sodium and phosphate restriction is usually necessary. Those children with persistent diarrhoea may require a semi-elemental feed. Fluid allowance depends upon overall fluid balance and whether the patient is being dialysed. Daily interpretation of the biochemical parameters

Table 11.1 Causes of acute renal failure

Pre-renal	*Acute hypovolaemia*
	Severe gastroenteritis
	Haemorrhage
	Third space losses e.g. burns, gastrointestinal surgery
	Hypoalbuminaemia e.g. nephrotic syndrome
	Peripheral vasodilation
	Sepsis
	Vasodilator drugs e.g. tolazoline
	Low cardiac output
	Cardiac failure
Renal	*Haemolytic uraemic syndrome*
	Acute glomerulonephritis
	Acute interstitial nephritis
	Drug hypersensitivity
	Severe pyelonephritis
	Nephrotoxins
	Antibiotics
	Antimitotic drugs
	Myoglobinuria, haemoglobinuria
	Vasculitis
	Polyarteritis
	Acute crystalline nephropathy
	Uric acid
	Oxalosis
	Post-ischaemic acute tubular necrosis (ATN)
	Bilateral renal vessel occlusion
	Renal artery/vein thrombosis
Post-renal	*Posterior urethral valves*
	Bilateral obstruction
	Pelviureteric or vesicoureteric junction
	Ureterocoele(s)
	Neurogenic bladder
	Stones

should be discussed with the medical and nursing staff so that the dietary prescription can be individualized for each child.

Nutritional Assessment in ARF will include:

- dietary history: this should be obtained from the parents/carers;
- growth parameters: height, if available, and weight plotted on a growth chart [7] will help determine a more accurate estimation of dry weight;
- fluid: allowances need to be determined;
- biochemical assessment: plasma levels of sodium, potassium, urea, creatinine, albumin, calcium and phosphate will be of particular relevance (see Table 11.3).

Methods of feeding

Enteral feeding

The child with ARF may initially take oral fluids willingly because of thirst. However, the majority of children fail to meet the necessary nutritional goals via the oral route. It is recommended that a fine bore nasogastric tube is passed routinely at the time of sedation for other procedures such as insertion of a peritoneal dialysis catheter or arterial line [5]. This allows the provision of prompt nutritional support, as anorexia, vomiting or refusal to take the nutritional prescription can complicate management.

A continuous 24 hour feed using an enteral feeding pump may be advantageous in the initial stages of treatment. As the oral intake improves, the transition from continuous to overnight feeding can help provide the remaining nutritional prescription until appetite has returned sufficiently and tube feeding can be withdrawn.

Total parenteral nutrition (TPN)

The parenteral route is only considered if enteral nutrition is not tolerated. Established hospital TPN regimens are not suitable for the child with ARF because of fluid restriction and electrolyte composition. The dietitian and medical staff must agree upon a suitable daily prescription to meet individual requirements. The use of high nitrogen, electrolyte free solutions can be considered (e.g. Vamin 18EF or 14EF) to allow for the provision of increased energy from carbohydrate and fat solutions (50% dextrose, Intralipid 20%) if fluid is limited. The flexibility of added electrolytes, on a daily basis, is also an advantage and will depend upon blood biochemistry. For most children parenteral nutrition is temporary with re-establishment of the enteral route as soon as possible.

Table 11.2 Nutritional guidelines for the child in acute renal failure (ARF)

	Energy* (kcal/kg body wt/day)	Protein (g/kg body wt/day)
Conservative management		
0–2 yr	95–150 (400–630 kJ)	1.0–1.8
Children/adolescents	Minimum of EAR for height age	1.0
Peritoneal dialysis		
0–2 yr	95–150 (400–630 kJ)	2.0–2.5**
Children/adolescents	Minimum of EAR for height age	1.0–2.5
Haemodialysis		
0–2 yr	95–150 (400–630 kJ)	1.5–2.1
Children/adolescents	Minimum of EAR for height age	1.0–1.8

EAR – Estimated average requirement (Dietary Reference Values, 1991) [9]

* These are guidelines which are rarely achieved in the acute stage because of fluid restriction

** If dialysis is prolonged, increased protein may be required

Nutritional considerations

Energy

Little is known about the energy requirements of infants and children with ARF [8]. The Estimated Average Requirement (EAR) for energy (DRV 1991) [9] for healthy children of the same chronological age can provide an approximate guideline (Table 11.2). Although such recommendations are unlikely to be achieved during acute treatment, it is important to provide the maximum energy intake tolerated within the fluid allowance. The prompt use of glucose polymers added to drinks of choice and flavoured according to preference, are recommended. A concentration of 1 kcal (4.2 kJ) per ml (25% carbohydrate concentration) should be encouraged, but will depend upon individual tolerance. Liquid glucose polymers may also be used but often require dilution to be acceptable to children. If fluid is severely restricted, ice cubes and lollies can be prepared with an energy-dense solution and offered at frequent intervals. Combined energy supplements of carbohydrate and fat or, alternatively, fat emulsions together with glucose polymers can also be considered (Table 11.4). These can be successfully added to infant formulas to increase the energy content. An energy density of 0.85–1 kcal (3.6–4.2 kJ) per ml of formula can be achieved in infants up to 6 months of age. Infants of 8–12 months of age should tolerate concentrations of

Table 11.3 Reference range guidelines for normal plasma values in childhood

	mmol/l
Sodium	132–142
Potassium*	3.0–6.6 (up to 1 month of age) 3.0–5.6 (after 1 month of age)
Bicarbonate	18–26
Urea	2.5–6.5
Calcium	2.1–2.6 (ionized calcium preferable if available)
Phosphorus*	1.2–2.8 (up to 1 month of age) 1.3–1.8 (after 1 month of age)
Albumin	34–45 (g/l)

* Age related

1.2–1.5 kcal (5–6.3 kJ) per ml without adverse effects.

Some children may have insulin resistance and hyperglycaemia can occur and be complicated by the absorption of glucose from the peritoneal dialysis fluid and the intake of high carbohydrate supplements. Insulin infusions should be considered to control blood glucose levels along with the dietary modification of carbohydrate.

Table 11.4 Nutritional supplements

Supplement	Suggested use
Energy	
Glucose polymers (powder) e.g. Maxijul, Polycal, Polycose	Add to infant formula, baby juice, cows' milk, water, squash, fizzy drinks, tea, milk, ice cubes and lollies
(liquid) e.g. Polycal Liquid, Maxijul, Hycal	Dilute with soda water, fizzy drinks of choice, squash (unless fluid restricted) Add to jelly
Fat emulsion e.g. Calogen	Add to infant formula, cows' milk
Combined fat and carbohydrate e.g. Duocal powder	Add to infant formula, cows' milk, nutritionally complete supplements
Protein	
Protein powders e.g. Protifar, Maxipro HBV	Add to infant formula, Liquid Duocal, modular energy components
Nutritionally complete	
Nutrison paediatric (2.7 g protein, 100 kcal, 58 mg phosphate, 80 ml water/100 ml)	For oral or supplementary tube feeding
Suplena (2.9 g protein, 200 kcal, 72 mg phosphate, 70 ml water/100 ml)	
Fortisip (5 g protein, 150 kcal, 50 mg phosphate, 79 ml water/100 ml)	
Nepro (6.9 g protein, 200 kcal, 72 mg phosphate, 70 ml water/100 ml)	

Protein

Protein intake should be reduced when treatment is first initiated and then gradually increased on dialysis where there is increased solute removal and possible protein losses. The Reference Nutrient Intake (RNI) values for protein [9] are not appropriate for the child with ARF and requirements will be determined for each child. The age and weight of the child and dialysis therapy, if implemented, will all need to be considered. Nutritional guidelines are shown in Table 11.2.

Nutritional supplements via the nasogastric route are frequently relied upon to meet protein requirements in the initial stages of treatment. For infants, the commercially available formulas, which are low in phosphate, are recommended and can be modified as required. For the older child there are a number of protein containing supplements available. Their composition of protein, phosphate and potassium need to be assessed prior to use.

If semi-elemental formulas or feeds are indicated they can be modified to meet individual requirements. Introduction should be gradual and delivery is usually by the nasogastric route. Once the child's appetite improves and protein intake is met by diet, energy supplemented drinks can then replace protein containing supplements.

Low protein products can contribute to the energy content of the diet. However on the grounds of their palatability most children either refuse them or don't take sufficient quantity to be of any value in the diet.

Fluid

The volume of fluid prescribed during conservative treatment is based upon insensible fluid requirements of 400 mls/m^2 body surface area/day or approximately 20 mls/kg body weight/day, with a 12% increase for each degree centigrade above 38.5°, and a reduction if the child is ventilated. Insensible losses should be added to the previous day's urine output to give the total daily fluid allowance.

If the child is being dialysed, the fluid prescription will be determined by monitoring the volume of fluid removed by ultrafiltration plus the insensible losses. Ideally fluid removal on dialysis should be flexibly managed to allow for increased 'nutritional space'.

Maximum nutrient intakes, using supplements, should be provided within the fluid allowance and divided equally throughout the day. It is important to remind medical and nursing staff that the fluid content of supplements is less than the prescribed volume (e.g. 100 mls of Nepro contains 70 mls of fluid).

Electrolytes

Initially, intakes of electrolytes such as potassium, sodium and phosphate are likely to be restricted. Plasma levels and the use of dialysis will dictate requirements thereafter.

All carers should be advised about potassium restriction so that rich sources are withdrawn. Citrus fruits and fruit juices, bananas, crisps and chocolate

Table 11.5 Potassium-rich foods and suggested alternatives

Rich potassium containing foods*	Suggested alternatives
Bananas, kiwi fruit, citrus fruits e.g. oranges, grapefruit, dried fruit e.g. raisins, tinned fruit in fruit juice	Apples, pears, tinned fruit in syrup
Fruit juices e.g. orange, apple, tomato Instant coffee and coffee essence Malted milk drinks e.g. Horlicks, Cocoa, drinking chocolate	Squash, Lucozade, lemonade, tea
Potato crisps and potato type snacks, nuts Salt substitutes Bovril, Marmite	Corn or rice snacks (take account of sodium content), sweetened popcorn, jam, honey, marmalade, syrup
Jacket potatoes, chips (oven and frozen), roast potatoes	Rice (boiled or fried), spaghetti, pasta, bread Boiled and/or mashed potato
Mushrooms, spinach, tomatoes, spaghetti in tomato sauce, baked beans	Carrots, cauliflower, swede, broccoli, cabbage
Chocolate and all foods containing it, toffee, fudge	Boiled sweets, jellies, mints, marshmallows
Chocolate biscuits	Biscuits – plain, sandwich, jam filled, wafer
Chocolate cake, fruit cake	Cake – plain sponge filled with cream and/or jam Jam tarts, apple pie, doughnuts
Milk, yoghurt, evaporated and condensed milk	Low protein milk substitutes e.g. double cream and water, Coffeemate, Coffee Compliment

* Allowance will depend upon individual assessment

Table 11.6 Phosphate-rich foods and suggested alternatives

Rich phosphate containing foods*	Suggested alternatives
Cows' milk (full cream, semi-skimmed, skimmed) Dried milk powder and other milk products	*Infants* Encourage infant formula e.g. SMA Gold, Nutrilon Premium, for at least 1–2 yrs *Children* Reduce intake, consider low protein milk substitute
Yoghurt, fromage frais, ice cream, custard made with milk	Reduce intake Custard made with double cream and water or milk substitute
Evaporated, condensed milk Single cream	Double cream, imitation cream
Cheese, e.g. Cheddar, processed cheese, cheese spread, Edam	Limit intake and/or encourage use of: cottage cheese (within protein allowance) or full fat cream cheese
Egg yolk	Meringues
Chocolate and chocolate containing foods, toffee, fudge	Boiled sweets, mints, dolly mixtures
Sardines, pilchards, tuna Baked beans	
Nuts, peanut butter Coca cola	Jam, honey, marmalade, syrup Squash, lemonade, Lucozade

* Allowance will depend upon individual assessment

are amongst the foods commonly brought into hospital by relatives. Advice on suitable low potassium alternatives should be given (Table 11.5). Limitation of sodium can be achieved by the avoidance of salted snacks and no added salt.

Phosphate restriction can be achieved in part when protein intake, particularly that of dairy products, is reduced (Table 11.6). Cows' milk is generally restricted or eliminated from the diet during the acute phase because of its high protein, phosphate and potassium content. Avoidance of cow's milk also reduces the potential cow's milk protein or lactose intolerance following the diarrhoeal prodrome in patients with HUS.

Micronutrients

Vitamin supplementation need only be considered if the dialysis treatment is prolonged. A general vitamin supplement (e.g. Abidec 0.6 mls daily) should be adequate for the majority of children as appetite improves. Iron supplementation may be indicated in some children during the recovery phase, particularly in those who had a poor diet history prior to the onset of the ARF.

Recovery phase

When the acute episode is over, and the child is passing urine, dialysis can be suspended and dietary restrictions can be gradually reduced. Attention to plasma electrolytes and intakes is essential as replacement therapy may be required if there are major losses during the diuretic phase.

Prior to discharge advice should be given on the gradual reintroduction of foods previously restricted as there are a number of children who vomit on returning home, when such foods are reintroduced quickly. The opportunity to educate the child and family about the principles of a well balanced diet should also be taken.

Some children may need to continue on energy and vitamin supplements for a short time. Their progress should be monitored in the clinic.

Outcome of ARF

The prognosis for children with ARF is generally very good. A small percentage of children with HUS and other causes of ARF may be left with impaired renal function and may require ongoing dietary advice.

NEPHROTIC SYNDROME

Nephrotic syndrome (NS) is characterized by heavy proteinuria (>40 mg/hr/m^2 body surface area or >200 mg/mmol creatinine in an early morning urine) leading to hypoalbuminaemia (<25 g/dl) and oedema.

The syndrome can be subdivided into three categories:

- congenital
- idiopathic (primary)
- secondary.

The majority of cases found in childhood are in the idiopathic category, so called minimal change nephrotic syndrome (MCNS). The syndrome is commonest in males (2:1) and characteristically affects the pre-school child. The cause of MCNS remains unknown, but is more prevalent in families with an atopic history of asthma, eczema and hay fever. If the child responds to corticosteroids then the prognosis is good and there are likely to be few long term dietary

problems [10]. However, children who relapse frequently and are steroid dependent may require ongoing dietary intervention to monitor and maintain nutritional status and prevent obesity. Growth failure remains an important issue in the long term management [11].

Nutritional issues in nephrotic syndrome

In previous years, high protein diets (3–4 g protein/kg body weight/day) were prescribed in the belief that the increased intakes of protein helped to restore serum protein pools [12]. However, animal studies have shown that although dietary protein augmentation increased albumin synthesis it had no significant effect upon serum albumin levels or muscle protein, as all of the additional ingested protein was catabolized to urea and excreted in the urine rather than used to promote growth [13]. The use of low protein diets have also been studied because of the additional concerns that high protein diets may accelerate the progression of human glomerulonephritis [14]. Although a decrease in albuminuria has been shown in animal studies [15], there remains the risk of malnutrition and poor growth particularly in childhood.

Both high and low protein diets are often impractical, resulting in additional family anxieties.

Nutritional assessment

The dietitian should be involved during the first hospitalization and obtain a detailed dietary history and chart growth parameters for both weight and height [7]. These can both help in the prediction of the child's acceptable dry weight and approximate nutritional requirements. Attention to fluid balance and plasma electrolytes is also important.

Nutritional management of NS

Energy and protein A balanced diet, adequate in both energy (EAR for children of the same chronological age) [9] and protein (1–2 g/kg body weight/day) should be adequate for most children. Energy intake may need to be reduced if the child gains weight rapidly.

Sodium Sodium intake is a major contributor to thirst and weight gain in children with nephrotic syndrome [16]. A 'no added salt' diet, particularly avoiding salted snacks, is recommended. Very low sodium diets and the use of specialist products are rarely necessary.

Fluid Both the restriction of fluid and the 'no added salt' diet are important in the initial oedematous phase.

Fats/oils Although diet is unlikely to reduce significantly the raised lipid levels commonly recognized in nephrotic patients, it is recommended that, as part of the initial general healthy eating advice, mono or polyunsaturated margarines and oils with a reduction of saturated fat intake should be advocated. This advice is more relevant for the child with a chronic nephrotic state who is resistant to steroid treatment.

Ongoing management

For most children the introduction of steroid therapy can stimulate appetite enormously and in practice the common dietary problem is the prevention of excessive weight gain [10]. Dietary advice to reduce the child's energy intake must be promptly initiated if obesity is to be prevented. Children will often feel hungry while on steroids and a reduction of between meal snacks such as biscuits, crisps, sweets, chocolate and fizzy drinks should be encouraged, with the substitution of suitable 'low calorie' alternatives. Healthy eating advice for all the family should be reinforced and a leaflet or booklet on healthy eating may be helpful.

Occasionally a child may require nutritional support because of prolonged anorexia or where there is evidence of malnutrition. Nutritional supplements taken orally or administered via a nasogastric tube should be considered.

Food allergy

Some reports have suggested that food hypersensitivity, particularly of milk and dairy products, may be involved in the aetiology of glomerular damage of both young and adult patients [17,18]. In those rare children who do not respond to treatment and who have a strong history suggesting food intolerance it may be of value to consider a trial of a few foods diet (page 155). This needs to be under close dietetic supervision.

Follow up

It is recommended that the dietitian should see all nephrotic patients at least once in clinic following discharge to monitor their clinical progress. Dietary guidelines should be reinforced to ensure that the diet is practical and not unnecessarily restrictive.

Psychosocial support

Naturally there is a great deal of concern and worry expressed by parents when they realize their child may have a chronic illness. Information about the management and treatment of nephrotic syndrome by means of a booklet (*Childhood Nephrotic Syndrome* [19]) is recommended. A parents' group may enable the sharing of experiences and be of great benefit to parents who feel they are struggling alone.

CONGENITAL NEPHROTIC SYNDROME

Congenital nephrotic syndrome (CNS) is rare and can present at birth or in the first few months of life. The proteinuria of up to 5 g/l is unresponsive to treatment, and may be associated with a deterioration in renal function. Unilateral or bilateral nephrectomy, dialysis and transplantation may be necessary in infancy. Such patients are likely to require intensive dietetic support and intervention.

Nutritional management of CNS

It is likely that fluid intake will be restricted allowing an intake equivalent to the child's insensible losses ($400 \, \text{mls/m}^2$ body surface area/day) plus the previous day's urine output. Sodium intake should also be reduced but this will depend upon blood biochemistry and fluid allowance. Energy intake should be maximized – 115–150 kcals (480–630 kJ)/kg body weight/ day – within the fluid allowed and a protein intake of 2–4 g/kg body weight/day may be indicated.

The infant who is breast fed is unlikely to meet dietary requirements and fluid balance may be difficult. Initially expressed breast milk (EBM) can be supplemented with protein and energy supplements. However, the medical staff and dietitian need to discuss the importance of ensuring adequate nutrition and fluid balance with the parents and supporting

Table 11.7 Causes of chronic renal failure in childhood

Cause	%
Chronic glomerulonephritis e.g. focal glomerulosclerosis	32
Reflux nephropathy and urinary tract malformation	22
Hereditary – familial e.g. Alport's syndrome	16
Renal hypoplasia/dysplasia	12
Other diagnosis e.g. Henoch-Schönlein purpura	12
Uncertain	6

European Dialysis and Transplant Association Registry, 1980

them in the possible decision to withdraw the infant from breast feeding. Infant formula may then be modified as required and normal weaning practices should be encouraged between four and six months of age.

Many infants are anorexic and require nutritional support via a nasogastric tube or by a gastrostomy button, which may be more appropriate when prolonged supplementary feeding is anticipated (page 29).

CHRONIC RENAL FAILURE

Chronic renal failure (CRF) may be recognized shortly after birth or can present later in life with growth failure and anorexia. It can proceed into end stage renal failure during childhood when dialysis and transplantation will be required [20].

The causes of chronic renal failure are shown in Table 11.7.

Management of CRF

Children with progressive CRF should be managed under the direction of a specialist centre where the dietitian is a member of the multidisciplinary team. Since CRF can have a profound effect upon growth and development, dietetic support is required long term. Dietary aims are to ensure adequate nutrition sufficient for growth while maintaining acceptable blood biochemistry and fluid balance. Individual dietary prescription must be practical if goals are to be achieved and compliance maintained. An understand-

ing of the psychosocial effects of feeding such children is as important as the nutritional advice. Although families may have to travel long distances to the unit, continuity of the dietetic education is essential. Regular telephone contact and visits to the home, nursery and school can be invaluable supportive measures. Infants with CRF present particular problems with anorexia and vomiting and nutritional support is now recognized to be important in management.

Most children with CRF pass through three stages of treatment:

- pre-dialysis or conservative management
- dialysis ⟨ peritoneal / haemodialysis
- transplantation.

Dialysis is seen as a 'holding' measure before renal transplantation although, unfortunately, some children may remain on dialysis for a prolonged period. There is an increasing trend to transplant children before dialysis is required (pre-emptive transplantation).

The stage of treatment and age of the child will influence the nutritional prescription. The overall principles of dietary management are discussed.

Chronic dialysis

Chronic peritoneal dialysis (CPD) is the preferred dialysis treatment in most centres [21] as it is technically easier than haemodialysis (HD) and the child can be managed at home. Generally, CPD allows a more liberal diet because of the continuous removal of wastes, electrolytes and fluid. *Continuous ambulatory peritoneal dialysis* (CAPD) involves three to four manual bag changes a day while *continuous cycling peritoneal dialysis* (CCPD) is performed automatically by a machine overnight. CCPD may be preferable, as it enables the child and family to be free of dialysis bag changes by day. Also compared with CAPD there may be less of a feeling of fullness as there is a smaller volume of dialysate in the abdomen during the day which could potentially depress appetite. *Haemodialysis (HD)* is an intermittent process lasting 3–6 hours, usually performed in hospital three times a week. Diet and fluid on HD is generally more restricted when compared with CPD to minimize the biochemical and fluid fluctuations between dialysis days.

Nutritional assessment in CRF

This will include the following.

Growth parameters

Weight and height in children, and weight, length and head circumference in infants should be regularly plotted on the appropriate chart [7] to monitor growth. Height velocity should also be recorded annually. The growth chart may also assist in determining the child's nutritional requirements as follows:

- interpretation of the child's height age (if below the third percentile) can be used as an initial value to determine acceptable baseline nutritional requirements
- if the child is within the percentile ranges for height, nutritional requirements can be based upon the recommendations for children of the same chronological age.

Midarm circumference (MAC), triceps skin fold (TSF) and subscapular skinfold (SSF) thicknesses may assist in assessing body protein and fat stores when compared with normal values. They should be carried out under a standard protocol, preferably by the same individual [22] but are perhaps more appropriate for research purposes than clinical application.

Food diaries

Food diaries using household measures, performed periodically for a three day period (including one weekend day) are useful to the dietitian when estimating individual requirements. Although not entirely reliable, the calculated daily nutrient intakes are a baseline on which to make further recommendations. The child's appetite and food choices can also be obtained from the diary which helps to devise a diet plan which is suitable for the child and family.

Biochemical assessment

Biochemical assessment of plasma urea, creatinine, albumin, sodium, potassium, calcium and phosphate levels are of particular relevance to the dietary prescription (Table 11.3). Reference range guideline values for plasma creatinine are shown in Table 11.8.

The glomerular filtration rate (GFR), if accurately

Table 11.8 Reference range guidelines for normal plasma creatinine values in childhood*

Age (yrs)	Plasma creatinine (μmol/l)
<5	<44
5–6	<53
6–7	<62
7–8	<71
8–9	<80
9–10	<88
10+	<106

* Ketones interfere positively
  Bilirubin interferes negatively

measured, will be used by the nephrologist to predict when dialysis is likely to be required.

Prescribed medications

Many of the prescribed medications are nutrition related (e.g. phosphate binders, sodium supplements, vitamins) and should be periodically reviewed by the dietitian as part of the dietary assessment. Problems with compliance, effect upon appetite and potential anxieties of the practicalities of taking the medications (e.g. at school) need to be identified and regimens adjusted accordingly. Families need to be updated about the medications and their relevance in the child's treatment.

Fluid balance

Fluid balance and assessment of the child's predicted dry weight is relevant to the dietary prescription. Fluid allowance will depend upon the aetiology of the renal disease and the child's native urine output. The fluid content of nutritional supplements and particular foods may need to be considered if fluid is restricted.

Dietary principles in CRF

The dietary aims in managing children with CRF require attention to:

- adequacy of energy intake
- regulation of protein
- fluid balance and electrolytes

Table 11.9 Nutritional guidelines for the child with chronic renal failure (CRF)

	Energy (kcal/kg body wt/day)	(kJ)	Protein (g/kg body wt/day)
Pre-dialysis			
Infants			
Preterm	120–180	500–750	2.5–3.0
0–0.5 yr	115–150	480–630	1.5–2.1
0.5–1.0	95–150	400–630	1.5–1.8
1.0–2.0	95–120	400–500	1.0–1.8
Children/adolescents			
2.0–puberty	Minimum of EAR for		1.0–1.5
pubertal	height age		1.0–1.5
post-pubertal			1.0–1.5
Peritoneal dialysis (CCPD/CAPD)			
Infants			
Preterm	120–180	500–750	3.0–4.0
0–0.5 yr	115–150	480–630	2.1–3.0
0.5–1.0	95–150	400–630	2.0–3.0
1.0–2.0	95–120	400–500	2.0–3.0
Children/adolescents			
2.0–puberty	Minimum of EAR for		2.5
pubertal	height age		2.0
post-pubertal			1.5
Haemodialysis			
Infants			
Preterm	120–180	500–750	3.0
0–0.5	115–150	480–630	2.1
0.5–1.0	95–150	400–630	1.5–2.0
1.0–2.0	95–120	400–500	1.5–1.8
Children/adolescents			
2.0–puberty	Minimum of EAR for		1.0–1.5
pubertal	height age		1.0–1.5
post-pubertal			1.0–1.5

EAR – Estimated average requirement (Dietary Reference Values, 1991) [9]

- regulation of calcium and phosphate
- adequacy of micronutrient intakes.

Each will be discussed separately and will depend upon age, stage of management and nutritional assessment.

Energy

The provision of adequate energy is essential to promote growth in all children with CRF, but is particularly important during the pre-dialysis stage of treatment and for children undergoing haemodialysis when protein intake is restricted. Nutritional guidelines are shown in Table 11.9.

High energy, low protein foods

These should be encouraged where possible e.g. sugar, glucose, jams, marmalade, honey, syrup. The use of poly or monounsaturated oils in cooking, or margarines spread on bread, toast or added to vegetables can also contribute quite significantly to the child's energy intake.

Energy supplements

In practice, these are relied upon to achieve the child's requirements, because of anorexia and in some cases fluid restriction. There are a number of supplements available (Table 11.4).

Combined fat and carbohydrate supplements (e.g. Duocal powder) can be successfully added to infant formula – 4–18 g of Duocal per 100 ml providing 0.8–1.5 kcal (3.3–6.3 kJ)/ml – and supplementary tube feeds and should be increased gradually. Liquid glucose polymers are more popular if diluted with a fizzy drink or squash but the volume allowed will depend upon fluid allowance. Powdered glucose polymers are useful for those children who drink plenty of water, squash or baby juice.

It is important to give a written and agreed prescribed daily intake of energy supplement. The use of measured scoops ensures better compliance at home and, should the child be admitted into hospital the prescription can be continued by the nursing staff. This practice also allows the dietitian more accurately to assess the child's intake.

Peritoneal dialysis and energy

Glucose is absorbed from the dialysis fluid during peritoneal dialysis and studies have shown an energy contribution of approximately 8 kcal (33 kJ)/kg body weight/day [23]. However, the strength of glucose concentration in the dialysate and duration of dwell time must be taken into consideration.

For children who require an additional energy supplement while undergoing CPD, it may be of value to consider using a nutritionally complete supplement (Table 11.4) in preference to a high carbohydrate supplement, particularly as protein requirements are generally increased and because of recognized raised triglyceride levels in children on CPD. Where possible the use of complex carbohydrate foods such as bread, potatoes and cereals should continue to be encouraged. It is recommended that fat intake should provide approximately 35% of the energy intake [24] but this will depend upon individual patients.

Protein

The recommended values (RNI) [9] for protein are not appropriate for the child with CRF as requirements vary and therefore the parameters of nutritional assessment will assist in the individual prescription of protein intake (Table 11.9).

Alterations to the protein intake should be made in conjunction with ensuring that the intake of energy is adequate. Particular attention to the plasma urea, albumin and phosphate levels will determine changes in management. Plasma urea levels should ideally be maintained at levels <20–25 mmol/l.

Conservative management

Protein intake is generally reduced during this stage of management to:

- minimize uraemia to urea levels <20 mmol/l
- preserve renal function which may delay the progression to end stage renal disease (ESRD), though this may not be relevant in the paediatric population [25,26]
- control hyperphosphataemia (phosphate intake is automatically reduced because of protein restriction).

Protein containing supplements are rarely required as most children usually receive sufficient protein from formula or diet.

Peritoneal dialysis

The protein requirements of children on CPD can be generally increased to allow for the reported dialysate losses of protein and albumin. However, the intake of cows' milk and other dairy products must be restricted if hyperphosphataemia is to be controlled. Most infants/children require supplements to meet recommended intakes (Table 11.4).

Peritonitis

The protein requirements of children during episodes of peritonitis or other intercurrent infections are increased. Serum albumin levels are likely to fall and increased intakes of prescribed supplements (protein and energy) should be encouraged as the majority of children will be anorexic. Supplementary tube feeding should be considered for those chidren who fail to take sufficient nutrition by the oral route.

Haemodialysis

The protein intakes of children undergoing HD

should be regulated to minimize fluctuations in pre-dialysis blood urea levels. Nutritional guidelines are shown in Table 11.9.

Protein intake from diet

Approximately 50% of the prescribed protein intake should be of high biological value (HBV). Cows' milk, eggs and other dairy produce should be limited because of their high phosphate content.

Protein Supplements

For infants, protein powders can be added to the commercially available infant formulas, which are low in phosphate. Additional energy supplements are required (Table 11.4). For infants more than 8 months of age, a nutritionally complete supplement can be considered, and is useful when fluid is restricted (Table 11.4). Some units have found Kindergen PROD (a specialized low phosphate infant formula) to be beneficial when serum phosphate levels have proved difficult to control. Additional sodium and potassium supplements may be required with the latter feed.

For children and adolescents, it is recommended that a nutritionally complete supplement, low in phosphate, is routinely prescribed on the commencement of peritoneal dialysis [27] (Table 11.4). Such supplements may also be required for children undergoing haemodialysis who fail to achieve recommended intakes. Prescribed supplements should be treated as a medication and if taken orally they are best taken in divided amounts (preferably after food) during the day or as a drink before bed.

Protein exchange lists

The use of protein exchange lists [28] is most appropriate when protein intake is either reduced (pre-dialysis) or regulated (haemodialysis). They are best adapted to include foods commonly consumed by each individual child, and should only be considered for those families who can interpret them confidently and practically. *Low protein foods* which are available on prescription (e.g. low protein bread and biscuits) can contribute to the total energy intake and can be encouraged for children whose protein intake is reduced. In practice the majority of children do not find them acceptable.

Fluid and electrolytes

Fluid

Many infants and young children in the early days of their disease pass copious amounts of dilute urine. While they are being managed conservatively there will be no need for fluid restriction. Individual fluid prescription can be devised by calculation of the insensible fluid losses ($400 \, \text{mls/m}^2$ body surface area/day) plus the volume of urine output from the previous day. When undergoing peritoneal dialysis the volume of fluid removed by ultrafiltration should also be added to the daily fluid allowance. Peritoneal dialysis will allow greater flexibility of fluid management in the oliguric or anuric child as the strengths of glucose solution used in the dialysis fluid can be varied to increase fluid removal. Care must be taken to ensure adequate fluid intake in those children who are polyuric.

Fluid balance in children on haemodialysis can be difficult as weight gain between dialysis sessions can be problematic and ideally, should not exceed 2–5% of the child's estimated dry weight [22]. *Accurate weighing* of patients with careful interpretation of the intake and output of fluids is important. The fluid content of nutritional supplements (Table 11.4) and foods which are fluid at room temperature, e.g. jelly, may need to be considered when fluid is restricted.

Education of both the child and parents together with written guidelines may improve compliance.

Sodium

Requirements will be determined by the:

- aetiology of the renal disease
- presence of hypertension and oedema
- stage of management and fluid restriction.

Prior to dialysis a 'no added salt diet' with avoidance of salted snacks may be recommended. However, these are some diseases which are associated with loss of sodium into the urine and supplements of sodium chloride or sodium bicarbonate are indicated. These should be taken with formula feeds/food, 3–4 times daily to maintain plasma levels.

In the child undergoing CPD the principles of a 'no added salt diet' should generally apply. If the child is hypertensive, oedematous or if fluid intake has to be regulated then careful attention to avoid increased sodium intake is important.

Infants are at risk of becoming hyponatraemic (Na <130 mmol/l) when increased strengths of dialysis glucose solutions (e.g. 2.27–3.86%) are required to increase the ultrafiltration of fluid, particularly as the dietary sodium intake of infants is normally low. Sodium intakes of 4–7 mmol/kg body weight/day may be required to maintain sodium balance.

On haemodialysis a 'no added salt' diet should be encouraged to reduce thirst and fluid intake. This may help in the control of interdialytic weight gain and hypertension. An intake of 1–3 mmol/kg body weight/day is usually acceptable.

Potassium

The dietary management of potassium is dependent upon the:

- aetiology of the renal disease
- glomerular filtration rate (GFR)
- stage of management and/or dialysis therapy.

The aim of management is to prevent:

Hyperkalaemia, which generally does not occur until the GFR is <5–10% of normal (however individual biochemical assessment will dictate requirements).

Possible causes of hyperkalaemia include a high dietary intake of potassium, catabolism (i.e. inadequate energy intake), antihypertensive drugs (e.g. Captopril) and constipation. A haemolysed blood sample will show a falsely high serum potassium level.

Hypokalaemia, which can occur in some renal tubular disorders such as cystinosis where potassium supplements are usually necessary, but will be withdrawn as renal function deteriorates. Other causes of hypokalaemia include: diuretics (e.g. frusemide) and anorexia.

Peritoneal dialysis, because of its more continuous removal of solutes, generally allows a moderate intake of potassium. However, care must still be taken to avoid the child indulging in potassium rich drinks and food. For example, squash instead of fruit juice to drink should be encouraged; crisps may be taken occasionally, but corn snacks are preferable (Table 11.5). Particular care should always be taken with infants and children who are anuric or anephric. As haemodialysis is intermittent, more careful dietary control will be necessary to minimize problems with hyperkalaemia (Table 11.5). If treats such as chocolate and crisps are allowed they should only be eaten in the first half an hour to an hour of dialysis. Hyperkalaemia can result in fatal cardiac arrhythmias; the dangers of hyperkalaemia must be explained and reinforced periodically during management. Ion exchange resins, e.g. calcium resonium may be required if serum potassium levels are dangerously high, but should only be used at a time of crisis.

Advice about potassium intake should be modified for each individual and discussed with the child and family. A photographic album of foods rich in potassium may be helpful. Intake needs to be reviewed at frequent intervals alongside blood biochemistry and dietary analysis.

Calcium and phosphate

The maintenance of normal serum calcium and phosphate biochemistry is crucial to achieve normal bone growth and to prevent renal osteodystrophy (a combination of both rickets and hyperparathyroidism). Abnormalities of bone mineral metabolism can be quite advanced before there are any significant changes in serum calcium, phosphate and alkaline phosphatase levels or evidence of changes on bone x-rays. Careful management early on in the treatment of CRF includes:

- dietary phosphate restriction
- prescription of a vitamin D analogue (1-alpha-hydroxycholecalciferol; 20–40 ng/kg body weight/day)
- phosphate binders.

Dietary phosphate restriction

Advice to reduce phosphate in the diet should apply throughout all the stages of CRF management (Table 11.6). Normal infant formulas, which are low in phospate, should be encouraged for infants for at least 1–2 years. Kindergen PROD, a specialized low phosphate infant formula, could be considered for those infants where phosphate control proves difficult on normal formulas. Thereafter, cows' milk may be introduced, but at an agreed amount for each individual child. Nutritional supplements should contain as little phosphate as possible and should be included within the dietary allowance. As a guideline phosphate should be restricted to:

<400 mg/day in infants;
400–600 mg/day in children <20 kg body weight;
<800 mg/day in children >20 kg body weight.

During the conservative stage of treatment or for children undergoing haemodialysis, phosphate intake will be reduced because of protein restriction. However, dietary restriction of phosphate may be difficult on peritoneal dialysis when protein intake is generally increased.

Vitamin D analogues

The prompt initiation of a vitamin D analogue, 1-alpha-hydroxycholecalciferol (Alfacalcidol) or 1,25-dihydroxycholecalciferol (Calcitrol), will help to control hyperparathyroidism by assisting the absorption of calcium in the small intestine. Therapy is based upon serum calcium levels and is reduced or suspended if calcium levels are above the normal range (>2.6 mmol/l).

Phosphate binders

Calcium carbonate is the first choice phosphate binder (aluminium hydroxide was formerly used, but has been implicated in bone and brain abnormalities). It is prescribed when dietary restriction can no longer control serum phosphate levels. Some of the available products are shown in Table 11.10.

The binders should be chewed and taken with meals. Alternatively, they can be crushed to a fine powder or used in solution. These can then be easily given to a bottle fed infant or added to an overnight feed, which often provides the major source of phosphate in those children requiring supplementary

Table 11.10 Phosphate binders

Phosphate binding preparation	Elemental calcium mg (mmol)	Dosage*/flavour**
Titralac Tablets	168 (4.2) (per tablet)	1–3 tablets tds/ mint
Calcium carbonate (10%) solution	200 (5.0) (per 5 mls)	5–15 mls tds
Calcichew	500 (12.6) (per tablet)	1 tablet tds/ orange
Settlers Tums	200 (5.0) (per tablet)	1–3 tablets tds/ cherry, orange, lemon

* Dosage will vary with individual dietary intake of phosphate
** Suggested flavours for children able to take orally

tube feeding. A proportion of the calcium from the phosphate binders is absorbed and may raise serum calcium levels. Low calcium dialysate may be indicated in some patients.

Micronutrients

Little is known about the micronutrient requirements of infants and children with CRF. The few recommendations made have been based upon reports from adult studies which may not be appropriate for the growing child. Children most at risk of possible micronutrient deficiencies are those who:

- are anorexic and are not receiving nutritional support
- remain on restricted diets for prolonged periods (i.e. are conservatively managed)
- have prolonged dialysis while awaiting transplantation
- have episodes of peritonitis
- are receiving erythropoietin.

Most children being managed *conservatively* will require a routine supplement when protein and potassium intakes are restricted. Accurate dietary assessment will help determine a suitable preparation to meet recommended reference nutrient intakes [9]. Ketovite tablets (2–3/day) will ensure intakes of vitamins C, E and the B complex, and are generally well tolerated. The kidney plays an important role in activating dietary vitamin D (cholecalciferol) from 25-hydroxycholecalciferol (this initial hydroxylation taking place in the liver) to 1, 25-dihydroxycholecalciferol in the kidney. Supplementation of vitamin D will be prescribed on an individual basis and will depend upon variable factors i.e. active bone disease and parathyroid gland activity. Activation of dietary vitamin D is reduced with progressive renal impairment. Supplementation of other vitamins will only be necessary if dietary intake is below RNI values. Iron supplementation may be required in some children. A comprehensive micronutrient supplement is necessary for children who remain on a restricted diet for a prolonged period.

Children undergoing dialysis require routine daily supplementation to meet RNI's [9] and to allow for the reported dialysate losses of micronutrients. As a guide the following vitamin intakes are currently recommended: C (50–100 mg); B6 (5–10 mg); and folate (0.5–1.0 mg), as reported in adult patients [29].

Vitamin A supplementation is not recommended unless the dietary intake (inclusive of nutritional supplements) is below RNI values, or if the child has been on prolonged dialysis to allow for the reported losses of vitamin A on CPD [30]. Vitamin D supplementation is recommended to maintain levels of other vitamin D metabolites such as 24, 25-hydroxy-vitamin D in children undergoing peritoneal dialysis [31]. Intakes of iron, copper and zinc have been reported to be below RNI values, despite adequate intakes of both protein and energy [27] and supplementation should be considered if serum levels are low. Children undergoing CPD (particularly those receiving erythropoietin) may have low serum iron levels and will require supplementation in excess of the RNI [32].

A vitamin preparation e.g. Ketovite tablets (2–3/day) and cholecalciferol (400 i.u. or 10 µg/day) may be adequate for most children who are consuming nutritionally complete supplements and are under regular dietetic review.

It is still of concern that some children undergoing prolonged or complicated dialysis may be at risk of both vitamin and trace mineral deficiencies. A comprehensive and palatable micronutrient supplement still needs to be developed for such patients.

Nutritional considerations for infants with CRF

Increasing numbers of infants are now receiving treatment for CRF due to improved expertise in dialysis techniques and renal transplantation. Although the ultimate goal for such children is a renal transplant, this is a more difficult procedure in the very small child and many centres prefer to promote the growth of the child to a size where the transplant operation will be easier and, hence, more successful. Optimal nutrition, with or without early dialysis, is therefore an essential requirement.

When diagnosis is first made there may be a period of conservative management to determine if renal function may improve or stabilize. Tube feeding may be indicated to achieve adequate nutrition for growth. For infants requiring dialysis, CCPD has become the preferred choice and, ideally, supplementary tube feeding programmes should be commenced at the initiation of dialysis. Nasogastric tubes are popular in many units [33]; however, gastrostomy feeding using a gastrostomy button device may be preferable in the long term [34]. Tube feeding undoubtedly reduces some of the parental pressures associated with oral feeding and is preferable to force feeding, which frequently results in vomiting and/or refusal of formula or food. Force feeding can have a deterimental affect on normal oral feeding behaviour in the long term [35].

Vomiting can be a persistent problem for some infants and feeding prescriptions should be monitored and altered appropriately. Medications to enhance gastric emptying such as Cisapride could be considered but are usually only beneficial in the short term. The use of a semi-elemental feed can be considered for those children with evidence of slow gastric emptying. Vomiting of a psychogenic nature may be responsible in some children, particularly those under stressful family circumstances [36].

Weaning should be encouraged at the usual time to develop and maintain normal oral feeding experiences. The hope is that following successful renal transplantation normal feeding will be resumed. In order to achieve a normal eating pattern at a later date, support from other renal team members, including an experienced speech therapist, is recommended [37]. Ongoing psychosocial support, with home visits whenever possible, is essential.

Nutritional support

Considerable reliance is placed upon supplements to meet nutritional requirements. If oral supplementation is unsuccessful then supplementary tube feeding should be considered. Discussion with the family and team members as to the most appropriate feeding route for each child should be implemented. The use of videos, photograph albums, booklets and dolls can assist in teaching and preparation.

Supplementary tube feeding should preferably be carried out overnight by means of an enteral feeding pump to allow oral feeding to be encouraged during the day. However, there are some infants and children who may require intermittent bolus feeds by day to maintain adequate intakes. Continuous 24 hour feeds, ideally delivered by a portable feeding pump, should only be considered if the latter regimens are not tolerated.

DIET FOLLOWING RENAL TRANSPLANTATION

The ultimate goal for the child with end stage renal

disease (ESRD) is a successful renal transplant to restore normal physiology and metabolic function without the aid of dialysis and dietary manipulation. Nutritional therapy remains as important aspect of treatment and the dietitian should continue to be involved with the ongoing management.

Initial management

Feeding can be commenced on the return of bowel sounds and if there are no complications the child will usually develop an appetite with improving renal function. Some children may require ongoing nutritional support, particularly those who have relied predominantly upon a supplementary feeding route prior to and when on dialysis. Children who experience acute tubular necrosis (ATN) following renal transplantation may require a further period of conservative management or dialysis therapy, with dietary prescription, until adequate renal function is achieved. Chronic rejection will result in the child returning to either conservative management or a dialysis programme with appropriate dietary intervention.

Although a renewed appetite is favourable in the initial stages of management, care must be taken to prevent excessive weight gain, which may lead to obesity in the long term. Both the child and family should be reminded of this early in treatment and follow appropriate dietary advice to prevent this from happening. The principles of a healthy eating, well balanced diet for all the family should be encouraged prior to discharge from hospital. The opportunity to advise about the benefits of exercise should also be taken. Hypertension may be present following transplantation and anti-hypertensive therapy may be required. Weight control and advice about a 'no added salt' diet as part of the healthy eating advice should be encouraged.

Hyperlipidaemia is evident in a large number of patients following transplantation and may put them at risk of developing premature cardiovascular disease [38]. The use of mono and polyunsaturated fats and oils, with reduction of the total fat intake, should be advised where possible.

Ongoing management

Following discharge from hospital frequent outpatient assessment to monitor renal function and growth pro-

vides an opportunity for the ongoing dietary advice about healthy eating. Hypophosphataemia due to a tubular leak may be noted on biochemical tests but rarely requires intervention.

Particular attention should be paid to those children who still require nutritional supplements, either orally or via a supplementary feeding route. A transition period to encourage the oral intake by reducing the overnight feed and/or day time boluses should be agreed with the parents and reviewed at clinic appointments. Visits to the nursery or school may be necessary to further implement the advised strategies. Once oral intakes are acceptable, supplementary feeding should be discontinued allowing the child to resume a normal diet. Some children may require iron supplementation despite an adequate intake from diet. Vitamin and/or trace mineral preparations may be required in those children whose micronutrient intakes are poor.

Adolescents

The prevention of rapid weight gain leading to obesity can be a difficult problem in this age group. The patient who was anorexic prior to transplantation may object to advice to reduce food intake to control body weight. Adolescent females who experience rapid weight gain and change of body image may be at risk of crash dieting and possible fasting to lose weight.

NEPHROGENIC DIABETES INSIPIDUS

The child with nephrogenic diabetes insipidus (NDI) presents with polyuria, polydypsia and often failure to thrive. Diagnosis is made by finding a low urine osmolality which does not respond to a water deprivation test or antidiuretic hormone replacement therapy. Treatment is generally with indomethacin and thiazides to try to reduce urine output, and hence the child's requirement for fluid.

Nutritional management of NDI

It is important to ensure that the child has free access to fluid [10] which, it is hoped, will be reduced on commencement of prescribed medications. The child's appetite may be poor because of frequent and large intake of fluids resulting in failure to thrive because of an inadequate nutritional intake. Supplements may be indicated in the initial management although once treatment has been established, it is likely that the child's appetite for food may significantly improve. A 'no added salt' diet will help to control the craving for fluids. Dietary assessment is necessary to ensure that the child is meeting recommended intakes for energy, micronutrients [9] and that protein intake is adequate (1–2 g/kg body weight/day).

RENAL STONES

Renal stones are relatively uncommon in children within the United Kingdom. Presentation is generally between 6 and 15 years of age and boys are affected twice as frequently as girls. Hypercalciuria is present in 40–60% of children with stones. Calcium is the most frequent component present in 90% of stones occurring in all children, although phosphate and oxalate are also present. Normal serum calcium with low to normal phosphate levels are characteristic [39].

Dietary management should include a diet history and 3 day food diary to accurately analyse dietary intake. In children with hypercalciuria calcium intake should be limited to the recommended intake for chronological age [9]. The level of calcium in the local water supply should be checked and if necessary deionised water may be indicated. Fluid intake should be encouraged to decrease the renal solute load and advice about suitable reduced sugar drinks to prevent dental caries should be given. Milk and milk products will usually need to be restricted.

HYPERCALCAEMIA

There are a number of causes of hypercalcaemia [40] which can be defined if the serum calcium is sustained at a level above 2.5 mmol/l with a normal serum phosphate level.

Infants who present with hypercalcaemia, e.g. William's syndrome, are anorexic, irritable and often constipated. Breast or formula milk is often refused in preference to water. A dietary assessment to determine the child's intake should be performed. Calcium intake should be reduced so as not to exceed recommended levels [9]. The prescription of a low calcium formula (e.g. Locasol) may be indicated and modified with energy supplements in the infant failing to thrive. It is also advisable to check the level of calcium in the local water supply and to use deionised water if necessary. Other rich sources of dietary calcium such as dairy produce should be limited.

REFERENCES

1 Feld LG, Springate JE Acute renal failure. In: Barakat AY (ed.) *Renal Disease in Children. Clinical Evaluation and Diagnosis*. New York: Springer Verlag, 1989: 269–285.

2 Brocklebank JT Renal failure in the newly born. *Arch Dis Childh*, 1989, **63** 991–994.

3 Milford DV, Taylor CM New insights into haemolytic uraemic syndrome. *Arch Dis Childh*, 1990, **65** 713–715.

4 Watson AR The management of acute renal failure. *Current Paediatrics*, 1991, **1** 103–107.

5 Coleman JE, Watson AR Nutritional support for the child with acute renal failure. *J Hum Nut Diet*, 1992, **5** 99–105.

6 Haycock GB Renal disease. In: McLaren DS, Burman D, Belton NR, Williams AF (eds.) *Textbook of Paediatric Nutrition*, 3rd edn. Edinburgh: Churchill Livingstone, 1991.

7 Tanner JM, Whitehouse RH Clinical longitudinal standards for height, weight, height velocity and stages of puberty. *Arch Dis Childh*, 1976, **51** 170–179.

8 Grupe WE Nutritional issues in acute renal insufficiency. In: Grand RJ, Sutphen JL, Dietz WH (eds.) Paediatric Nutrition, Therapy and Practice. Stoneham, Mass: Butterworths, 1987.

9 Department of Health Report on Health and Social Subjects No 41. *Dietary Reference Values for Food, Energy and Nutrients for the United Kingdom*. London: HMSO, 1991.

10 Haycock GB Renal disease. In: McLaren DS, Burman D, Belton NR, Williams AF (eds.) *Textbook of Paediatric Nutrition*, 3rd edn. Edinburgh: Churchill Livingstone, 1991.

11 Rees L *et al*. Growth and endocrine function in steroid sensitive nephrotic syndrome. *Arch Dis Childh*, 1988, **63** 484–490.

12 Blainey JD High protein diets in the treatment of the nephrotic syndrome. *Clin Sci*, 1954, **13** 567–581.

13 Al-Bander H, Kaysen GA Ineffectiveness of dietary protein augmentation in the management of nephrotic syndrome. *Paediatr Nephrol*, 1991, **5** 482–486.

14 Brenner BM, Mayer TW, Hostetter TH Dietary protein intake and the progressive nature of kidney disease. *New Eng J Med*, 1982, **307** 652–659.

15 Feehally J, Baker F, Walls J Dietary manipulation in experimental nephrotic syndrome. *Nephron*, 1988, **50** 247–252.

16 Grupe WE Nutritional issues in glomerular damage In: Grand RJ, Sutphen JL, Dietz WH (eds.) *Paediatric*

nutrition, Theory and Practice. London: Butterworths, 1987.

17 Genova R *et al.* Food allergy in steroid resistant nephrotic syndrome. *Lancet,* 1987, **i** 1315–1316.

18 Lagrue G, Laurent J, Rostoker G, Lang D Food allergy in idiopathic nephrotic syndrome. *Lancet,* 1987, 277.

19 Paediatric Renal Unit *Childhood Nephrotic Syndrome.* Nottingham: Nottingham City Hospital Trust, 1988.

20 Watson AR Disorders of the urinary tract. In: Levine MI (ed.) *Jolly's Diseases of Childhood* 6e. Oxford: Blackwell Scientific Publications, 1991: 226–268.

21 Balfe JW *et al.* The use of CAPD in the treatment of children with end stage renal disease. Perit Dial Bull, 1981, **1** 35.

22 Nelson P, Stover J Principles of nutritional assessment and management of the child with ESRD. In: Fine RN, Gruskin AB (eds.) *End Stage Renal Disease in Children* Philadelphia: WB Saunders, 1984.

23 Balfe JW Peritoneal dialysis. In: Holliday MA, Barratt TM, Vernier RL (eds.) *Paediatric Nephrology* 2nd edn. Baltimore, MD: Williams & Wilkins, 1987.

24 Salusky IB The nutritional approach for paediatric patients undergoing CAPD/CCPD. In: Khanna R (ed.) *Advances in Peritoneal Dialysis: Selected Papers from 10th Annual Conference.* Toronto: University of Toronto Press, 1990.

25 Wingen AM *et al.* Multicentre randomized study on the effect of a low protein diet on the progression of renal failure in childhood: one year results. *Miner Electrolyte Metab* 1992, **18** 303–308.

26 Kist-van Holthe tot Echten JE *et al.* Protein restriction in chronic renal failure. *Arch Dis Childh,* 1993, **68** 371–375.

27 Coleman JE, Watson AR Vitamin, mineral and trace element supplementation of children on chronic peritoneal dialysis. *J Hum Nut Diet,* 1991, **4** 13–17.

28 Francis D *Diets for Sick Children. Protein-and sodium-modified diets for renal, liver and other conditions in infants and children.* Oxford: Blackwell Scientific Publications 4th edn, 1987.

29 Kopple JD, Blumenkrantz MJ Nutritional requirements for patients undergoing continuous ambulatory peritoneal dialysis. *Kidney Int,* **24**(Suppl 16), 295–302.

30 Vahlquist A *et al.* Vitamin A losses during continuous ambulatory peritoneal dialysis. *Nephron* 1985, **41** 179–193.

31 Watson AR *et al.* Renal osteodystrophy in children on CAPD: A prospective trial of 1-alpha-hydroxycholecalciferol therapy. *Child Nephrol Urol,* 1988, **9** 220–227.

32 Coleman JE, Watson AR Micronutrient supplementation in children on continuous cycling peritoneal dialysis. In: Khanna R (ed.) *Advances in Peritoneal Dialysis: Selected Papers from 12th Annual Conference.* Toronto: University of Toronto Press, 1992.

33 Conley SB Supplemental (NG) feedings of infants undergoing continuous peritoneal dialysis. In: Fine RN (ed.) *Chronic Ambulatory Peritoneal Dialysis (CAPD) and Chronic Cycling Peritoneal Dialysis (CCPD) in Children.* Boston. 1987: 263–269.

34 Coleman JE, Watson AR Gastrostomy buttons: the optimal route for nutritional support in children with chronic renal failure. *J Ren Nutr,* 1992, **2**(3) 21–26.

35 Warady BA *et al.* Nutritional and behavioural aspects of nasogastric tube feeding in infants receiving chronic peritoneal dialysis. In: Khanna R (ed.) *Adv in Perit Dial.* Univ of Toronto Press, 1990, **6** 265–268.

36 Gonzalez-Heydrich J, Kerner JA, Steiner H Testing the psychogenic vomiting diagnosis: four paediatric patients. *Am J Dis Childh,* 1991, **145** 913–916.

37 Kamen RS Improved development of oral-motor functions required for normal oral feeding as a consequence of tube feeding during infancy. In: Khanna R (ed.) *Advances in Peritoneal Dialysis: Selected Papers from 10th Annual Conference.* Toronto: University of Toronto Press, 1990.

38 Drukker A *et al.* Hyperlipidaemia after renal transplantation in children on alternate day corticosteroid therapy. *Clin Nephrol,* 1986, **26**(3) 140–145.

39 Teotia M, Teotia SPS Paediatric nephrolithiasis. In: Wickham JEA, Buck AC (eds.) *Renal Tract Stone. Metabolic Basis and Clinical Practice.* Edinburgh: Churchill Livingstone, 1990.

40 Levine M Metabolic disorders. In: Levine MI (ed.) *Jolly's Diseases of Childhood* 6e. Oxford: Blackwell Scientific Publications, 1991.

CHAPTER 12

The Cardiothoracic System

CONGENITAL HEART DISEASE

The incidence of congenital heart disease (CHD) is approximately 8 in every 1000 live births. It is the largest single group of congenital abnormalities and accounts for approximately 30% of the total. Eight lesions make up 80% of cases; the most common which are ventricular septal defect, patent ductus arterosis, atrial septal defect and tetralogy of Fallot.

Congestive heart failure (CHF) describes a set of symptoms and clinical signs which show myocardial dysfunction and cardiac output inadequate to meet the metabolic demands of the body. In infants and children it may be caused by increased cardiac workload. Congenital heart disease is the cause of most congestive heart failure during infancy and childhood. Severe anaemia may also produce congestive heart failure at any age.

Malnutrition and growth retardation are both commonly associated with congenital heart disease and congestive heart failure during infancy [1–6]. Although early total surgical correction of the congenital heart lesion may be the optimal treatment for affected infants, in practice not all complex defects are correctable during the neonatal period.

The prolonged nutritional deficits and secondary growth disturbances related to heart defects in infants not undergoing early operative correction may ultimately result in increased surgical risks. It is therefore important that wherever possible nutritional deficits are corrected [7]. Many factors may contribute to reduced growth and poor weight gain in infants and children with congenital heart disease. Some or all of the following factors may be involved:

- fatigue on feeding leading to low total intake
- fluid restriction
- poor absorption
- increased metabolic expenditure
- early satiety
- anorexia
- frequent infections
- frequent use of antibiotics affecting gut flora.

All of these factors will compromise the nutritional adequacy of the child's dietary intake. It is often necessary therefore to manipulate the diet so that a higher concentration of nutrients are obtained from the amount of feed being taken.

Intestinal function in children with CHD

The intestinal function of children with CHD and CHF has been assessed by a number of studies [8,9,10]. The main findings in these studies were that some of the cardiac infants exhibited mild absorptive abnormalities, mild steatorrhoea, bile salt loss, delayed gastric emptying, excessive enteric protein loss. The studies concluded that no consistent pattern of gastrointestinal abnormalities was detectable. The mild gastrointestinal defects found were felt to be unrelated to the type or severity of the cardiac lesion, but were thought to be severe enough to be of potential nutritional significance. All of the studies concluded that, if sufficient energy was provided, weight gain and linear growth could be achieved. Yahov et al. [11] found a good correlation between energy intake and weight gain in all their study patients; however a constant weight gain was observed in all patients only when energy intake exceeded 170 kcals (710 kJ)/kg/day. Below this the most severely nutritionally depleted infants continued to lose weight.

Feeding the infant with cardiac abnormalities

Both carbohydrate and fat can be used to increase the energy density of an infant formula to allow increased energy without an increase in the volume of feed taken.

Concentrating feeds for infants who are fluid restricted and/or failing to thrive

In normal circumstances infant formula powder should be made according to the manufacturer's instructions (13% solution for most infant formula in this country). To provide more energy and nutrients in a smaller volume, feeds may be concentrated using a 15% solution, providing 75 kcals/100 ml (314 kJ/100 ml) (page 8). If this feed is well tolerated it may then be possible to add additional carbohydrate and fat. Table 12.1 shows a comparison of the energy and protein obtained from standard infant formula and fortified infant formula fed at increasing volumes, illustrating the volumes and concentration of feed necessary to facilitate growth in infants with CHD.

A high to very high energy feed may be needed to achieve adequate weight gain and appropriate catch up growth in infants with CHD. The concentration and energy increases to the feed should be done slowly over a number of days in order to achieve a maximum tolerance, particularly when concentrations of carbohydrate are over 12% and fat over 5%.

Concentration, energy density and fluid volume can be increased as shown in Table 12.2.

If no weight gain is being achieved at the above concentration when fed at 150 ml/kg and it is not possible to increase the volume of feed given, then a further gradual increase in energy density of the feed should be undertaken. Carbohydrate should be increased by 0.5% glucose polymer/day up to 15% concentration, and fat (using long chain triglycerides) by 0.5% LCT emulsion/day up to 6% concentration. The final feed provides an energy density of 1.2 kcal/ml (5 kJ/ml). It may be necessary to reduce the energy density of the feed if it is not being absorbed, significant aspirates are being obtained or the infant develops diarrhoea. When the infant is once more absorbing the feed or diarrhoea has settled, then energy density should gradually be increased again.

Table 12.1 A 3 month old infant with a congenital cardiac defect, weight 3.5 kg: Plan for increase in volume, concentration and energy density of feeds

	Energy (kcals)	(kJ)	Protein (g)

1 Feeding 100 ml/kg

Total fluid intake 360 ml
Feeding 45 ml × 3 hourly × 8 feeds

		(kcals)	(kJ)	(g)
a) 360 ml standard infant formula	=	233	974	5.3
per kg	=	66	276	1.5
EAR** per kg	=	100	418	1.8
Suggested requirement per kg	=	140+	585	3→4.5
b) 360 ml fortified infant formula	=	355	1484	6.5
per kg	=	101	422	1.8
EAR per kg	=	100	418	1.8
Suggested requirement per kg	=	140+	585	3→4.5

2 Feeding 120 mls/kg

Total fluid intake 440 ml
Feeding 55 ml × 3 hourly × 8 feeds

		(kcals)	(kJ)	(g)
a) 440 ml standard infant formula	=	286	1195	6.6
per kg	=	81	339	1.8
EAR per kg	=	100	418	1.8
Suggested requirement per kg	=	140+	585	3→4.5
b) 440 ml fortified infant formula	=	429	1793	7.8
per kg	=	122	510	2.2
EAR per kg	=	100	418	1.8
Suggested requirement per kg	=	140+	585	3→4.5

3 Feeding 150 mls/kg

Total fluid intake 520 ml
Feeding = 65 ml × 3 hourly × 8 feeds

		(kcals)	(kJ)	(g)
a) 520 ml standard infant formula	=	341	1425	7.8
per kg	=	97	405	2.2
EAR per kg	=	100	418	1.8
Suggested requirement per kg	=	140+	585	3→4.5
b) 520 ml fortified infant formula	=	514	2149	9.4
per kg	=	147	614	2.7
EAR per kg	=	100	418	1.8
Suggested requirement per kg	=	140+	585	3→4.5

a) Standard 13% infant formula
b) 15% infant formula + glucose polymer to 12% CHO
    + LCT* emulsion to 5% fat

* Long chain triglyceride
** Estimated average requirement (Dietary Reference Values 1991) [12]

Table 12.2 Increasing concentration, energy density and fluid volume in infant feed on a daily basis

	Fluid ml/kg	Feed	kcal/kg	kJ/kg
Day 1	120 ml	15% infant formula	91	380
Day 2	120 ml	15% infant formula 1% glucose polymer	96	401
Day 3	120 ml	15% infant formula 1% glucose polymer 1% LCT emulsion	101	422
Day 4	140 ml	15% infant formula 1% glucose polymer 1% LCT emulsion	118	493
Day 5	140 ml	15% infant formula 2% glucose polymer 1% LCT emulsion	124	518
Day 6	150 ml	15% infant formula 2% glucose polymer 1% LCT emulsion	132	551
Day 7	150 ml	15% infant formula 2% glucose polymer 2% LCT emulsion	140	585
Day 8	150 ml	15% infant formula 3% glucose polymer 2% LCT emulsion	145	606

Methods of feed administration

The cardiac infant will commonly fail to complete feeds offered orally. This may be due to fatigue brought on by the effort of sucking, anorexia or experiencing a feeling of early satiety. If an infant is regularly failing to complete feeds one of the following strategies should be employed:

- offer smaller, more frequent feeds orally;
- complete feeds via nasogastric tube if necessary;
- give small frequent bolus feeds via nasogastric tube;
- top up small frequent day time feeds with continuous feeds overnight via an enteral feeding pump;
- give feeds continuously over 24 hrs via an enteral pump.

There have been a number of studies looking at the efficacy of methods of feed administration in infants

with CHD. Schwarz *et al.* [12] compared oral feeding, oral daytime feeds plus 12 hours continuous nasogastric feeding overnight, and 24 hours continuous nasogastric feeding in a small group of infants with CHD and CHF. For all patients the feed used was fortified to an energy density of 1 kcal/ml (4.2 kJ/ml). During the five months of the study only the group of infants receiving 24 hour continuous nasogastric feeds achieved intakes in excess of 140 kcal/kg/day (585 kJ/kg/day).

Vanderhoof *et al.* [7] studied a small group of children with complex congenital heart lesions who were all given feeds continously via a nasogastric tube. These children had all failed to achieve adequate weight gain despite the use of orally administered fortified feeds. Continuous feeding was instigated using the same fortified feeds as had been offered orally. Energy intake and weight measurements were obtained at weekly or monthly intervals. Both mean daily energy intake and mean daily weight gain were greater after initiation of continuous nasogastric feeding. Heymsfield *et al.* [13] suggested that continuous feeding caused a smaller rise in basal metabolic rate and heart rate than occurs after bolus feeds.

Sodium supplementation of infant feeds

Some infants with CHD may be failing to gain weight on an energy intake in excess of 140 kcal/kg (585 kcal/kg). These infants may need to have their feeds supplemented with sodium. A 24 hour urine sodium balance should be done to establish urinary sodium losses. Once the level of sodium loss is known the level of sodium supplementation should be discussed with the medical staff. It should be remembered that an infant feeding 150 ml/kg of a standard infant formula would be receiving 0.9 mmols Na/kg (the reference nutrient intake for sodium for an infant aged 0–3 months is 1.5 mmols Na/kg [14].

CHYLOTHORAX

Chylothorax is the accumulation of chyle in a pleural cavity from an internal lymphatic fistula; this may be unilateral or bilateral. The origin of the fistula can be congenital, obstructive or traumatic.

The loss of protein, fats and fat soluble vitamins in chylothorax, if unchecked, would invariably lead to serious metabolic deficit.

Methods of treating chylothorax

This condition can be treated conservatively using a diet containing a minimal amount of long chain triglyceride [15,16]; or a surgical repair of the fistula can be performed [16,17].

The aim of conservative treatment is to reduce the lymph flow and so allow the fistula to heal naturally. The transport of ingested fats is the principal function of thoracic duct lymph. A diet containing a minimal amount of long chain triglyceride greatly reduces the lymph flow. After hydrolysis in the intestinal lumen, dietary fats are absorbed as glycerol and fatty acids. In the mucosal cells, long chain fatty acids (12 or more carbon atoms) are reesterified to triglycerides, and pass into the lymph as chylomicra. Medium chain fatty acids (6–10 carbon atoms), however, do not undergo resynthesis and pass directly into the portal vein where they are transported in the form of 'free fatty acids' bound to albumin [18].

In man, dietary fat is mainly composed of long chain triglyceride (LCT). Medium chain triglyceride (MCT) does not constitute more than a minor proportion of normal dietary fats (Fig. 12.1).

The flow of lymph in the thoracic duct can be increased by up to ten times its resting volume following a high fat meal. A lesser but definite increase in flow is seen after ingestion of a balanced meal containing protein, carbohydrate and fat [19].

Dietary treatment of chylothorax

Minimal LCT Diet A general guide is to give not more than 1 g of long chain triglyceride per year of life – up to a maximum of 4 to 5 g LCT per day.

Addition of MCT The addition of medium chain triglyceride to the diet increases the energy value and palatability.

Vitamin and Mineral supplementation Since a wide range of foods must be either excluded from the diet or taken in reduced quantities, it is essential to check the vitamin and mineral content of the diet, giving supplements as necessary.

Minimal LCT feed for the infant with chylothorax

The feed should be nutritionally adequate and contain a minimum amount of LCT. The feeds available at the present time are:

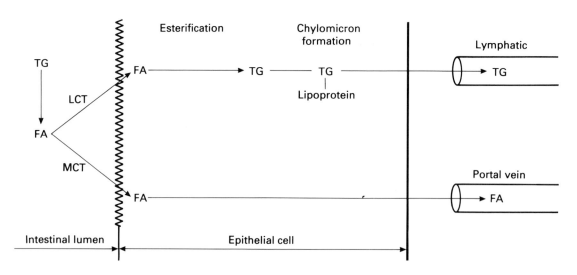

FA = Fatty acid
TG = Triglyceride

Fig. 12.1 Scheme of the pathways of absorbtion of LCT and MCT

- skimmed milk powder (SMP) based feed
- MCT Pepdite 0–2
- Portagen.

An alternative feed, which is being evaluated at the present time, is Monogen.

Skimmed milk powder based feed

This is a modular feed with skimmed milk powder providing a minimal fat protein source. To produce a nutritionally adequate infant feed carbohydrate, a suitable fat source, and minerals and vitamins must be added. An example of such a feed is shown in Table 12.3.

Once the full strength feed is tolerated, weight gain should be reviewed. It may be necessary to increase the energy density of the feed to facilitate weight gain. This should be done by gradual daily increments of glucose polymer and MCT emulsion. A total of 12% carbohydrate and 4% fat as MCT should be tolerated. It is suggested that carbohydrate be increased in 1% daily increments and MCT be increased in 0.5% daily increments.

The following points should be considered:

A skimmed milk powder which is fortified with vitamins A and D should be used to make this feed. The feed may still be too low in vitamin D and supplementation with mothers' and children's vitamin drops A, D, C (supplied under the Welfare Food Scheme) which provide 7 µg vitamin D may be necessary.

This feed, when taken as the sole source of nutrition, does not provide sufficient folate and supplementation will be necessary. 0.1 ml Lexpec should be given daily.

The copper content of this feed is 87 µg/100 kcals. This is marginally in excess of the EEC directive (91/321/EEC), which gives the desired minimum copper content of infant formula as 20 µg/100 kcals and the desired maximum as 80 µmols/100 kcals.

Monogen

Monogen is a nutritionally complete whey based infant formula. The fat sources are fractionated coconut oil and walnut oil. The standard dilution for use as infant formula is 17.5%. The product is not yet available on prescription.

Table 12.3 A three month old infant presents with a chylothorax (weight 4 kg, feeding 150 ml/kg)

	Na mmol	K mmol	Energy kcal	Energy kJ	CHO g	Protein g	LCT g	MCT g
35 g skimmed milk powder	8.3	14.2	122	510	18.5	12.5	0.2	–
45 g Caloreen	0.8	0.1	180	752	45	–	–	–
25 ml Liquigen	0.4	0.2	104	435	–	–	–	12.5
7 g Paediatric Seravit + water to 600 ml	–	–	21	89	5.3	–	–	–
Totals	9.5	14.5	427	1786	68.8	12.5	0.2	12.5
per 100 ml	1.6	2.4	71	298	11.5	2.1		2.1
per kg	2.4	3.6	107	447		3.1		

Day 1	Day 2	Day 3
17 g SMP	35 g SMP	35 g SMP
20 g Caloreen	40 g Caloreen	40 g Caloreen
6 ml Liquigen	12 ml Liquigen	18 ml Liquigen
2 g Paed Seravit water to 600 ml	3 g Paed Seravit water to 600 ml	5 g Paed Seravit water to 600 ml

Aims in constructing feed – 3 g protein per kg
 – 70 kcals per 100 ml (293 kJ per 100 ml)
 – 10% carbohydrate concentration

The feed should be gradually increased as shown to the full concentration

Table 12.4 Nutritional content per 100 ml standard dilution Monogen

Energy	70 kcals (293 kJ)
Protein equivalent	2 g
Carbohydrate	12 g
Fat – MCT	1.86 g
– LCT	0.14 g

Table 12.5 A comparison of the % energy derived from linoleic and alpha-linolenic acids in current minimal LCT feeds

	% Energy from C18:2	% Energy from C18:3
SMP based feed	0.01	0.01
MCT Pepdite 0–2	4.2	0.1
Portagen	3.4	0.07
Monogen	1.1	0.25

MCT Pepdite 0–2

MCT Pepdite 0–2 is a nutritionally complete infant formula. It has been used in very young infants with chylothorax where whole unmodified cows' milk protein was felt to be inappropriate or where an infant has developed a lactose intolerance. It has a higher LCT content than Monogen, 17% of the fat being present as LCT. This level of LCT may not be low enough to adequately reduce chyle flow in some infants.

Portagen

Portagen is a non-modified casein based formula. It is an adult formula, for which the manufacturers give an alternative dilution to enable it to be used for infants. It contains 7% of fat as LCT; 25% of the carbohydrate is present as sucrose which may not be well tolerated by many cardiac infants. It has a high vitamin A content at 238 μg per 100 kcals. The EEC directive (91/321/EEC) gives the desired maximum for vitamin A in an infant formula to be 180 μg per 100 kcals.

Essential fatty acids

Essential fatty acids (EFAs) in phospholipids are important for maintaining the function and integrity of cellular and subcellular membranes. They also participate in the regulation of cholesterol metabolism, being involved in its transport, breakdown and ultimate excretion. It has been postulated that in infants there may be a specific dietary requirement for these longer chain fatty acids during rapid brain development [20]. A deficiency state arising from an inadequate intake of linoleic acid has been demonstrated in children [21]. Although a specific deficiency state arising from inadequate dietary alpha-linolenic acid has not been demonstrated in healthy humans, it is regarded as a dietary essential [21]. It has been recommended that the neonate requires 1% of energy intake from linoleic acid (C18:2) and 0.2% of energy

from alpha-linolenic acid (C18:3) [14]. Table 12.5 gives a comparison of EFA content of feeds used in the treatment of infants with chylothorax.

If using any of the minimal LCT feeds shown in Table 12.5 other than Monogen, supplementation with a source of EFA is necessary. This should be done using walnut oil. The fatty acid content of this oil will provide linoleic and alpha-linolenic acids in the required quantity and ratio, with a minimum of LCT. Walnut oil contains 61 g linoleic and 12 g alpha-linolenic acids per 100 g.

EFA supplementation in a SMP based feed

The addition of 0.8 ml walnut oil to the feed illustrated in Table 12.3 would supply EFA to the required quantity and ratio, at the same time providing the minimum amount of LCT.

This would give a total of:

1%   energy from linoleic acid
0.2%   energy from alpha-linolenic acid.

As the energy in the feed increases it will be necessary to increase EFA supplementation proportionately.

Minimal LCT weaning diet

The following foods contain minimal LCT and can be introduced as weaning solids:

- puréed vegetables e.g. potato, carrots, swede, green beans
- puréed fruit e.g. pears, apples, banana, peaches
- puréed boiled rice mixed with minimal fat milk
- proprietary baby rice reconstituted with minimal fat milk
- tins and jars of baby foods containing less than 0.2 g of LCT per 100 g. These are mainly the fruit based tins and jars. (Other dried packet baby foods,

Table 12.6 Sample day's menu for a toddler on a minimal LCT diet

Minimal LCT milk (MLM)

60 g skimmed milk powder	
35 ml Liquigen	Provides 500 kcals (2090 kJ)
30 g glucose polymer	22 g protein
8 g Paediatric Seravit	0.8 g LCT
+ water to 600 ml	

Use throughout the day as drink and mixed with appropriate food

Breakfast	10 g Rice Krispies + 60 ml MLM
	A drink of MLM
Mid AM	A drink of MLM
	2 MCT biscuits
Lunch	80 g baked beans + 50 g MCT chips
	50 g very low fat fromage frais
	A drink of fruit squash + glucose polymer
Mid PM	A drink of MLM
	Meringue
Supper	40 g white fish steak fried in MCT oil
	Fat-free mashed potatoes plus 2 teaspoons Liquigen
	40 g vegetables
	50 g very low fat ice cream
Bedtime	A drink of MLM

Total LCT intake for the day = 2 g

tins and jars contain too much LCT and should be avoided.)

Even when solids are introduced to the diet of the infant, a minimal LCT milk formula will continue to form a major part of his nutritional intake providing energy, protein, vitamins and minerals. A sample day's menu for the toddler on a minimal LCT diet is given in Table 12.6.

The mimimal LCT milk can be flavoured with Nesquik powder, fruit Crusha syrups or low fat chocolate flavour topping. It can also be used on breakfast cereals, to make custard or cereal puddings. Extra energy can be added to the diet by increasing the concentration of glucose polymer in the milk or by using 10–15% solution of glucose polymer to make up fruit squash. Further energy can be given by the addition of Liquigen to suitable food such as mashed potatoes.

Table 12.7 Free foods for minimal LCT diet

All fruits fresh, tinned or frozen (except olives and avocado pear)
All vegetables, fresh, tinned or frozen
Sugar, honey, golden syrup, treacle, jam, marmalade
Jelly and jellied sweets such as Jelly Tots, Jelly Babies, wine gums or fruit pastilles
Boiled sweets, mints (not butter mints)
Fruit sorbets, water ices, ice lollies
Meringue, egg white, Rite diet egg replacer
Spices and essences
Salt, pepper, vinegar, herbs, tomato ketchup, most chutneys, Marmite, Oxo, Bovril
Fruit juices, fruit squashes, Crusha fruit flavouring syrups, Nesquik fruit flavouring powder, chocolate flavour topping, bottled fruit sauces.
Fizzy drinks, lemonade, cola, Lucozade

Feeding the older child and adolescent with chylothorax

Aiming to keep LCT intake to a minimum necessitates the exclusion of many foods including animal and vegetable fats such as butter, lard, margarine and vegetable oils. It also makes it necessary to strictly limit or exclude protein foods which have a high fat content such as meat, fatty fish, full fat milk, cheese and eggs. All cakes, pastry, and biscuits made with LCT fats must also be avoided.

The diet relies on skimmed milk fortified with carbohydrate and MCT as a source of energy, protein, minerals and vitamins. MCT can be added to the diet in the form of MCT oil or MCT emulsion. The use of MCT oil allows fried foods to be included in the diet, such as fried fish, chips and crisps. MCT oil and MCT emulsion can both be used in baking, cakes, biscuits, pastry. All these foods are valuable sources of energy and can greatly enhance the acceptability of the diet to the patient. Recipes for MCT biscuits and Liquigen pastry are available from the author, Marion Noble, at her place of work (see Contributors list at the front of this volume). Table 12.7 lists foods containing minimal LCT which can be used freely in the diet. The weights and fat contents of foods which can be used to construct a day's meals containing minimal LCT for the child or adolescent with chylothorax are given in Table 12.8.

The final diet may contain 40–70 g MCT, depending on the age and energy requirement of the patient. This would be gradually introduced over a period of 7–10 days in order to avoid abdominal discomfort.

Table 12.8 LCT content of foods suitable for use in minimal LCT diet

Food	Weight of serving (g)	LCT Content (g)
Breakfast cereals		
Cornflakes	25	0.2
Frosties	45	0.2
Sugar Puffs	25	0.2
Special K	25	0.2
Cocopops	25	0.2
Ricicles	45	0.2
Weetabix (2 biscuits)	40	0.8
Bread		
White bread, large thin cut loaf	25	0.4
Matzos	20	0.2
Crumpets, toasted	25	0.5
Dairy foods		
Reduced fat cottage cheese	45	0.6
Very low fat yoghurt	45	0.1
Very low fat fromage frais	50	0.2
Condensed milk, skimmed, sweetened	50	0.5
Very low fat ice cream	50	0.2
Fish		
Grilled white cod steak	70	0.8
Grilled white haddock fillet	60	1.0
Steamed whiting	100	0.9
Grilled/steamed smoked fish	100	0.6
Prawns – peeled	80	1.4
Fish finger, 1	25	1.8
Fish cakes (Findus cod), 2	120	0.6
Meat and poultry		
Roast turkey, light meat	70	1.0
Roast chicken, light meat	50	2.0
Roast lamb, lean	25	2.0
Roast beef, lean topside	45	2.0
Beef, lean silverside	40	2.0
Tinned ham	20	0.8
Legumes, pasta, rice		
Baked beans in tomato sauce	200	1.0
Tinned spaghetti in tomato sauce	125	0.5
White rice, boiled	140	0.4
White pasta, boiled	120	0.9

A day's meals for a 14 year old boy with chylothorax is shown in Table 12.9, and Table 12.10 gives a nutritional analysis of the diet.

REFERENCES

1 Webb JG, Kiess MC, Chan Yan CC Malnutrition and the heart. *Canad Med Ass J*, 1986, **135** 753–759.

Table 12.9 Day's meals for a 14 year boy with chylothorax (Aim: 4–5 g LCT per day)

Daily milk allowance

Fortified skimmed milk (FSM)

   100 g skimmed milk powder
   100 g glucose polymer
   50 ml Liquigen
   + water to 1000 ml

20% Glucose polymer solution

   40 g glucose polymer
   + water to 200 ml

1000 ml FSM provides: 950 kcals (3971 kJ), 36 g protein, 1.3 g LCT.

Breakfast	25 g Cornflakes 120 ml orange juice and glucose polymer Apple
Mid AM	Glass of FSM + Meringue + 2 MCT biscuits

Lunch	70 g roast turkey (light meat only)
	150 g mashed potatoes +
	  15 ml Liquigen
	60 g carrots
	120 g tinned fruit
	+ 120 ml custard made with FSM
	Glass fruit squash made with
	  glucose polymer solution

Mid PM	250 ml FSM + 1 sachet strawberry Build-up + Banana + 2 MCT biscuits
Supper	200 g baked beans + 100 g MCT chips Apple pie made with MCT pastry + 100 g very low fat fromage frais
Bedtime	Glass of FSM
Vitamin supplementation	6 Cow & Gate Supplementary Vitamin tablets + 5 ml Ketovite liquid

2 Bougle D *et al*. Nutritional treatment of congenital heart disease. *Arch Dis Childh*, 1961, 799–801.

3 Naeye RL Organ and cellular development in congenital heart disease and in alimentary malnutrition. *J Pediatr*, 1965, Sept 447–458.

4 Krieger I Growth failure and congenital heart disease: energy and nitrogen balance in infants. *Am J Dis Childh*, 1970, **120** 497–504.

5 Pittman JG, Cohen P The pathogenesis of cardiac cachexia. *N Engl J Med*, 1964, **271** 403–409.

6 Mehrizi A, Drash A Growth disturbance in congenital heart disease. *J Pediatr*, 1962, **61** 418–422.

7 Vanderhoof JA, Hofsschire PJ, Baluff M *et al*. Continuous enteral feedings: an important adjunct to the

Table 12.10 Nutritional analysis of minimal LCT diet for a 14 year old boy showing comparison with current dietary reference values

			DRV#
Energy	(kcal)	2700 (11.3 MJ)	2200 (9.2 MJ)
Protein	(g)	87	42
LCT	(g)	5	
Na	(mmol)	100	70
K	(mmol)	130	80
Ca	(mmol)	42	25
Fe	(µmmol)	300	200
Vitamin D	(µg)	13	10
Vitamin A	(RE*µg)	1200	600
Vitamin C	(mg)	165	35

* Retinol equivalent
\# Dietary Reference Values [14]

management of complex congenital heart disease. *Am J Dis Childh*, 1982, **136** 825–827.

8 Sondheimer JM, Hamilton JR Intestinal function in infants with severe congenital heart disease. *J Pediatr*, 1978, **92** 572–578.

9 Cavell B Gastric emptying in infants with congenital heart disease. *Acta Paediatr Scand*, 1981, **70** 517–520.

10 Davidson JD *et al.* Protein-losing gastroenteropathy in congestive heart failure. *Lancet*, 1961, **1** 899.

11 Yahov J *et al.* Assessment of intestinal and cardiorespiratory function in children with congenital heart disease on high calorie formulas. *J Pediatr Gastroenterol Nutr*, 1985, **4** 778–785.

12 Schwarz SM *et al.* Enteral nutrition in infants with congenital heart disease and growth failure. *Pediatr*, 1990, **86**(3) 368–373.

13 Heymsfield SB, Hill JO, Evert M Energy expenditure during continuous intragastric infusion of fuel. *Am J Clin Nutr*, 1987, **45** 526–533.

14 Department of Health Report on Health and Social Subjects No 14. *Dietary Reference Values for Food Energy and Nutrients for the United Kingdom*. London: HMSO, 1991.

15 Cooper P, Paes ML Bilateral chylothorax. *Brit J Anaes*, 1991, **66** 387–390.

16 Puntis JWL, Roberts KD, Handy D How should chylothorax be managed? *Arch Dis Childh*, 1987, **62** 593–596.

17 Stringer G, Mercer S, Bass J Surgical management of persistent postoperative chylothorax in children. *Canad J Surg*, 1984, **27** 543–546.

18 Bessone LN, Ferguson TB, Burforoth TH Chylothorax: collective review. *Ann Thor Surg*, 1971, **12**(5) 527–545.

19 Issalbacher KJ, Senior ED Mechanisms of absorption of long and medium chain triglycerides. In *Medium Chain Triglycerides*. Philadelphia: University of Pensylvania, 1968.

20 Crawford MA, Sinclair AJ Nutritional influences in the evolution of mammalian brain. In: Elliot T, Knight J (eds.) *Lipids, Malnutrition and the Developing Brain*. Amsterdam: Elsevier, 1972.

21 Hansen AE *et al.* Eczema and essential fatty acids. *Am J Dis Childh*, 1947, **73** 1–18.

FURTHER READING

Gracey M, Burke V, Anderson CM Medium chain triglycerides in paediatric practice. *Arch Dis Childh*, 1970, **45** 445–452.

Kosloke AM, Martin LW, Schubert WK Management of chylothorax in children and medium chain triglyceride feedings. *J Ped Surg*, 1974, **9** 365–371.

Ramos W, Faintuch J Nutritional management of thoracic duct fistula. A comparative study of parenteral versus enteral nutrition. *J Parent Ent Nutr*, 1986, **10**(5) 519–521.

CHAPTER 13

The Immune System

FOOD ALLERGY AND INTOLERANCE

Food allergy and intolerance is a poorly understood, controversial area to which many symptoms have been attributed and which it will be hard to define until more is known about its pathogenesis [1]. Food intolerance has been described as a reproducible, unpleasant reaction to a food which can occur even when the food is eaten unknowingly (blind). Food aversion, on the other hand, is a psychological intolerance or avoidance caused by emotions associated with food and which does not occur when the food is given in a disguised form [2].

MECHANISMS RESPONSIBLE FOR FOOD INTOLERANCE

A variety of mechanisms are responsible for food intolerance some of which are well understood and are listed below, but others remain as yet obscure:

- some food intolerance occurs as a result of enzyme deficiencies such as lactase deficiency or disorders of amino acid or intermediary metabolism e.g. phenylketonuria. Such intolerances are discussed elsewhere in this book
- alternatively, some foods may have an unpleasant pharmacological effect, e.g. caffeine in tea, coffee and kola nuts; vasoactive amines in cheese and wine; phenylethylamine in chocolate
- some foods such as shellfish and strawberries contain histamine-releasing agents which cause adverse reactions
- the best known type of food intolerance is food allergic disease where an abnormal immune response occurs after eating certain foods.

FOOD ALLERGY OR INTOLERANCE

The pathogenesis of many symptoms which have been shown to be related to food intolerance is either poorly understood or completely unknown. Food allergic disease and other forms of intolerance which may or may not have an immunological component are discussed.

The symptoms of food allergy or intolerance may come on quickly or slowly. An immediate reaction can occur when the subject has been exposed to a very small amount of the provoking food and is often associated with antibodies of the immunoglobulin E (IgE) class (Table 13.1). There is generally no doubt about which food is provoking problems and radioallergosorbent tests (RASTs) or skin prick tests will often show the presence of IgE antibodies to the foods concerned.

Reactions to foods may also develop slowly after hours or days and only when a considerable amount of the provoking food has been consumed [3]. When the symptoms are insidious it may be difficult, if not impossible, to identify the provoking foods. RAST and skin prick tests are unhelpful and association with foods may not be clearcut.

Table 13.1 lists the many symptoms which have been attributed to food allergy or intolerance although some of these are more firmly established as being food related than others. With the exception of IgE mediated (often immediate) reactions, an immunological component to food intolerance can often not be established. However, it is possible that at least some of the symptoms listed in Table 13.1 may be related to other immune reactions such as antigen-antibody formation (Gell and Coombs type III reaction) or cell-

Table 13.1 Symptoms sometimes attributed to food intolerance

Quick onset	Mostly slow onset
Anaphylaxis	Diarrhoea/abdominal pain/bloating
Angioedema	Failure to thrive
Urticaria	Post gastroenteritis enteropathy
Vomiting	Eczema/skin rashes
Rhinitis	Asthma
Colic	Migraine
	Epilepsy with migraine
	Hyperactivity/behaviour disorder
	Rheumatoid arthritis/joint pains

NB The association of food with those symptoms below the line is more controversial

mediated immune reactions (type IV) [4]. Despite lack of knowledge regarding the pathophysiology of the symptoms listed, there are two factors which draw them together. First, it is not unusual for sufferers to have not one but several of the symptoms listed. Second, the same shortlist of foods always seem to be the most common culprits.

DIAGNOSIS OF FOOD ALLERGY OR INTOLERANCE

Although small bowel biopsy may be a useful diagnostic tool for gastrointestinal food allergy or intolerance, dietary manipulation is the mainstay for both diagnosis and treatment. Other diagnostic tests have been described to identify specific intolerances but their efficacy is either the source of much difference of opinion or has not been validated.

The dietary manipulations involved

The dietary manipulations used for diagnosis are broadly similar whatever the symptoms may be. They may not only help to establish a diagnosis but also exclude a diagnosis that has been wrongly made. Since restricted diets require considerable effort on the part of the family, a number of points must be considered before a diet is embarked upon:

(1) Are the clinical symptoms severe enough to warrant a diet? For example a child with eczema

should not be put on a diet unless he has failed to respond to optimum topical treatment.
(2) Is the child or parent motivated and able to adhere to the diet? Non compliance renders the diet trial a waste of time.
(3) Unless a relationship with food seems very likely from diet history, other disease should be excluded before embarking on a diet trial, particularly if symptoms are very severe (e.g. headaches).

The diagnosis and treatment of food allergy or intolerance by diet involves three phases of dietary manipulation. The first comprises an appropriate diagnostic elimination diet which should be used for between two and six weeks. The length of time will depend on frequency of symptoms, degree of restriction of diet and type of symptoms involved (improvement in gastrointestinal symptoms may occur within a day or two whereas improvement in eczema may take a week or two). If successful, this diet will result in significant relief of the symptoms. The second phase involves a series of open reintroductions to identify provoking foods. The third phase is the adherence to a maintenance diet excluding foods that have caused problems.

Attention must always be paid to nutritional adequacy during these dietary manipulations. The initial diagnostic diet may not be adequate and supplements particularly of vitamins and calcium may be used (see Table 13.4, later). However, this initial diet is used for only a short time and it can be argued that supplements are unneccesary at this stage. Indeed, highly food-intolerant children may be adversely affected by the supplements themselves. The important thing is that close attention is paid to adequate nutrition during the reintroduction phase so that the final maintenance diet is adequate and supplements are incorporated if necessary.

Throughout the period of dietary manipulations, and for at least a week before any diet starts, it is extremely useful for the parent (or patient) to keep a symptom score diary. It is then possible to be reasonably objective about change in severity of symptoms. Physical symptoms can be listed at the end of each day and a numerical score can be inserted for each one (e.g. 0 for no symptoms and 1 to 3 for symptoms which are mild, moderate or severe). Where attention deficit and hyperactivity are concerned it is useful to use a shortened form of the Conner's scale (Table 13.2) [5].

Table 13.2 Short form of Conner's Scale for hyperactivity

Observation date . . .	Degree of activity			
	Not at all	Just a little	Pretty much	Very much
Restless or overactive				
Excitable, impulsive				
Disturbs other children				
Short attention span				
Constantly fidgeting				
Inattentive, easily distracted				
Demands must be met immediately				
Cries often and easily				
Mood changes quickly and drastically				
Temper outbursts, explosive and unpredictable behaviour				

Phase 1. Initial diagnostic diet

A full diet history is mandatory before embarking on a diet and may indicate possible provoking foods. It is not uncommon for parents to jump to the wrong conclusions as to which foods affect their child and intolerance to foods eaten several times every day such as wheat or milk may go completely unnoticed. Keeping a food diary for some weeks before starting a diet may provide a baseline, but seldom adds useful information about suspect foods which has not been revealed by diet history. A diagnostic elimination diet should avoid disliked foods and foods which are craved or eaten in large amounts. The initial diet may exclude one or a large number of foods. The choice of diet is a matter of clinical judgement taking into account age, severity and frequency of symptoms and whether diets have already been tried. There are four main types of diet – a simple exclusion diet, an empirical diet, a few foods diet or an elemental diet.

Simple exclusion diet

When reactions are quick it is easy to identify the provoking food. The food may be nutritionally unimportant, e.g. nuts. All sources of the provoking food must be removed from the diet. Sometimes quick reactions happen with staples such as cows' milk; an alternative to milk must be considered and is mandatory in infants. Quick reactions to food can be the most severe and are occasionally life threatening, so complete avoidance is vital.

Empirical diet

An empirical diet is used where allergy or intolerance is suspected, but the causative agents are not known. Here, some of the most commonly provoking foods are avoided. In under one year olds the most frequent offender is cows' milk-based infant formula or cows' milk itself, so a cows' milk protein-free diet is frequently used. The most common provoking foods in children are cows' milk, egg, wheat, rye, chocolate, citrus and other fruits, nuts, fish and some additives.

A diet avoiding milk and egg is recommended by several centres for children with severe eczema and the recommendations variously suggest also avoiding beef, chicken, fish and some food additives. The additional avoidance of nuts and all fruit except bananas has been advocated by some workers in this field [6].

Alun Jones, Workman and Hunter, working with adults suffering from irritable bowel syndrome, published their empirical diet in the popular press and recommended it for other symptoms as well as gastrointestinal ones [7]. This diet avoids cows' milk, egg, all grains except rice, potatoes, chocolate and some food additives. This diet does allow sheep's and goats' milk which is not generally a good idea as there is immunological cross reactivity between the proteins of mammalian milks.

An elimination diet, aimed at adults attending the Middlesex Hospital in London, published by the Good Housekeeping Institute suggests avoiding all grains, milk, egg, chocolate, citrus fruit and some food additives [8]. This is recommended for any symptoms which might be related to food intolerance. A very similar diet was described by Rowe *et al.* in 1959 [9] for the diagnosis and treatment of food induced asthma.

As far as additives are concerned, those most commonly cited as being potential problems are: artificial colours (azo, coal tar and erythrosine dyes) (E102–E155); benzoate preservatives (E210–E219), sulphur dioxide preservatives (E220–E224), and nitrite preservatives (E249–E252). However, there are reports of intolerance to some of the natural colours [10]. Foods containing the above additives usually also contain flavours and these should not be assumed to be inert. Antioxidants BHA and BHT have also been implicated but they are less commonly found in manufactured foods these days. It is advisable for an empirical 'additive free' diet to exclude artificial colours; benzoate, sulphur dioxide, nitrite/nitrate preservatives; food flavours where possible. This will automatically exclude major sources of natural colours.

There is evidence that urticaria may sometimes be provoked by aspirin and this has been used as an argument for removing fruits and vegetables containing natural salicylates from the diet. A self help group also suggests that hyperactive children may be affected by these foods. The only available analysis of the salicylate content of fruits and vegetables has been carried out by Swain and Truswell and it is not clearcut which foods should be avoided on such a diet [11]. Intolerance to fruits should not be assumed to be due to salicylate content. Many food intolerant children are affected by some fruits but can manage others which contain salicylates.

Empirical diets can have their problems when excluded foods are inadvertently replaced by others which are also capable of causing reactions. For example, a child on a milk free diet may drink soya milk or orange juice instead which can also cause problems. Failure to respond to an empirical diet does not rule out the possibility of food intolerance. More restricted diets therefore have a role to play.

Few food diet

There are considerable difficulties in teaching people how to avoid a large number of foods. It is easier to decide on which foods the child can eat and teach the diet in terms of which foods are allowed rather than concentrating on those which are forbidden. This is the basis for the few food diet which has been constructed in different ways choosing those foods least likely to cause problems. Three to four weeks is the longest time one should consider using a very restricted diet although improvement may occur in a shorter time.

The simplest few food diet to have been described consists of lamb, pears and spring water only but a

Table 13.3 Two examples of Few Food diets

Under two year olds require a nutritionally adequate milk substitute. This diet should not be used for longer than four weeks

A	B
Turkey	Lamb
Cabbage, sprouts, broccoli, cauliflower	Carrots, parsnips
Potato, potato flour	Rice, rice flour
Banana	Pear
Soya oil	Sunflower oil
Calcium and vitamins (see Table 13.4)	Calcium and vitamins
Tap water	Tap water

Possible additions: whey-free margarine, sugar for baking
Possible variations: bottled water; rabbit instead of above meats; peaches and apricots, melon, pineapple instead of above fruits

small child cannot be expected to adhere to this for three weeks. Diets using one meat, one carbohydrate source, one fruit, one vegetable have been used [12]. If no improvement occurs a second diet containing a different set of foods can be used (Table 13.3) [13,14]. In extreme circumstances one could include rarely eaten foods such as rabbit, venison, sweet potatoes, buckwheat [15]. Children under approximately two years old need a nutritionally adequate hypoallergenic milk substitute or formula.

Since the above diets are extremely rigorous, less restricted diets have been used which make adherence much less of a problem (Table 13.4) [16,17,18]. A similar diet is described by Bock *et al.* [19]. However, it is very difficult to find a completely different set of foods for a second attempt if the first is not helpful. It is necessary, therefore, to monitor progress closely and change or further restrict the diet during the third or fourth week in an attempt to achieve eventual success.

The acceptability of the few food diet depends greatly on the dietitian's advice as regards planning menus, giving ideas for main meals and recipes for baking with permitted flours [20]. Ideas for packed lunches should be given as most school canteens cannot cope adequately with such a restricted diet. For vegetarians one would have to allow a larger range of vegetables including pulses. The dietitian should keep in touch with the family and be available by telephone during this time. Cost of the diet may be a problem and should be discussed with the family. Recipes for use with a few food diet are available from

Table 13.4 Less restricted Few Food diet

This diet should be used for no more than four weeks. Under two year olds require a nutritionally adequate substitute for milk

Choose two foods from each food group

Meat	Lamb, rabbit, turkey, pork
Starchy food	Rice, potato, sweet potato
Vegetables	Broccoli, cauliflower, cabbage, sprouts (brassicas) Carrots, parsnips, celery Cucumber, marrow, courgettes, melon Leeks, onions, asparagus
Fruit	Pears, bananas, peaches and apricots, pineapple

Also included: Sunflower oil, whey free margarine
Plain potato crisps
Small amount of sugar for baking
Tap or bottled water
Juice and jam from allowed fruits
Salt, pepper and herbs in cooking

A calcium (300–400 mg/d) and vitamin supplement is advisable:
calcium gluconate effervescent 1 g × 3 daily; or calcium lactate 300 mg × 6 daily; or Sandocal 400 × 1 tablet daily.
Abidec 0.6 ml daily

the author, Christine Carter, at her place of work (see Contributors list at the front of this volume).

Few food diets (and empirical diets) are generally carried out in the home environment. It is important that the child's lifestyle is not altered otherwise changes in symptoms could be attributed to factors other than change in diet. For example, children with eczema may be affected by contact with or inhalation of substances so if they improve on a diet in hospital, this improvement may be due to change in the environment alone. Medication should not be changed for a few weeks prior to, or during, the dietary manipulations for the same reasons. Children on regular medication, such as anticonvulsants, should remain on these but be changed on to colour/additive free versions where possible. Attention should be paid to nonfood items which may be consumed by a small child such as toothpaste (white toothpaste should be used), chalks and paints.

Hypoallergenic formula only

Hypoallergenic or semi-elemental formulas can occasionally be justified for children who have not responded to a restricted diet, but this treatment should be very much a last resort as suitable products do not have a good taste and tube feeding may be necessary to achieve adequate nutrition. This will involve a hospital admission. Suitable products are listed in Tables 6.13 and 6.15. These formulas have been used mainly for children with severe eczema [21] and aslo to obtain remission in Crohn's disease. There is a difference of opinion as to why an elemental feed achieves remission of Crohn's disease (page 75).

Hypoallergenic formulas for infants

The hypoallergenic or semi-elemental formula is the diet of choice for an infant with possible cows' milk protein intolerance. There are a variety of such infant formulas available where the protein has been highly hydrolysed, although the degree of hydrolysis varies somewhat as does the source of protein (Tables 6.13, 6.15). Many studies have shown the efficacy of these hydrolysates in treating cows' milk protein allergy or intolerance, but most of the studies have been carried out with Nutramigen and Pregestimil (which are the most highly hydrolysed, with peptide sizes not above 1200 Daltons) and Alfare as these products have been on the market the longest. Rugo *et al.* compared six different hydrolysates in children with immediate IgE mediated cows' milk allergy and found that the casein hydrolysates had the least residual allergenic activity using both *in vivo* and *in vitro* measures [22]. However, all the products listed in Table 6.13 are being routinely used to treat infants with cows' milk protein allergy or intolerance. Some of the more recent products which are not quite as highly hydrolysed do have a slightly better taste, which may make them more acceptable to some children. The problem with all these products, however, is their palatability and although the infant will accept them quite readily, children over approximately one year of age often do not.

It should not be assumed that the hydrolysate formulas will be tolerated and anaphylactic reactions have been described with both whey and casein hydrolysates [23]. Highly allergic infants may tolerate one and not another of these products. They should be introduced to the child under carefully controlled conditions in hospital. An amino acid based formula (Neocate) could be tried if hydrolysates are not tolerated.

There are lower degree hydrolysates available in some European countries made by Nestlé under the brand name HA (e.g. Beba HA) and in the United States and Canada (Good Start HA, Carnation).

These are intended for prophylactic use rather than treatment; they are not available in the UK. Unlike the high degree hydrolysates, Good Start HA contains a considerable proportion of peptides with molecular weight above 1500 Daltons. For comparison, the majority of whole cows' milk proteins have molecular weights between 15 000 and 24 000 Daltons although the molecular weights of serum albumin and immunoblobulins (which contribute less than 5% of the total protein) are far greater than this. The majority of whole soy proteins have molecular weights between 180 000 and 600 000 Daltons.

Infant formulas based on soy protein isolate have been available without a doctor's prescription for many years and no doubt have been used inappropriately on a large scale, without medical supervision, for vague symptoms. The use of a soy formula by clinicians for infants with cows' milk protein intolerance has decreased because of an increasing number of reports that it can provoke adverse reactions including enteropathy [24,25]. Although the soy formula is therefore not recommended for gastro-enteropathic food intolerance, its use may be justified for atopic infants with cows' milk protein allergy. This, however, is a controversial issue. Other reasons for not dismissing soy based infant formulas are that they are cheaper than hydrolysates and they have a better taste.

Hydrolysate formulas (or possibly soy formulas in some instances) should be used to treat infants with cows' milk protein allergy or intolerance who are bottle fed. Solely breast fed infants who develop symptoms of food allergy may benefit from some restriction of the mother's diet.

Other mammalian milks, ewes' and goats' milk, are not suitable for infants with cows' milk protein intolerance as they are not nutritionally adequate and their proteins can be as highly sensitizing as cows' milk protein. They can sometimes be introduced into the diet of an older child who has benefited from an initial diagnostic diet and is known to be cows' milk intolerant as a single open reintroduction. In such cases raw fresh milk should be boiled to minimize bacterial contamination.

Which diagnostic diet to use?

It is sometimes suggested that an empirical diet should be tried first, with a steadily increasing set of restrictions if it does not result in relief of symptoms [26] (Table 13.5). When the diet history indicates multiple intolerances, or if diets have already been tried, the

Table 13.5 Diagnostic procedure for the identification of suspected food allergy or intolerance

Stage 1	Stage 2	Stage 3	Stage 4
Avoid:	*Avoid:*	*Foods allowed:*	*Hospital admission*
Dairy products	Dairy products	Lamb or rabbit	Vivonex *
Egg	Egg	Cabbage	(unflavoured)
	Chicken	Carrots	or glucose
	Game	Celery	and
	Pork	Lettuce	electrolytes
	Offal	Rhubarb	+ distilled
	Fish	Sugar	water + sago
	Shellfish	Treacle	
	Fruit (except rhubarb and banana)	Syrup	
		Salt	
	Vegetables (except those listed in stage 3)	Sago	
		Tomor margarine	
		Water	
	Chemical additives	Tea (without milk)	
	Alcohol		
	Herbs/spices		
	Nuts		

From Hathaway and Warner [26]

* No longer available in the UK

few food diet may be the preferred first step. The most important thing about a prescribed diet however, is that it should be practical for the patient. There is no point in prescribing sago or rhubarb for children who dislike such foods. Diets should be prescribed for the individual. It must be remembered that although any food is capable of causing problems, a wide variety of symptoms can be caused by the most common provoking foods.

The few food diet is most difficult to perform in children between one and two years of age. Many of these children are still reliant on milk for a significant proportion of their nutritional intake and should ideally take one of the hydrolysate formulas. Unfortunately these are often refused.

Phase 2. Reintroduction of foods

The parent of a child who has experienced significant relief of symptoms on a diet will usually want to carry on with it. Young infants who were suffering severe

Table 13.6 Open reintroduction of foods

Each food should be given in normal quantities daily for a week before being allowed freely in the diet. A test dose may be recommended initially. The order of reintroduction depends on the patient's preference and on which foods were avoided initially

Oats	Porridge oats, Scottish oatcakes, home made flapjacks (if sugar is already allowed)
Corn	Sweetcorn, home made popcorn, cornflour, maize flour, cornflakes if malt is tolerated
Meats	Try meats (including offal) singly, e.g. chicken, beef, pork
Wheat	Wholemeal or unbleached white flour for baking, egg-free pasta, Shredded Wheat, Puffed Wheat
Yeast	Pitta bread; ordinary bread (this usually also contains soya)
Rye	Worth trying if wheat is not tolerated; pure rye crisbread; pumpernickel
Cows' milk	Fresh cows' milk, cream, butter, plain yoghurt, milk containing foods with tolerated ingredients e.g. rice pudding. Try cheese separately later
Cows' milk sustitute	If cows' milk is not tolerated try substitutes one by one. Infant soya formula or infant hydrolysate formula. Ewes' milk, goats' milk for over one year olds (boiled or pasteurized). Supermarket liquid soya milk with additional calcium
Egg	Use one whole fresh egg per day for test period. It may be preferred to begin with small amounts of egg in baking
Fish	Fresh or fresh frozen (not smoked, battered etc.) e.g. cod, herring etc. If one type is not tolerated others may be. Try shellfish separately later
Tomatoes	Fresh tomatoes, canned and puréed tomatoes, ketchup
Peas/beans	These include peas, green beans, kidney beans, lentils, baked beans in tomato sauce if tomato is tolerated
Orange	Pure orange juice, oranges, satsumas. If oranges are tolerated all citrus fruit probably is too
Sugar	Use ordinary sugar on cereal, in drinks and baking. Some parents comment that small amounts are tolerated whereas larger amounts are not
Chocolate	Try only if sugar is tolerated. If diet is milk-free, use milk-free chocolate. Cocoa powder in drinks and cooking
Carob	Carob confectionery can be tried if chocolate is not tolerated. Check other ingredients – it may contain milk or soya

Table 13.6 *Continued*

Tea/coffee	Add milk if this is already in the diet
Peanuts	Plain or salted peanuts (not for under four year olds) peanut butter. Beware of peanut (arachis) oil in patients who have immediate severe reactions to peanuts
Other nuts	Try singly or mixed
Malt	Malt/malt flavouring is present in most breakfast cereals. Try Rice Krispies if rice is tolerated etc.
Nitrite/nitrate	Corned beef if beef is tolerated, ham and bacon if pork is tolerated
Sodium benzoate	Supermarket lemonade provided other ingredients are tolerated
Sodium glutamate	Stock cubes, gravy mixes, flavoured crisps, provided the other ingredients are tolerated
Sodium metabisulphite	Some squashes, sausages provided the other ingredients are tolerated, dried fruit
Vitamins Minerals	These may be given if needed to enhance nutritional adequacy and introduced singly to test tolerance

Other foods e.g. fruit and vegetables can be introduced gradually as desired. Manufactured foods such as ice cream, biscuits can be introduced taking into account known sensitivities. Many additives e.g. colours, flavours will be introduced as mixtures in manufactured foods such as sweets and canned/bottled drinks. For children with multiple cereal intolerances, flours such as buckwheat, soya, gram (chickpea), wheatstarch may be tried. Some of the special dietary products for gluten-free and low protein diets may be suitable but other ingredients must be checked (they are not strictly prescribable for food allergy)

symptoms and failure to thrive before changing the milk they were feeding should not be challenged with cows' milk or cows' milk based formula in the near future. Nine to twelve months may elapse to allow the child to thrive. Risk of a severe reaction lessens as the child matures.

In an older child, if the inital diet avoids several foods, these should be reintroduced singly in order to identify those which provoke symptoms. Each new food may be tried in a small test quantity and then given in normal amounts every day for a week. If symptoms do not recur the food may then be incorporated freely into the diet. A guide to reintroduction of foods is given in Table 13.6. The order of reintroduction should depend on the child's or parent's preferences with the aim being for nutritional adequacy.

It is not unusual to find that children with multiple symptoms and intolerances react differently to different foods in terms of both speed and type of reaction. Immediate and delayed reactions can occur in the same individual.

Where there is a risk of an immediate severe reaction to a food reintroduction, that food should be either avoided or only given under supervision in hospital. Fatal immediate reactions, although rare, do happen [27], and even late anaphylactic reactions have been reported [28]. Infants are especially at risk and milk introductions are best performed under medical supervision. As already discussed, even the hydrolysate formulas have been known to cause severe reactions in the very sensitive infant.

Phase 3. Maintenance diet

The maintenance diet has been achieved when the introduction of all foods has been attempted and the child is on the fullest diet possible. Nutritional adequacy is paramount and supplements are sometimes necessary. Children without milk or a nutritionally adequate substitute will need a calcium supplement [29].

Occasionally children are adversely affected by so many foods that a satisfactory maintenance diet is difficult to achieve. For them it may be possible to avoid foods causing severe symptoms but allow food causing minor problems on a rotational basis.

Where common provoking foods such as milk have to be avoided, information regarding manufactured foods free of these items can be obtained in booklet form from the British Dietetic Association. The information is provided by the Food Intolerance Databank at the Leatherhead Food Research Association. To date, only some of the large supermarket chains have participated so its limited content is not useful to some parents. Some supermarkets provide their own 'free from' booklets. Parents should be instructed to look at labels on manufactured foods in order to avoid the necessary foods.

Where diet does not completely control symptoms a trial of Nalcrom (sodium cromoglycate, Fison's Ltd) may be indicated. Nalcrom may also be useful as a prophylactic measure before occasional planned breaks in a diet [30].

Since children often lose their intolerances over a period of time, attempts should be made every 6–12 months to reintroduce avoided foods (particularly if they are staples such as milk or wheat). In fact this may happen in an unsupervized way as the result of an accidental or deliberate break in the diet.

CONFIRMATION OF FOOD ALLERGY OR INTOLERANCE

Confirmation within research studies has usually involved double blind placebo controlled provocations. The use of a nasogastric tube for blind provocations is too invasive a procedure for use outside research projects.

Sampson has used up to 8 g of dehydrated encapsulated food in challenges and symptoms occurred within two hours of ingestion [31]. Bock *et al.* have published a manual where double blind, placebo-controlled challenges are described [19]. They deal mainly with immediate IgE related allergy and recommend both the use of encapsulated food and, especially for children, dried or fresh foods disguised in other food (e.g. apple sauce). Alun Jones *et al.* [32] and Egger *et al.* [14–18] found that adverse reactions often occurred after intervals varying between a few hours and several days and after a considerable amount of the food had been eaten. Where staple foods such as milk and wheat are concerned large amounts of food may be needed to produce a response. Blind provocations with encapsulated foods are likely to be unsuitable for slow onset food intolerance because they contain too little of the provoking food. Unfortunately, it is in the more controversial areas of possible food intolerance such as hyperactivity and migraine where intolerance is described as coming on over as long a period as several days. In such cases blind challenges are the only way of confirming food intolerance but can be very difficult, if not impossible, to carry out. Pearson *et al.* [33] studied adults with multiple symptoms including psychiatric disorder and showed the value of proof by blind challenge as several patients reported reaction to the placebo. Bentley *et al.* [34] studied patients with the irritable bowel syndrome; food sensitivity could only be confirmed by double blind food provocation in three out of 27 adults who also had associated atopic disease. In both these studies, blind provocation tests were performed with dried encapsulated food or in fresh food (e.g. cows' milk disguised in soya milk). Patients were given three provocation preparations and three placebos in random order and one presumes that only one dose of each was given. It could be that some patients did not react because they were not given a sufficient quantity of the provocation.

Before embarking on a double blind placebo-controlled provocation test attention should be given to the following points:

(1) The required amount of provoking food should first be established during open reintroduction together with the duration of the provocation. These findings should be applied to the double blind procedure. This is extremely important as one needs to ensure enough of the food is given, but on the other hand, one cannot risk giving too much in very sensitive individuals. Indeed, it could be argued that severe immediate reactions should not be tested by a double blind procedure.

(2) The provoking food must be hidden in other food and this (the placebo and excipient) must be food which has shown to be tolerated by the child in the amounts which are to be used.

(3) A challenge performed during a quiescent phase of the disease may give a different result from a challenge performed at another time (e.g. urticaria).

(4) The placebo must be indistinguishable from the provoking agent.

(5) The provoking food should possibly be given in the same form as that which caused relapse on open reintroduction. For example dried powdered milk cannot necessarily be substituted for doorstep cows' milk as heat treatment is known to affect its allergenicity [35].

(6) When dealing with children, the material must be palatable or it will be refused. Many children will not swallow capsules.

(7) The child must not break his diet during the period of blind provocation or placebo. Those who are subject to allergic reactions to food may also react to inhaled substances or skin contact. Such a reaction during a blind food provocation may remain undetected and give spurious results.

(8) The possibility that particular foods only provoke symptoms under certain circumstances is rarely considered despite published reports of food-dependant, exercise-induced anaphylaxis. Perhaps there are parallels to this in other forms of food intolerance that we are, as yet, unaware of.

(9) The administration of three provocations and three placebos will be impossible to achieve with a slow onset of food intolerance where each preparation may have to be given for several days.

Double blind food provocations, especially for slow onset food intolerance, are very time consuming and probably have little place outside the research field. The paediatric dietitian cannot be expected to find time to organize such things routinely. He or she may be asked to arrange blind provocations where the diagnosis is suspect and children are on very restricted diets. In such cases the dietitian should be given full information regarding the diet and suspected intolerances so that a decision can be made regarding the feasibility of providing material for such a provocation. Whether this is best performed as an outpatient or an inpatient should also be discussed beforehand. It is important to have some idea of how long it might take for the child to relapse on a blind provocation so that an admission can be properly planned.

SOME PROBLEMS WITH DIETARY TREATMENT

Since this is a poorly understood and controversial area of dietetics it is perhaps not surprising that there is a wide range of views amongst the medical profession as to the value of dietary treatment. Parents who feel that diet plays a role in their child's illness should have the opportunity to discuss in an unbiased fashion the possibilities of dietary treatment. It is the lack of sympathetic approach which leads to a self-imposed diet or self-referral to a practitioner who may not have adequate expertise.

Many children are already on a diet when referred and such diets are usually, at least partially, ineffective (hence the referral). Whatever the prejudices of the professionals involved, the question of diet must be discussed as the child may be on an inadequate and inappropriate diet [36]. It must be remembered that, although some children may be on unnecessary diets, others may benefit dramatically from the correct diet. The need for the medical profession to deal more adequately with these problems has been discussed by David [37]. The role of the dietitian is to assist in maintaining helpful diets, broaden the diet as much as possible and encourage people to abandon unhelpful diets. An open minded approach is necessary. Occasionally parents will not take advice and in exceptional cases the restrictions imposed by the parent on the child may be regarded as a form of child abuse [38].

DIETARY TREATMENT OF SPECIFIC SYMPTOMS

So far the dietary treatment of food allergy or intolerance has been discussed generally as many sufferers have multiple symptoms and the same foods tend to be the most common provokers whatever the symptoms. However it is useful to discuss some of the symptoms separately.

Eczema

Atherton has written a comprehensive review on the subject of diet and eczema [39]. There is a role for diet both in treating the eczema and also the non-eczematous food-allergic symptoms which may also be present. However, more than nine out of ten children with eczema will respond to topical treatment and do not require dietary intervention [39]. It is possible that the younger the child the more likely it is that diet will help.

Empirical diets have been discussed and should avoid, for a trial period of a few weeks only, egg and cows' milk (and other mammalian milks) together with some additives and any foods already suspected. Failing this, a few food diet may be tried (for 3–4 weeks) for very severe eczema where parents are highly motivated, although Pike *et al.* [15] found that only a few sufferers benefited. Semi-elemental formulas for children should be very much a last resort [21]. For infants the feed of choice is a hydrolysate formula. Soya formula may be used, but failure to respond does not rule out food intolerance.

Attempts to confirm diet responsiveness by double blind provocation are not without problems. Sampson [31] used small amounts of encapsulated food and obtained reactions within two hours although these may have been of an urticarial not an eczematous nature. Perhaps eczema itself, if diet related, is exacerbated by larger amounts of food after a longer time. This has been discussed by David at greater length [40]. Double blind provocations under such circumstances are hard to achieve [15].

Attention deficit disorder and hyperactivity (ADDH)

Of all the symptoms discussed in this chapter, the question of diet and ADDH is the most controversial. The results of many studies aimed at testing Feingold's

hypothesis indicate that only a few hyperactive children respond to the elimination of food additives from their diets. Problems with methodology and interpretation of these studies have been discussed by Taylor [41]. Two controlled studies by Egger *et al.* [16] and Kaplan *et al.* [42] have looked at a possible relationship between food (not just additives) and behaviour. There are indications from this work that the idea that food can affect behaviour should be taken seriously although the proportion of children who might benefit is not known. Although food additives may adversely affect hyperactive children, foods can do so also and the most common provoking foods are the same as those which cause food allergy or intolerance generally. It is not always possible to carry out a trial of diet as older children (over 8 years or so) may be completely out of control and non-compliant.

Many hyperactive children have cravings and bizarre eating habits and the first line of approach may be to enforce a more 'normal' diet. Naturally, any improvement may be due to firmer parental control rather than anything else. An 'additive free diet' may also serve the same purpose. However, to look into the possibility of food intolerance properly, one must use an empirical or few food diet as described. This should only be attempted where the problems are severe as the difficulties of adhering to the diet can easily become worse than the behaviour problem it is supposed to be treating. It must be stressed to parents that this is a little researched area and that diet may not be the answer for their child. Other treatments such as behaviour modification or even medication may be more effective. However, parents of children with severe behavioural problems who wish to try the dietary approach should be given the opportunity to do so otherwise they will be tempted to experiment with diet unsupervised.

Migraine and epilepsy

Children with severe migraine have been shown to benefit from diet [14]. If migraine attacks are fewer than one per week it is difficult to use the dietary approach. If symptoms are infrequent, three weeks observation on a diet would not be long enough to assess a change in number of attacks and the reintroduction phase can become very muddled. However, for children with severe frequent migraine who have not responded to medication, a diet trial is a worthwhile procedure.

It is not uncommon for children with migraine to have other symptoms and epilepsy may be one of these [14]. Some children who have epilepsy and migraine respond to diet with respect to both these symptoms whereas children with epilepsy alone do not [17]. As with migraine the dietary approach cannot be tried unless fits are frequent. A trial of diet for such children who have not responded to conventional treatment is worth considering.

Rheumatoid arthritis

There is some evidence that some adults with rheumatoid arthritis benefit from diet [43]. There is no reason why this approach should not be tried in children whose parents have noticed foods affecting their child and wish to try a diet. Although the role of diet is far from clear, a supervized diet trial which is abandoned if ineffective is preferable to allowing families to experiment with diet alone.

PREVENTION OF FOOD ALLERGY OR INTOLERANCE

Parents of newborn infants at risk of developing food allergy or intolerance because of a family history of allergy will request advice as to how to feed their children in an attempt to prevent symptoms developing.

Results of numerous prevention studies comparing the value of breast versus bottle feeding are conflicting [44,45] probably because they were not properly randomized and were not well controlled for variables such as age of weaning, exposure to pets, tobacco etc. However, the following guidelines have been put forward by Cant despite the need for more research in the area in order to give practical advice to families [44]:

(1) It is not worth suggesting that lactating mothers restrict their own diets unless the breast fed child develops symptoms or unless the mothers have had a previous child who developed allergic disease whilst being exclusively breast fed. At that stage the mother should try a milk and possibly egg free diet (and take a calcium supplement). This should be abandoned if it does not help after two weeks.

(2) The mother should breast feed exclusively for at least four and possibly six months. Any supplementation should be preferably with a hydrolysate formula rather than a soya milk, although hydrolysates are not prescribable for prophylactic use.

(3) The relationship between weaning and the development of food allergic disease has been little studied but Cant and Bailes [46] suggested a system of introducing one food group at a time and leaving the most common provoking foods until last. They suggested breast feeding until six months with regular weight checks and a varied maternal diet with plenty of fluids. At six months a supplement of 0.3 ml Abidec and 2.0 ml Niferex iron supplement should be given. Foods should then be introduced in the following order:

- milk free baby rice
- puréed root vegetables: potatoes, carrot, parsnip, swede, turnip
- puréed fruit: apple, pear, banana (not citrus fruit until 9 months)
- other vegetables; peas, beans, lentils etc.
- other cereals (not wheat until 8 months)
- lamb, turkey and then other meats
- fish (not until 10 months)
- cows' milk products, ordinary infant formula (not until 10 months). If breast milk has diminished before that a supplementary feed will be needed as infant soya formula or hydrolysate
- eggs (not until one year).

HIV AND AIDS

Human immunodeficiency virus (HIV) is the virus that causes acquired immune deficiency syndrome (AIDS). The infection may be transmitted vertically from an infected mother to child, via blood or blood products or by sexual intercourse. The Center for Disease Control (CDC), USA, has classified paediatric HIV into three main groups – indeterminate, asymptomatic and symptomatic (Table 13.7) [47]. Indeterminate classification applies to children under 18 months still carrying maternal HIV antibodies. Without another manifestation of HIV, serology alone cannot diagnose these children as HIV infected. By

Table 13.7 CDC classification of paediatric HIV infection

P–0 Indeterminate infection

P–1 Asymptomatic infection:
  A Normal immune function
  B Abnormal immune function
  C Immune function not studied

P–2 Symptomatic infection:
  A Non-specific signs and symptoms
  B Progressive neurological disease
  C Lymphocytic interstitial pneumonia
  D Secondary infectious disease
  E Secondary cancer
  F Other diseases possibly due to HIV

Table 13.8 Reported paediatric HIV cases until January 1992

Transmission route	Infected	Indeterminate	Negative
Vertical	133	174	137
Blood products	262		
Total	395	174	137

January 1992, 706 HIV positive children in the United Kingdom were reported to the Communicable Disease Surveillance Centre (CDSC) (Table 13.8) [48].

Paediatric HIV infection differs from the adult infection in a number of ways. The incubation period is shorter with a higher mortality rate. Bacterial infections and lymphocytic pneumonia are more common and Kaposi's sarcoma, malignancies and some opportunistic infections, e.g. toxoplasmosis, are rare. Chronic growth and developmental problems are a complication of the disease itself. Frequent infections, fevers, diarrhoea, neurological and social problems result in malnutrition, and can affect both adults and children alike.

COMPLICATIONS ASSOCIATED WITH AIDS

Common infections

Pneumocystis carinii pneumonia (PCP) is the most common and often the first opportunistic infection to appear in the paediatric patient. PCP is characterized by a dry cough, shortness of breath and increased respiratory rate. Severe coughing causes fatigue and limits oral intake. Lesions in the mouth and oesophagus caused by recurrent or long episodes of candidiasis make sucking, chewing and swallowing painful. Bottle and food refusal is common.

Diarrhoea

Diarrhoea in patients with AIDS is associated with altered gut immunity, opportunistic infections and nutrient malabsorption. The main pathogens isolated include cryptosporidium, cytomegalovirus (CMV), salmonella and other food-borne bacteria [49]. Cryptosporidium interferes with intestinal brush border function causing nutrient malabsorption. Patients experience large bouts of watery diarrhoea about eight times a day, nausea, vomiting and fatigue leading to rapid weight loss. Dehydration occurs quickly and parenteral hydration is necessary. CMV infection is one of the final complications of AIDS present in most patients at death. Disseminated CMV causes numerous (up to 30) small volume bowel movements a day. Severe weight loss is common although treatment with Ganciclovir increases appetite and promotes body cell mass repletion [50].

Patients with symptomatic disease are more likely to acquire Salmonella, Listeriosis and other food borne pathogens. Food preparation and hygiene advice should be given to parents and carers.

HIV encephalopathy

In Europe 20–30% of HIV infected children develop neurological abnormalities [51]. Sucking, swallowing and hand to mouth co-ordination may be affected. Close collaboration with a speech therapist experienced in feeding problems ensures appropriate foods are offered which meet the child's nutritional requirements.

DIET THERAPY

Children with asymptomatic HIV infection may not meet daily nutritional requirements even in the presence of a good appetite and access to food. It has been demonstrated that severe progressive malnutrition occurs in adult AIDS patients, with lowest lean body masses occurring in those close to death [52]. It has been estimated that these patients have an estimated 14% additional energy requirement above estimated average requirement (EAR), and protein requirements should be increased by 10% per degree Celsius of fever. Some centres have reported increasing dietary protein intake in children by 50–100% to maintain nitrogen balance [53]. In addition, the child still has increased requirements to allow for adequate growth.

Attention to diet early in the disease may prevent weight loss and promote growth. Diet therapies used in the treatment of the problems previously outlined are shown (Table 13.9). During periods of acute illness, enteral or parenteral feeding may be necessary.

Breast feeding

The European Collaborative Study has estimated the risk of transmitting HIV through breast feeding as 28% depending on the mother's stage of HIV infection [54]. In developed countries, the World Health Organization discourage HIV infected women from breast feeding when a safe alternative is available [55]. In developing countries the risks of bottle feeding outweigh the risk of HIV transmission through breast milk, so breast feeding is the preferred method of feeding in these infants.

Social problems

Many HIV infected children in the UK come from intravenous drug using families. Associated poor housing facilities, irregular meal times, food shortages and ill parents lead to poor nutrition. Advice on appropriate foods for facilities, food hygiene and food programmes should be available.

Drug nutrient interactions

In children with symptomatic HIV infection, Zidovudine (AZT) is a proven effective antiviral therapy. It delays neurological deterioration, increases appetite and promotes growth [56]. The value of AZT in asymptomatic patients is being assessed. AZT, like other drugs used to treat HIV and its associated infections, can interact with nutrients and food intake (Table 13.10).

Table 13.9 Dietary intervention in paediatric HIV patients [53]

Symptomatic problem	Primary intervention	Secondary intervention
Diarrhoea/ malabsorption	Decrease insoluble fibre Decrease high osmolar fluids Lactose restriction Minimal fat restriction (when steatorrhoea present)	Elemental diet Parenteral nutrition
PCP	Small frequent meals High protein/high energy	Gastrostomy
Candida	Soft, cold, non-irritating food Avoid hot, coarse food	
Anorexia	High energy/nutrient-dense feeds Small, frequent meals Child choose and prepare food	
Neurological problems	Thickened feeds Puréed foods Finger foods	Overnight nasogastric feeding

Table 13.10 HIV drug nutrient interactions

Medication	Use	Possible interaction
AZT [56]	Inhibits HIV replication	Nausea/vomiting Abdominal pain B12 deficiency
Dideoxyinosine (ddI) (on clinical trial, USA, [57])	Inhibits HIV replication	Pancreatitis
Co-Trimoxazole [58] (Bactrim, Septrin)	PCP	Megaloblastic anaemia Nausea/vomiting
Pentamidine Isethionate (inhaled), [59,60]	PCP	Altered taste Nausea/vomiting Hypoglycaemia Hypocalcaemia
Ganciclovir [51]	CMV	Diarrhoea/vomiting Gastric ulceration (rare) Promotes body cell mass repletion
Fluconazole [61] and Ketocanazole [62]	Candida	Nausea/vomiting
Amphotericin	Severe Candida	Nephrotoxic (Hypokalaemia, hypomagnesia) Diarrhoea

SCID

Severe combined immunodeficiency (SCID) is a disorder characterized by profoundly defective cellular (T lymphocyte) and humoral (B lymphocyte) immunity. The condition is usually inherited, but similar clinical symptoms can arise secondary to cancer therapy, retroviral infections or as part of the acquired immune deficiency syndrome (AIDS). X-linked, autosomal and sporadic forms can occur, resulting in a 4:1 male to female ratio of occurrence. In 1988 the frequency of SCID was estimated at 1 in 50 000 births [63].

In the most severe form, infants present at 4–8 months of age with recurrent infections, diarrhoea, failure to thrive and vomiting. These symptoms are unresponsive to conventional therapy and, if untreated, the condition is invariably fatal within the first year of life. The only treatment is a matched or mismatched bone-marrow transplant (BMT). The success rate of HLA-identical transplants has improved considerably over the last 10 years from about 40% to more than 90% [64]. The best results are achieved in infants who are well nourished and free of infection when transplanted. In future, the use of gene therapy to treat certain types of SCID may become routine.

DIETETIC MANAGEMENT

Before transplantation

The dietary management of these children will depend on their symptoms at presentation and the mode of treatment chosen. Newborn babies with SCID have a normal gut but the onset of infections, such as rotavirus, can disrupt the integrity of the mucosal surface. An assessment of the extent of gut damage from a jejunal biospy is not usual practice because of the risk of gut organisms entering the circulation during the procedure, leading to septicaemia. Some units use non-absorbable antibiotics if a biopsy or endoscopy is indicated, to reduce the risk of acquiring secondary gut infections.

Infants who are breast fed appear to have more resistance to infections, so a delay in introduction of normal infant formulas seems prudent. For infants with persistant diarrhoea, extensively hydrolysed protein feeds, e.g. Pregestimil or Nutramigen, may be more efficiently absorbed and so promote weight gain.

Prior to treatment, infants with SCID may have increased energy and protein requirements. This can be due to both malabsorption and to the demands imposed by recurrent infections. Energy and protein supplementation of feeds and/or tube feeding may then be necessary.

Infants receiving unmatched transplants need immunosuppressive conditioning therapy for about 10 days pre-transplant, to ablate recipient haemopoietic and lymphoid stem cell populations. This often disrupts the rapidly dividing mucosal cells of the gut and mouth leading to poor tolerance and acceptance of oral feeds and diet. Local anaesthetic sprays are sometimes helpful if an infant is experiencing oral pain. Where possible some oral feeding should continue, even if most of the nutrition is being provided parenterally. This will preclude the loss of the sucking reflex and also minimizes gut atrophy. To protect against oral infections such as Candida or Herpes, antifungal agents are usually given pre and post-transplant. In addition, in neutropenic post-transplant patients, prophylactic antibacterial mouth washes are used.

After transplantation

Post-transplant the patient is nursed in isolation with a filtered air system to protect against environmental pathogens. 'Clean diet' precautions are imposed to reduce the risk of food borne pathogenic organisms infecting the immunoincompent infant (page 19). Empirically, most units will feed infants a pasteurized extensively hydrolysed feed or breast milk at this time. Expressed breast milk needs to be tested for microbial contamination to ensure that the infant does not receive a high bacterial load. Most centres are very cautious with feeding post-transplant, as diarrhoea leading to an infected nappy area and perianal abcess can be life threatening.

Clean precautions are lifted once bacterial resistance has increased. This may take between three weeks and six months with neutrophil counts used as indicators (e.g. a neutrophil count of $>1.0 \times 10^9/l$).

During immunological reconstitution, food intolerances may appear but usually subside over 12 months. For this reason, as a precaution post-transplant, a diet avoiding milk and egg (and sometimes gluten) is imposed. The timing of the re-introduction of these potential antigens is usually dictated by immune function; gluten is introduced first followed by milk and finally egg. A successful transplant outcome will not necessitate further dietetic involvement.

REFERENCES

Food allergy and intolerance

1 Cant AJ Food allergy in childhood. *Human Nutr: Appl Nutr*, 1985, **39A** 277–293.

2 Lessof MH (Chairman) Joint Report of the Royal College of Physicians and the British Nutrition Foundation. Food Intolerance and Food Aversion. *J R Coll Physicians*, 1984, **18**(2) 84.

3 Ford RPK *et al*. Cow's milk hypersensitivity: immediate and delayed onset clinical patterns. *Arch Dis Childh*, 1983, **58** 856–862.

4 Coombs RRA, Gell PGH Classification of allergic reactions responsible for clinical hypersensitivity and disease. In: Gell PGH, Coombs RRA, Lachman PJ (eds.) *Clinical Aspects of Immunology*. Oxford, London, Edinburgh, Melbourne: Blackwell Scientific Publications, 1975.

5 Conners CK Rating scales for use in drug studies with children. *Psychopharmacology Bulletin* (Special Issue Pharmacotherapy with Children), 1973, **9** 24–28.

6 Price ML. The role of diet in the management of atopic eczema. *Human Nutr: Appl Nutr*, 1984, **38A** 409–415.

7 Workman E, Hunter J, Alun-Jones V *The Allergy Diet*. London: Martin Dunitz, 1984.

8 Ambasna C *Cookery and Eating for Food Allergy and Intolerance*. London: Good Housekeeping Institute, National Magazine House, 1992 (rpt).

9 Rowe AH *et al*. Bronchial asthma due to food allergy alone in ninety five patients. *J Am Med Assoc*, 1959, **169** 104–108.

10 Young E *et al*. The prevalence of reaction to food additives in a survey population. *J R Coll Physicians*, 1987, **21**(4) 241–247.

11 Swain R, Truswell AS Salicylates in foods. *J Am Diet Assoc*, 1985, **85**(8) 950–960.

12 Minford AMB *et al*. Food intolerance and food allergy in children: a review of 68 cases. *Arch Dis Childh*, 1982, **67** 742–747.

13 Atherton DJ Dietary treatment in childhood atopic eczema. *Proceedings of the Second Food Allergy Workshop 1983*. Oxford: The Medicine Pub Foundation, 1983: 109–110.

14 Egger J *et al*. Is migraine food allergy? *Lancet*, 1985, **2** 865–869.

15 Pike MG *et al*. Few food diets in the treatment of atopic eczema. *Arch Dis Childh*, 1989, **64** 1691–1698.

16 Egger J *et al*. Controlled trial of oligoantigenic diet treatment in the hyperkinetic syndrome. *Lancet*, 1985, **1** 540–545.

17 Egger J *et al*. Oligoantigenic diet treatment of children with epilepsy and migraine. *J Pediatr*, 1989, **114** 51–58.

18 Egger J *et al*. Effect of diet treatment on enuresis in children with migraine or hyperkinetic behaviour. *Clinical Pediatr*, 1992, **31** 302–307.

19 Bock SA *et al*. Double blind, placebo-controlled food challenge (DBPCFC) as an office procedure: A manual. *J Allergy Clin Immunol*, 1988, **82** 986–997.

20 Carter CM *et al*. A dietary management of severe childhood migraine. *Human Nutr: Appl Nutr*, 1985, **39A** 294–303.

21 Devlin J *et al*. Elemental diet fot refractory atopic eczema *Arch Dis Childh*, 1991, **66** 93–99.

22 Rugo E *et al*. How allergenic are hypoallergenic formulae? *Clin Experimental Allergy*, 1992, **22** 635–639.

23 Schwartz H *et al*. Cow milk protein hydrolysate formulas not always 'hypoallergenic'. *J Pediatr*, 1991, **119** 839–840.

24 Taitz LS Soy feeding in infancy. *Arch Dis Childh*, 1982, **57** 814–815.

25 Perkkio M *et al*. Morphometric and immunohisto-chemical study of jejunal biopsies from children with intestinal soy allergy. *European J Pediatr*, 1981, **137** 63–69.

26 Hathaway MJ, Warner JO Compliance problems in the dietary management of eczema. *Arch Dis Childh*, 1983, **58** 463–464.

27 Sampson A *et al*. Fatal and near fatal anaphylactic reaction to food in children and adolescents. *N Eng J Med*, 1992, **Aug** 380–384.

28 David TJ Anaphylactic shock and elimination diets for severe atopic eczema. *Arch Dis Childh*, 1984, **59** 983–986.

29 Devlin J *et al*. Calcium intake and elimination diets for severe atopic eczema. *Arch Dis Childh*, 1989, **64** 1183–1193.

30 Edwards AM Diet and sodium cromoglycate in the management of food allergic disorders. *Proceedings of the Second Food Allergy Workshop 1983*. Oxford: The Medicine Publ Foundation, 1983: 95–97.

31 Sampson HA Role of immediate food hypersensitivity in the pathogenesis of atopic dermatitis. *J All and Clin Immunol*, 1983, **71** 473.

32 Alun Jones V *et al*. Food intolerance: a major factor in the pathogenesis of irritable bowel syndrome. *Lancet*, 1982, **2** 1115–1117.

33 Pearson D *et al*. Food allergy. How much in the mind? *Lancet*, 1983, June, 1259–1261.

34 Bentley S *et al*. Food hypersensitivity in irritable bowel syndrome. *Lancet*, 1983, Aug, 295–297.

35 McLaughlin P *et al*. Effect of heat on the anaphylactic sensitising capacity of cows milk, goats milk and various infant formulae fed to guinea pigs. *Arch Dis Childh*, 1981, **56** 165–171.

36 David TJ *et al*. Nutritional hazards of elimination diets in children with atopic eczema. *Arch Dis Childh*, 1984, **59** 323–325.

37 David TJ The overworked or fraudulent diagnosis of food allergy and food intolerance in children. *J R Soc Med*, 1985, **78**(Suppl 5) 21–30.

38 Warner JO, Hathaway MJ Allergic form of Meadows syndrome (Munchausen by proxy). *Arch Dis Childh*, 1984 **59** 151–156.

39 Atherton DJ Diet and atopic eczema. *Clinical Allergy*, 1988, **18** 215–228.

40 David TJ. Dietary treatment of atopic eczema. *Arch Dis Childh*, 1989, **64** 1506–1509.

41 Taylor E Toxins and allergens. In: Rutter M, Casaer P (eds.) *Biological Risk Factors for Psychosocial Disorders*. New York: Academic Press, 1992.

42 Kaplan BJ *et al*. Dietary replacement in preschool-aged hyperactive boys. *Pediatrics*, 1989, **83** 7–17.

43 Darlington LG *et al*. Placebo-controlled, blind study of dietary manipulation therapy in rheumatoid arthritis. *Lancet*, 1986, **1** 236–238.

44 Cant AJ Diet and prevention of childhood allergic disease. *Human Nutr: Appl Nutr*, 1984, **38A** 455–468.

45 Zeiger RS *et al*. Effectiveness of dietary manipulation in the prevention of food allergy in infants. *J Allergy Clin Immunol*, 1981, **78** 224–238.

46 Cant AJ, Bailes JA How should we feed the potentially allergic infant? *Human Nutr: Appl Nutr*, 1984, **38A** 474–476.

HIV and AIDS

47 Center for Disease Control Classification system for IIIV infection in children under 13 years of age. *MMWR*, 1987, **36** 225–230.

48 Public Health Laboratory Service AIDS & HIV-1 antibody reports – United Kingdom. *Communicable Disease Review*, 1992, **2**(12) 55–56.

49 Kotler DP Diarrhoea in AIDS: diagnosis and management. *Medical Times*, 1989, **177**(3) 101–108.

50 Kotler DP Body cell mass repletion during Ganciclovir treatment of CMV infections in patients with AIDS. *Arch Intern Med*, 1989, **149** 901–905.

51 Epstein CG *et al*. Neurological manifestations of HIV. *Pediatrics*, 1986, **78** 678–687.

52 Kotler DP, Gaety HP Enteropathy associated with the acquired immunodeficiency syndrome. *Ann Intern Med*, 1984, **101** 421.

53 Bentler M, Stanish M Nutritional support of pediatric patients with AIDS. *J Am Diet Ass*, 1987, **87**(4) 488–491.

54 European Collaborative Study Risk factors for mother-to-child of HIV-1. *Lancet*, 1992, **339** 1007–1012.

55 Global Programme on AIDS. Consensus statement from the WHO/UNICEF consultation on HIV transmission and breast feeding. *Weekly Epidemiol Rec*, 1992, **67** 177–184.

56 Pizzo PA *et al*. Effect of continuous intravenous infusion of zidovudine (AZT) in children with symptomatic HIV infection. *N Eng J Med*, 1988, **319** 889–896.

57 Bristol-Myers USA *Videx (Didanosine): Full Prescribing Information*.

58 Wharton JM Trimethoprin-sulfamethoxazole or pentamidine for *pneumocystis carinii* pneumonia in the acquired immunodeficiency syndrome. *Ann Intern Med*, 1986, **105** 37–44.

59 Pearson RD, Hewlett EL Pentamidine for the treatment of pneumocystis carinii pneumonia and other protozoal diseases. *Ann Intern Med*, 1985, **105** 782–786.

60 Anderson R Adverse reactions associated with pentamidine isethionate in AIDS patients: recommendations for maintaining therapy. *Drug Intel Clin Pharm*, 1986, **20** 862–868.

61 Sugar AM, Saunders C Oral fluconazole as suppressive therapy of disseminated cryptococcus in patients with acquired immunodeficiency syndrome. *Am J Med*, 1988, **85** 481–489.

62 Lake-Bakaar G Gastropathy and ketoconazole malabsorption in the acquired immunodeficiency syndrome (AIDS). *Ann Intern Med*, 1988, **109** 502–504.

SCID

63 Ryser O, Moreel A, Hitzig WH Primary immunodeficiencies in Switzerland: first report of the national registry in adults and children. *J Clin Immunol*, 1988, 479–488.

64 Fischer AMD, Griscelli CMD Severe combined immunodeficiencies. *Current Opinion in Pediatrics*, 1990, **2** 920–925.

FURTHER READING

Brostoff J, Challacombe SJ (eds.) *Food Allergy and Intolerance*. London: Baillière Tindal, 1987.

Downing D, Davies S 'Allergy: Conventional and Alternative Concepts.' A Critique of the Royal College of Physicians of London's Report. *J Nutr Med*, 1992, **3** 331–349.

Royal College of Physicians of London Committee on Clinical Immunology and Allergy. *Allergy: Conventional and Alternative Concepts*. Report of the Committee. London: Royal College of Physicians, April 1982.

CHAPTER 14

Ketogenic Diet for Epilepsy

Epilepsy is a common disorder which is a symptom of cerebral dysfunction; it is classified according to the type of manifestations produced, but these categories should not be regarded as separate disease entities. A convusion or other epileptic manifestation is thought to occur when there is a sudden disorganized discharge of electrical activity from a group of neurones producing symptoms ranging from sensory abnormalities to convulsive movements and unconsciousness. In children it presents typically as myoclonic epilepsy (massive violent muscular contractions that can co-exist with other types of fits). Drug therapy is often difficult.

THE KETOGENIC DIET

The ketogenic diet was first used as a treatment in 1921 [1]. It aims to mimic the effects of fasting, using fat as the major energy source leading to the production of ketone bodies. It is effective for myoclonic, focal and temporal lobe epilepsy. The exact mode of action has still to be elucidated [2,3].

The ketogenic diet is often the last line of treatment for children with intractable epilepsy. When high levels of anticonvulsants have proved unsuccessful the ketogenic diet can provide an alternative, or it can be used with a prescribed drug regimen. A ketogenic diet may also be useful if anticonvulsant drugs cause unpleasant side effects [4].

CRITERIA FOR PATIENT SELECTION

The diet appears to be most succesful in children with myoclonic epilepsy, major motor epilepsy (grand mal) and minor motor epilepsy. Children aged from 6 months to 16 years have been shown to be receptive to

this type of treatment, although greater success has been described in the younger age range [5].

The regimen is a difficult one and the implications of the diet should be explained to parents; there must be considerable committment from the parents and the dietitian, and parents should express a willingness to co-operate before the diet is constructed. This diet should be commenced in hospital with appropriate monitoring and teaching and usually requires an admission of up to five days.

PRACTICAL MANAGEMENT

(1) A diet history should be taken to obtain meal patterns, food preferences and current energy intake. Very fussy eaters are unlikely to be able to comply with the dietary restrictions, as are children who dislike fatty foods.

(2) Details of current fluid intake should be sought; a high intake (more than 1–1.5l daily) is contraindicated on this regimen.

(3) It is often advisable to begin with a short fast (about 12 hours) before commencing the diet, so that ketosis is more readily achieved.

(4) Restricted foods both in the hospital and at home should be weighed.

(5) No sweet foods or sugar are allowed.

(6) No foods other than those on the diet sheet are allowed.

(7) Unrestricted foods are listed in Table 14.1. Sufficient unrestricted foods must be available within the diet to provide bulk and alleviate hunger.

Table 14.1 Unrestricted foods in ketogenic diets

Drinks	Tea and coffee (no milk or sugar), sugar-free drinks, diabetic squash, mineral water **Do not use drinks containing sugar, glucose or fructose**
Salad vegetables	Celery, chicory, cucumber, lettuce, spring onion, tomato, watercress
Green vegetables	Broccoli, brussel sprouts, cabbage, carrots, cauliflower, courgettes, green and runner beans, leeks, marrow, mushrooms, onions, peppers, spinach **Potato, peas, beans and lentils are restricted**
Fruit	Rhubarb, stewed without sugar
Flavourings	Salt, pepper, herbs, spices, vinegar, oil and vinegar dressing, beef extracts, yeast extract, Worcester sauce, food essences and colourings, gelatine and sugar-free jelly
Artificial sweeteners	Aspartame and saccharine based sweeteners **Do not use sweeteners containing sucrose, glucose, lactose or fructose**

(8) The fat intake should be spread fairly evenly throughout the day; this is particularly important if a special milk is used.

(9) Snacks in between meals should be discouraged as they impair ketone production.

(10) In regimes using medium chain triglyceride (MCT) emulsion (Liquigen Table 1.6) the Liquigen should be diluted with at least an equal volume of other fluid.

(11) MCT should be introduced gradually to avoid abdominal discomfort and diarrhoea. In small children this may be in 5–10 g (10–20 ml Liquigen) increments. Older children may tolerate a more rapid introduction, giving one quarter strength feeds on day 1, half strengh on day 2, three quarters on day 3 and full strength on day 4.

(12) A full vitamin and mineral supplement (e.g. Forceval Junior Capsules plus calcium) must be given to ensure that nutritional requirements are met.

(13) All medicines and tablets should be carbohydrate free.

WHICH KETOGENIC DIET?

The same principle is common to all regimens, in that they are high in fat, low in protein and carbohydrate. All calculations are based on the child's actual body weight unless the child is obese, when it may be preferable to use the ideal weight for height to prevent exacerbation of the obesity [6].

Three types of diet can be used:

- the 4:1 classical ketogenic diet
- medium chain triglyceride diet
- John Radcliffe diet and GOS diet.

Classical ketogenic diet

This diet is reported to give the most favourable results, but it is very restrictive and requires a large amount of dietetic involvement in terms of calculations, monitoring, patient support and motivation of the family to adhere to the diet [7]. The diet contains a ratio of 4 g fat to each 1 g protein and carbohydrate combined; in children under the age of 18 months a ratio of 3:1 may be used. Children on this diet are unlikely to achieve a normal height or weight velocity, although there will be a compensatory growth spurt when the diet is discontinued. The dietary energy content is 75 kcal/kg and the protein content is 1 g/kg body weight.

Calculation of daily amounts

If the patient's weight is W kg then:

$$\text{Energy content (kcal)} = 75 \times W$$

4:1 ratio
$$\text{Fat content (g)} = 7.5 \times W$$
$$\text{Protein content (g)} = W$$
$$\text{Carbohydrate content (g)} = 0.875 \times W$$

3:1 ratio
$$\text{Fat content (g)} = 7.25^* \times W$$
$$\text{Protein content (g)} = W$$
$$\text{Carbohydrate content (g)} = 1.44^* W$$

* rounded to two decimal places

Table 14.2 Example of a calculation of a 4:1 classical ketogenic diet for a patient of weight (*W*) 31.4 kg

Nutrient	Quantity per day	Quantity per meal (daily amount ÷ 3)
Energy	75 *W* kcal = 75 × 31.4 = 2355 kcal	
Fat	7.5 *W* g = 7.5 × 31.4 = 235.5 g	78.5 g
Protein	*W* g = 31.4 g	10.5 g
Carbohydrate	⅞ *W* g = $\frac{7 \times 31.4}{8}$ = 27.5 g	9.2 g

Construction of the diet

- When the quantity of protein, fat and carbohydrate has been calculated the totals are divided into three to give the amounts for each meal (see Table 14.2).
- Meals are calculated which provide the necessary proportions of protein, fat and carbohydrate.
- To provide variation in the diet other 'whole' meals can be calculated which contain the required amounts of nutrients and one whole meal can be exchanged for any other whole meal.
- 10 ml double cream or 10 ml Calogen (Table 1.6) can be utilized instead of 5 g fat within any whole meal if this is more palatable.

Medium chain triglyceride diet

Medium chain triglycerides (MCT) have been shown to be more effective at reducing fits in lower quantities than long chain fats. The MCT diet is calculated using the desired energy intake for the child's age and size.

Calculation of MCT diet

60% of total energy is derived from MCT; the remainder of the energy allowance can be distributed in two ways:

(1) 60:11:19:10 – MCT oil: (saturated fat: carbohydrate + protein).
(2) 60:40 – MCT oil: (saturated fat + carbohydrate + protein).

Construction of the diets

- Both of these diets are practically interpreted through the inclusion of a specific quantity of skimmed milk plus MCT oil in the form of Liquigen (MCT/water emulsion, SHS); the remainder of the diet is given in the form of exchanges.
- MCT oil is used for cooking.
- For the MCT 1 diet protein exchanges based on one egg (6 g protein + 6 g fat) or 50 g meat (12 g protein + 10 g fat) are used to ensure the correct amount of protein. Carbohydrate is regulated by a 10 g carbohydrate exchange system (Table 14.3).
- For the MCT 2 diet the 40% of the energy intake that is derived from protein, fat and carbohydrate is interpreted by 100 kcal exchanges (Table 14.4). It is important that 2–3 exchanges which include protein are taken.

Modification of these diets because of practical difficulties has resulted in the development of other regimens.

John Radcliffe diet

This is a variation of the MCT diet, but is easier to manage practically. The calculation is based on the daily energy intake required for the child, with 30% energy being provided from MCT and 30% from other fat which may be of vegetable or animal origin.

Calculation of daily amounts

Energy intake for the day should be apportioned as follows:

30:30:11:19:10 – MCT oil:double cream:fat from foods:carbohydrate:protein

Construction of the diet

- Skimmed milk is used as the medium for incorporating MCT oil or Liquigen into the diet and an allowance for this is made before calculating the rest of the diet.

Table 14.3 6 g protein and 10 g carbohydrate exchanges for ketogenic diets

6 g protein exchanges (each contains 6 g fat)	10 g carbohydrate exchanges
30 g meat	20 g wholemeal bread
40 g fish, white, fried in oil	10 g unsweetened breakfast cereal
50 g egg	15 g semi-sweet biscuit
30 g cheese, hard	20 g crisps
	50 g boiled potato
	25 g chips
	100 g apple or pear
	50 g banana
	100 ml natural orange juice

Table 14.4 15 g fat and 100 kcalorie exchanges for ketogenic diets

Each of the following contains 15 g fat	Each of the following contains 100 kcalories
20 g butter or margarine	150 ml whole cows' milk
15 ml oil	300 ml skimmed milk
30 ml double cream	25 g Chedddar-type hard cheese
2 egg yolks or 2 standard eggs	20 g Stilton or cream cheese
60 ml single cream	200 g natural yoghurt
20 ml mayonnaise (not salad cream)	60 g ham or gammon
	40 g cooked meat or bacon
	50 g chicken, turkey or veal
	20 g salami-type sausage
	30 g English sausage
	30 g beefburger
	100 g steamed/baked white fish
	50 g fatty fish
	40 g fried fish finger
	45 g bread
	30 g unsweetened breakfast cereal
	85 g cooked pasta
	80 g boiled rice
	125 g boiled potato
	85 g potato mashed with butter and milk
	115 g jacket potato with skin
	65 g roast potato
	40 g chips
	20 g crisps
	155 g baked beans in tomato sauce
	200 g eating apple
	125 g banana
	160 g grapes
	280 g orange
	250 ml natural orange juice
	270 g pear

- The amount of double cream required is calculated; 10 ml double cream can be exchanged for 5 g other fat (e.g. butter).
- Fat used in cooking is not included in the calculations provided the energy intake is not excessive.
- Protein foods are counted using 6 g protein exchanges (see Table 14.3); 6 g fat is assigned to each 30 g meat (1 protein exchange).
- Carbohydrate foods are counted using a 10 g exchange system (Table 14.3), avoiding high sugar foods or those with a significant protein content.
- If the total number of protein and/or carbohydrate exchanges are not consumed this is acceptable, provided the estimated protein requirement is met and weight loss does not occur.
- A combined protein and carbohydrate exchange can be calculated for foods that are not on the exchange list, allowing greater flexibility.

An example of the John Radcliffe diet is given in Table 14.5.

The Great Ormond Street diet

This is an alternative version of the MCT diet, based on fat and energy exchanges. The child's energy requirement is derived from 30% MCT, 30% long chain fat, counted as 15 g fat exchanges and 40% from other foods, counted as 100 kcal exchanges.

Construction of diet

The diet is composed of four parts:

- an allowance of Liquigen so that MCT = 30% energy intake
- 15 g fat exchanges = 30% energy intake (Table 14.4)
- 100 kcalorie exchanges = 40% energy intake (Table 14.4)
- free foods (Table 14.1).

The diluted Liquigen can be flavoured with artificial sweetener, coffee, tea, low calorie squash, spices (e.g. cinnamon), flavouring essencs (e.g. vanilla) or an allowance of skimmed milk can be calculated. Fat present in the calorie exchanges is not counted as part of the fat allowance.

An example of this type of diet is shown in Table 14.6.

Table 14.5 Example calculation of John Radcliffe diet, based on a desired intake of 1500 kcal

	Fat (g)	Protein (g)	Carbohydrate (g)
25 g skimmed milk powder	0.3	9.1	13.2
100 ml double cream	48.0	1.5	2.0
4 protein exchanges	24.0	24.0	0.0
5 carbohydrate exchanges	Tr	Tr	50.0
	24.3	34.6	65.2

MCT oil = 450 kcal = 50 ml MCT oil
From calculation:

MCT oil	= 50 ml × 8.3 (1 g MCT = 8.3 kcal)	= 450 kcal	= 30%
Fat from double cream	= 48.0 g × 9 (1 g fat = 9 kcal)	= 433.8 kcal	= 29%
Saturated fat	= 24.3 g × 9 (1 g fat = 9 kcal)	= 218.7 kcal	= 14.5%
Protein	= 34.6 g × 4 (1 g protein = 4 kcal)	= 138.4 kcal	= 9.2%
Carbohydrate	= 65.2 g × 4 (1 g CHO = 4 kcal)	= 260.8 kcal	= 17.3%
		151.7 kcal	

Total daily intake in 24 hours from calculation

   4 protein exchanges
   5 carbohydrate exchanges
   25 g skimmed milk powder plus water to 250 ml
100 ml Liquigen
100 ml double cream or 50 ml double cream and
   25 g other fat (e.g. butter, margarine)

SPECIAL OCCASIONS

Diabetic foods are generally not allowed (with the exception of sugar-free drinks), as they make a significant energy contribution to the diet. Diabetic chocolate can be allowed very occasionally (e.g. Christmas, Easter, birthday) provided that only a small amount (30 g) is consumed on any one day. Sugar-free diabetic fruit gums can be used occasionally.

    Party suggestions include eclairs (without chocolate topping) filled with cream, sugar-free plain cake (sponge cake recipe omitting the sugar), jelly made with sugar-free squash and gelatine.

    If food taken on a special occasion exceeds the

Table 14.6 Great Ormond Street ketogenic diet

Estimated energy requirement – 1500 kcalories	
55 g MCT = 110 ml Liquigen (diluted to 220 ml with water)	= 457 kcal
3.5 × 15 g fat exchanges	= 473 kcal
6 × 100 kcal calorie exchanges	= 600 kcal
Total	= 1530 kcal

Breakfast	40 ml Liquigen drink	
	1 calorie exchange	– 30 g breakfast cereal
	1 fat exchange	– 60 ml single cream
Mid AM	40 ml Liquigen drink	
Lunch	40 ml Liquigen drink	
	2 calorie exchanges	– 50 g chicken
		– 115 g jacket potato
	1 fat exchange	– 20 g butter for potato
	free vegetables	– cauliflower
Mid PM	40 ml Liquigen drink	
Tea	40 ml Liquigen drink	
	2 calorie exchanges	– 155 g baked beans
		– 20 g crisps
	1 fat exchange	– 2 eggs, scrambled
	free vegetables	– tomatoes and mushrooms
Bedtime	20 ml Liquigen drink	
	1 calorie exchange	– 25 g bread
		– 60 g banana
	½ fat exchange	– 10 g butter

dietary allowances, it must be counterbalanced by the addition of extra cream or MCT.

KETOGENIC ENTERAL FEEDS

Enteral feeds should be based on the same total and percentage nutrient content as the oral diet.

    On the classical diet double cream or Calogen will form the basis of the feed; on regimens containing MCT, Liquigen will be used. Protein and carbohydrate can either be added using skimmed or whole milk, or separate protein and carbohydrate modules (e.g. Maxipro and glucose polymer). It is important that a complete vitamin, mineral and trace element supplement (e.g. Paediatric Seravit) is included in the feed.

ACUTE ILLNESS

Give frequent drinks of carbohydrate-free liquids (e.g. sugar-free lemonade) for 24–48 hours. If the child is ill for more than 24 hours then medical advice should be sought.

It is important that intravenous dextrose is not given unless absolutely essential, as it can provoke convulsions. A low blood sugar in itself is not an indication for intravenous dextrose.

It is usually necessary to stop the fat and/or the MCT for a short period of time, particularly if the child is vomiting. If the child is unwell but is able to eat, then use exchanges with smaller bulk. If the child is unable to eat, give drinks such as milk or unsweetened fruit juice but avoid concentrated sugary drinks, while remaining within exchanges.

Slowly restart protein and carbohydrate or calorie exchanges after 24 hours, beginning with one quarter of the normal allowances. Exchanges can be increased over the next four days. At the same time reintroduce fat/MCT. If Liquigen is used a half strength dilution should be given initially, building up to full strength over 2–3 days. Where diarrhoea is a problem it may be necessary to begin with one quarter strength and build up over 4–5 days.

MONITORING

The diet is monitored by regular testing of urinary ketone levels, the overall aim being to produce a ketone level in the region of 3.9–7.8 mmol/l. If an initial starvation period is not instigated prior to the commencement of the diet then testing for ketones should not be carried out until the diet has been followed for at least 10 days.

Testings should be undertaken twice a day; variations are usually seen with trace to small readings (1.5 mmol/l) in the morning and moderate (3.9 mmol/l) to large (7.8–15.7 mmol/l) in the afternoon. In babies where a specimen cannot be collected the test can be done on a wet nappy, although the result is less accurate. A record of ketone levels should be kept as they can be correlated with seizure patterns. A sudden fall in urinary ketones is often an indication of illness or the initial stages of an infection; ketones will reappear on recovery.

If ketone levels are low or absent then the following points need to be checked:

(1) That diet is being strictly adhered to – i.e. the prescribed number of foods is not exceeded, sweet or sugary foods are not being consumed, sugar-containing drugs have not been prescribed.
(2) The last intake of fat and/or MCT should not be consumed too early in the day – fat and MCT should be spread throughout the day; it may be neccessary to give fat/MCT immediately before sleep to achieve a positive morning result.
(3) Excess fluid should not be consumed – it may be neccessary to impose a daily restriction of 1000 ml total.

If none of these factors apply the diet needs to be adjusted and the carbohydrate content reduced, either by reducing carbohydrate or calorie exchanges.

DURATION AND DISCONTINUATION OF THE DIET

The diet should be followed for a minimum of three months, although insurmountable problems may result in its earlier cessation.

The diet is designed for children with intractable epilepsy and should not be considered a diet for life. The optimum duration of the diet is unknown and often the duration will be self-determined by the level of compliance. Research has shown any period between six months and four years as being of benefit to the child.

If the diet is continued for more than a few months it is necessary to re-evalute energy and nutrient requirements regularly (six monthly) and to adjust the diet accordingly. Anticonvulsant therapy may have been reduced during the period of the diet and the family may be reluctant to relax the diet.

When the decision is made to discontinue it is imperative that the dietary restrictions be released slowly over a 5–10 day period; the length of time taken should be determined by the length of time the child has been on the diet. A sudden increase in dietary carbohydrate or a drop in ketone levels can precipitate seizures and this is potentially dangerous.

The following steps to relax the diet are suggested:

- reduce fat by 5 g (10 ml emulsion) each day until normal levels are reached
- increase protein until normal size portions are reached
- introduce unrestricted cows' milk after seven days

- introduce increased quantities of carbohydrate foods after seven days, avoiding concentrated sugars

If at any stage the seizures reappear or become more severe, food consumption should revert to a stage where control was acceptable. Once the child is stable the relaxation of the diet should be resumed at a slower rate.

CONCLUSION

Ketogenic diets have a valuable role to play in the control of seizures in children with intractable epilepsy. They are however, complex diets to institute and follow and must only be contemplated where close medical and dietetic supervision is available.

REFERENCES

1 Wilder RM The effects of ketonuria on the course of epilepsy. *Mayo Clin Bull*, 1921, **2** 307.
2 Schwartz R, Aynsley-Green A, Bower BD Clinical and metabolic aspects of ketogenic diets. *Res Clin Forums*, 1980, 2(2) 63–74.
3 Schwartz Ruby M, Boyes S, Aynsley-Green A Metabolic effects of three ketogenic diets in the treatment of severe epilepsy. *Developmental Med Child Neurol*, 1989, **31** 152–160.
4 Bower BD *et al.* The use of ketogenic diets in the treatment of epilepsy. *Topics in Perinatal Medicine*. London: Pitman, 1982.
5 Schwartz RH *et al.* Ketogenic diets in the treatment of epilepsy; short term clinical effects. *Developmental Med Child Neurol*, 1989, **31** 145–151.
6 Eaton J Epilepsy. In: Thomas B (ed.) *Manual of Dietetic Practice*. Oxford: Blackwell Scientific Publications, 1988: 489–497.
7 Livingston S Dietary treatment in epilepsy. In: *Comprehensive Management of Epilepsy in Infancy, Childhood and Adolescence*. Springfield: Charles C Thomas, 1977: III, 378–405.

Inborn Errors of Metabolism

CHAPTER 15

Disorders of Amino Acid Metabolism, Organic Acidaemias and Urea Cycle Defects

DISORDERS OF AMINO ACID METABOLISM

PHENYLKETONURIA

Phenylketonuria (PKU) is a group of recessively inherited disorders characterized by deficiency of the liver enzyme phenylalanine hydroxylase which is necessary for the breakdown of the essential amino acid phenylalanine to tyrosine (Fig. 15.1). Plasma phenylalanine concentrations rise while tyrosine levels are normal or low. Abnormal metabolites are excreted in the urine.

Classical PKU, where phenylalanine hydroxylase activity is very low or absent, was first described by Folling in 1934 [1]. Many different mutations of the phenylalanine hydroxylation gene have now been identified [2] which correlate with the degree of phenylalanine hydroxylase activity. On normal protein intakes of 2–3 g/kg body weight/day infants with classical PKU have plasma phenylalanine levels usually exceeding 1200 µmol/l; in milder forms, although the enzyme block is less complete, phenylalanine levels are persistently above 400 µmol/l. Untreated, classical PKU can cause mental retardation, seizures and defects in pigmentation [3,4].

Since 1968 all infants in the United Kingdom are screened for PKU between the 6th and 14th day of life using the Guthrie technique [5]. The incidence in the UK is 1 in 10 000 live births, whilst in Ireland there is a much greater incidence of 1 in 4500.

Some 1–2% of patients with PKU have a defect of pterin metabolism rather than phenylalanine hydroxylase deficiency [6]. Tetrahydrobiopterin (BH4) is required as a co-factor for the hydroxylation of phenylalanine, tyrosine and tryptophan (Fig. 15.1). There may be a defect in either the synthetic pathway or in recycling of BH4. Patients often present with hyperphenylalaninaemia in association with progres-sive neurological damage, due to deficiency of catecho-lamines and serotonin resulting from the impaired synthesis of L-dopa and 5-hydroxytryptophan. Treat-ment involves control of hyperphenylalaninaemia and correction of amine deficiency.

In addition, where there is a defect in recycling of BH4 due to a deficiency of dihydropteridine re-ductase, folate metabolism is impaired and folate supplementation is required [7]. The dietary treatment of pterin defects is similar to that of classical PKU, but a more generous intake of phenylalanine can be tolerated. It is standard practice in most centres to exclude a defect in pterin metabolism in infants with hyperphenylalaninaemia.

Principles of dietary management

PKU is treated by a low phenylalanine diet which should be introduced as early as possible, certainly by 20 days of life. Dietary phenylalanine intake is reduced so that phenylalanine concentration can fall within the plasma reference range of 120–360 µmol/l. Phenylalanine is an essential amino acid and should not be completely removed from the diet for any length of time. The formation of tyrosine from phenylalanine is severely limited and an adequate dietary intake must be supplied, 100–120 mg/kg body weight/day is recommended [8].

In order to achieve optimal control children with classical PKU need to avoid foods of high phenylalanine content such as meat, fish, cheese, eggs, nuts, textured vegetable protein and soya. Phenylalanine is provided in the diet by a measured intake of foods of a lower protein content such as cereals, potato and some vegetables. In the UK a

Clinical Paediatric Dietetics

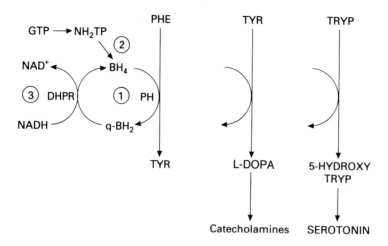

DHPR = Dihydropteridine reductase
PH = Phenylalanine hydroxylase
GTP = Guanosine triphosphate
NH₂TP = Dihydroneopterin triphosphate
BH₄ = Tetrahydrobiopterin
q-BH₂ = Quinoid-dihydrobiopterin
NAD = Nicotinamide adenine dinucleotide

1 Classical PKU
2 ⎫ Defects in tetrahydrobiopterin
3 ⎭ metabolism

From McLaren DS *et al.* (eds.) *Textbook of Paediatric Nutrition*, 3e. Edinburgh: Churchill Livingstone, 1991. By kind permission.

Fig. 15.1 Hydroxylation of phenylalanine (phe), tyrosine (tyr) and tryptophan (tryp)

system of 50 mg phenylalanine exchanges is used to measure these foods, i.e. the weight of food which provides 50 mg phenylalanine (Table 15.1). When phenylalanine analysis of foods is not available, 1 g protein is assumed to contain 50 mg phenylalanine.

Fruits and vegetables which have a very low phenylalanine content are traditionally taken without measurement (Table 15.2), but this practice is undergoing review. It is important to assess the contribution of these foods to the phenylalanine content of the diet in children with classical PKU. Other foods that have negligible phenylalanine content (such as sugar, sweetened drinks, butter, vegetable oils) are allowed freely, and are useful energy sources (Table 15.3). Manufactured low protein foods are essential for both provision of adequate energy and variety in the diet. These include bread, biscuits, flour, pasta. Most are approved by the Advisory Committee on Borderline Substances for prescription on FP10 (Table 15.4).

The diet must contain adequate protein for growth. The degree of restriction of phenylalanine needed to control phenylalanine levels within the safe range (120–360 μmol/l) limits the intake of natural protein to below minimum requirements for growth. A protein substitute free from phenylalanine, with added tyrosine, is essential. Generous quantities of the protein substitute are recommended both because of its synthetic nature and the competitive inhibition of phenylalanine transport across the blood brain barrier by other amino acids [9]. Guidelines for amino acid and protein requirement are provided in Table 15.5. The intake of protein substitute is divided evenly between main meals. A variety of products of differing composition are available (Table 15.6).

Phenylalanine restriction also limits the intake of most vitamins and minerals and a supplement becomes necessary. The nutritionally complete protein substitutes provide enough vitamins and minerals if taken in adequate quantities. Pure amino acid mixtures require full supplementation; 8 g Aminogran Mineral Mixture plus Ketovite, 3 tablets and 5 ml liquid, is commonly used. Paediatric Seravit, or For-

Table 15.1 Basic list of 50 mg phenylalanine exchange foods for PKU or 1 g protein exchange foods for low protein diets

	Metric weight (g)
Cow & Gate Premium	90 ml (70 ml = 1 g protein)
SMA Gold/Farley's First Milk/Aptamil	60 ml (65 ml = 1 g protein)
Cows' milk	30 ml
Single Cream	40 ml
Double Cream	60 ml
Vegetables	
Potatoes:	
raw	50
boiled	55
mashed and milk free	55
roast	35
chips	25
chips, frozen oven baked	30
tinned, new (drained contents)	65
baked, flesh and skin	25
baked, flesh only	45
crisps	15
Peas, frozen boiled	15
Petit pois, frozen boiled	20
Mange-tout peas, boiled	30
Brussel sprouts, boiled	35
Brussel sprouts, frozen boiled	30
Broccoli tops, boiled	30
Spinach, boiled	45
Sweetcorn kernels and baby corn, drained canned	35
Asparagus	60
Sweet potato, boiled	40
Yam, boiled	60
Parsnip, boiled	65
Heinz baked beans in tomato sauce	20
Banana, raw without skin	100
Cereals	
Cornflakes, Weetaflakes	10
Rice Krispies	15
Frosties	20
Sugar Puffs	15
Weetabix	10
Shredded Wheat	10
Ready Brek	10
Oatmeal (raw) and rolled oats	10
Rice (raw) white or brown	15
Rice (boiled) white or brown	45
Farley's Rusk	15

Weight of food given is equal to 50 mg phenylalanine. Foods should be weighed after cooking unless otherwise stated

Table 15.2 Fruits and vegetables of negligible protein content

Fruit

Angelica	Guavas	Passion fruit
Apples	Kiwi fruit	Paw paw
Apricots (not dried)	Kumquats	Peaches (not dried)
Bilberries	Lemons	Pears
Blackberries	Limes	Pineapple
Cherries	Loganberries	Plums
Clementines	Lychees	Pomegranate
Cranberries	Mandarins	Quince
Currants	Mango	Raisins
Damsons	Medlars	Raspberries
Figs (not dried)	Melons (all types)	Rhubarb
Fruit Salad	Mulberries	Strawberries
Gooseberries	Mixed peel	Sultanas
Grapes	Nectarines	Tangerines
Grapefruit	Olives	
Greengages	Oranges	

Vegetables

Artichoke	Courgette	Onion
Aubergine	Cucumber	Parsley
Beans (French/green)	Endive	Peppers (red and green)
Beansprouts	Fennel	Pumpkin
Cabbage	Gherkin	Radish
Capers	Ladies fingers	Spring greens
Carrots	Leek	Swede
Cauliflower	Lettuce	Tomato
Celeriac	Marrow	Turnip
Celery	Mushrooms	Watercress
Chicory	Mustard and cress	

ceval Junior Capsules together with a calcium supplement, are good alternatives.

Foods which contain the artificial sweetener aspartame (Nutrasweet) – such as fizzy drinks, squashes, desserts and the table top sweetener Canderel – must be avoided as aspartame is derived from a dipeptide composed of phenylalanine and the methyl ester of aspartic acid.

Newly diagnosed infant with PKU

If on routine screening blood phenylalanine levels exceed 400 µmol/l a quantitative estimation of plasma phenylalanine is performed to confirm a diagnosis of PKU. The dietary treatment will depend on this plasma phenylalanine concentration. Infants whose blood phenylalanine concentrations exceed 600 µmol/l in the presence of a normal or low plasma tyrosine, whilst receiving a normal protein intake (2–

Table 15.3 Foods of negligible protein content

Fats	Butter
	Margarine
	Lard, dripping, solid vegetable fat
	Vegetable oils
Sugar and starches	Cornflour, custard powder, sago, tapioca
	Vegetarian jelly, agar agar
	Sugar, glucose
	Jam, honey, marmalade, golden syrup, treacle
	Boiled sweets
Drinks	Flavoured fizzy drinks e.g. Lucozade, lemonade, Coca Cola
	Squash, cordials, Ribena
	Fruit juice
	Tonic water, soda water, mineral water
Miscellaneous	Salt, pepper, herbs, spices, pure mustard powder, vinegar
	Baking powder, bicarbonate of soda, cream of tartar
	Food essences and colourings
	Tea, coffee
Manufactured foods	(see Table 15.4)

Table 15.4 Low protein manufactured products

Food item	Manufacturer
Breads	
Juvela – vacuum packed	Scientific Hospital Supplies
Loprofin – vacuum packed – canned	Nutricia Dietary Products
Ultra – canned, white	Ultrapharm
Flour	
Aproten	Ultrapharm
Ultra	Ultrapharm
Tritamyl	Procea
Mixes	
Aproten – cake – bread	Ultrapharm
Juvela	Scientific Hospital Supplies
Rite Diet – bread – cake	Nutricia Dietary Products
Loprofin	Nutricia Dietary Products
Biscuits	
Aproten – crispbread – sweet	Ultrapharm
Ultra – sweet	Ultrapharm
DP – cookies	Nutricia Dietary Products
Juvela – cookies	Scientific Hospital Supplies
Loprofin – wafers – cracker – cookies	Nutricia Dietary Products
Pasta	
Aproten – various shapes	Ultrapharm
Loprofin – various shapes	Nutricia Dietary Products
Rite Diet LP Spaghetti* (canned)	Nutricia Dietary Products
Rice	
Aglutella	Ultrapharm
Low protein milks (contain significant amount of phenylalanine)	
Milupa lpd	Milupa
Loprofin PKU Long Life	Nutricia Dietary Products
Sno Pro	Scientific Hospital Supplies
Egg replacers	
Loprofin Egg Replacer	Nutricia Dietary Products
Loprofin Egg White Replacer*	Nutricia Dietary Products
Ener-G Egg Replacer*	General Designs
Protein Free High Energy Bar	
Duobar	Scientific Hospital Supplies
Fat Products	
Calogen LCT Emulsion	Scientific Hospital Supplies
Duocal (liquid and powder)	Scientific Hospital Supplies

* Not prescribable

3 g/kg/day), should start a low phenylalanine diet. Infants whose phenylalanine levels are between 400–600 μmol/l require further monitoring before deciding whether or not dietary treatment is necessary.

If blood phenylalanine levels are between 600 and 1000 μmol/l, complement feeds of phenylalanine-free formula are given in addition to breastmilk or normal infant formula. If phenylalanine levels are greater than 1000 μmol/l, the phenylalanine source (whether breast milk or infant formula) is stopped for a short time to achieve a rapid fall in plasma phenylalanine level. A decrease of between 300 and 600 μmol/l per day is normal during this period. An infant formula free from phenylalanine must be given. Ideally plasma phenylalanine levels should be measured daily to monitor the rate of decrease and to prevent possible phenylalanine deficiency.

Following confirmation of diagnosis it is important that parents are counselled by a paediatrician and dietitian about the disease, genetics, prognosis and dietary treatment. Ideally children with PKU should be treated in centres that have special interest in metabolic disease.

Table 15.5 Guidelines for amino acid and protein requirements in classical PKU (per kg actual body weight)

Age in years	Supplement of amino acids (g)	Total protein and amino acids (g)
0–2	3	3 to 4
2–6	3 to 2	3.5 to 2.5
6–10	2 to 1.5	2.5 to 2.0
10–14	1.5 to 1	2 to 1.5
Over 14	1	1.5 to 1.0

Breastfeeding the infant with PKU

Whilst the infant is having only the phenylalanine-free formula, the breast feeding mother expresses to maintain lactation. Breast feeding is recommended when the phenylalanine level is less than 600 μmol/l. Table 15.7 provides guidelines for an initial breast feeding regimen.

Plasma phenylalanine levels are controlled by giving a measured volume of the phenylalanine-free formula before five to six breast feeds. The infant then breast feeds on demand. Any additional feeds required

throughout the 24 hours are breast feeds alone. For the first two weeks it may be necessary to do blood tests twice a week whilst phenylalanine levels are stabilizing. The volume of phenylalanine-free formula given is altered according to plasma levels of phenylalanine. If the plasma phenylalanine levels fall below 120 μmol/l the total volume of phenylalanine-free formula is reduced so that the infant will demand more breast milk. If plasma phenylalanine levels are above 360 μmol/l the volume of formula is increased (Table 15.8).

Introduction of solids to the breast fed infant

Solids are introduced at the usual time between 4 and 6 months of age. Phenylalanine-containing solids are introduced first. Initially one 50 mg phenylalanine exchange (e.g. 10 g Farex weaning food or 15 g Farley's rusk) is given before the feed, followed by the usual volume of phenylalanine-free formula. The baby can then breast feed to appetite. The quantity and range of 50 mg exchange foods is gradually increased and given before a second and third feed. If the infant still appears to be hungry after the breast feed, a few teaspoons of low phenylalanine puréed fruits and

Table 15.6 Low phenylalanine protein substitutes

Composition per 100 g	Amino acids (g)	Phenylalanine (mg)	Energy (kcal)	(kJ)	Carbohydrate (g)	Fat (g)
Infants						
XP Analog	15.5	Nil	462	1936	54	23
Lofenalac	15 (equivalent protein nitrogen × 6.25)	80	460	1930	59.6	18
Minafen*	12 (equivalent protein nitrogen × 6.25)	<20	509	2124	47.9	31
Children						
Albumaid XP*	40	<10	320	1350	50	Nil
Aminogran Food Supplement**	100	Nil	400	1675	Nil	Nil
XP Maxamaid	30	Nil	300	1260	51	<0.5
PK AID III**	93.2	Nil	326	1387	4	Nil
PKU2	80.1	Nil	298	1265	7.5	Nil
Phenyl-free	20	Nil	405	1710	66.0	6.8
Adolescence and pregnancy						
XP Maxamum	47	Nil	290	1226	34	<0.5
PKU 3	81.6	Nil	286	1214	3.4	Nil

* Needs vitamin supplement e.g. Ketovite 3 tablets plus 5 ml liquid
** Needs complete vitamin and mineral supplement e.g. Paediatric Seravit

Table 15.7 Initial breast feeding guidelines for infant with PKU

Initial phenylalanine level μmol/l (i)	Breast feeds	Phenylalanine-free formula
400 to 600	On demand	30 ml × 3
600 to 1000	On demand	30 ml × 5
1000 to 2000	Nil 1–3 days* On demand thereafter	150–200 ml/kg for 1–3 days thereafter 45 ml × 5
>2000	Nil 3–5 days* On demand thereafter	150–200 mls/kg for 3–5 days thereafter 60 ml × 5

(i) Quantitative plasma phenylalanine for confirmation of diagnosis
* Mother expresses to maintain lactation

Table 15.8 Guide to blood phenylalanine monitoring of breast fed infants with PKU

Blood phenylalanine level μmol/l	Phenylalanine-free formula	Breast feeds
<120	Decrease by 75 ml (÷ 15 ml × 5)	On demand – baby should take more
120 to 360	No change	On demand
>360	Increase by 75 ml (÷ 15 ml × 5)	On demand – baby should take less

Table 15.9 Initial bottle feeding guidelines for infant with PKU

Initial phenylalanine level μmol/l	Infant formula	Phenylalanine-free formula
400 to 600	On demand	30 ml × 3
600 to 1000	50–70 mg phenylalanine/kg from infant formula	On demand
1000 to 2000	Nil 1–3 days thereafter 50 mg phenylalanine/ kg from infant formula	150–200 ml/kg for 1–3 days thereafter on demand
>2000	Nil 3–5 days thereafter 40–50 mg phenylalanine/kg from infant formula	150–200 ml/kg for 3–5 days thereafter on demand

Table 15.10 Guide to monitoring plasma phenylalanine of bottle fed infants with PKU

Phenylalanine level μmol/l	Infant formula	Phenylalanine-free formula
<60	Increase by 50–100 mg phenylalanine	On demand
60 to 120	Increase by 50 mg phenylalanine	On demand
120 to 360	No change	On demand
360 to 600	Decrease by 25–50 mg phenylalanine	On demand
>600	Decrease by 50–100 mg phenylalanine	On demand

vegetables can be given at the end of the feed. As the quantity of 50 mg exchange foods is increased, the intake of breastmilk naturally declines and eventually solid food will completely replace breast milk.

Bottle feeding the infant with PKU

When the plasma phenylalanine level has fallen to below 600 μmol/l phenylalanine is reintroduced to the diet as a whey-based infant formula. The quantity of infant formula given depends on the initial plasma phenylalanine level, usually starting with 40–70 mg phenylalanine per kg body weight. Table 15.9 gives guidelines on the initial feeding regimen. The pre-scription of infant formula is divided evenly between 5–6 feeds and fed first. Afterwards the phenylalanine-free formula is given to appetite, and at any susequent feeds the baby demands. An alternative is to mix both formulas together, but the infant must then take the full volume of feed to ensure that all the prescribed phenylalanine is given.

The quantity of infant formula is altered according to the plasma phenylalanine levels. If plasma phenyla-lanine levels are less than 120 μmol/l the infant for-mula is increased; when greater than 360 μmol/l, it is decreased (Table 15.10).

Introduction of solids to the bottle fed infant

The first solids offered contain negligible phenyla-lanine e.g. puréed fruit such as apple or crushed low protein biscuits mixed with cooled, boiled water to a smooth paste. A few teaspoons are introduced after the bottle feeds to appetite. Once the infant is happily taking solids, a 50 mg phenylalanine exchange of food is given before the bottle feeds to replace one exchange of formula milk. Gradually all formula milk is replaced with solid food.

Administration of protein substitute

Between five and six months of age, whether breast or bottle fed, the infant requires additional amino acids as the contribution of amino acids from the phenylalanine-free formula declines. Aminogran (10 g Food Supplement and 2.7 g Minerals, dispensed in handy scoop measures) is mixed with either water and milk shake flavouring or concentrated fruit juice to make a smooth paste. The paste is fed from a spoon, initially one teaspoon is given before a feed once a day. The infant is praised and never forced to take this unpalatable preparation. The quantity given is gradually increased to one teaspoon three times per day. A drink is given at the same time to dilute this hyperosmolar mixture. Current practice is to provide 3 g amino acids per kg body weight per day for the first two years of life [8]. As the volume of phenylalanine-free formula declines, the quantity of Aminogran is increased to provide the amino acid requirements (Table 15.5). If insufficient Aminogran is taken from the spoon, it can be added to the bottle of phenylalanine-free formula. Complete vitamin supplementation (Ketovite – 5 ml liquid plus three tablets) is necessary when the infant is having less than 450 ml of the phenylalanine-free formula.

A fluoride supplement should be given at this age if the local water supply is not fluoridated, because the high sugar content of the diet increases the risk of dental caries.

As the infant matures it is important to introduce new consistencies and flavours to the diet, progressing from smooth purées to mashed and chopped foods. Finger foods should be introduced at about 8 months of age. Suitable finger foods include low protein biscuits or pieces of low protein fruit and vegetables. Table 15.11 provides a sample menu for a 7–9 month old infant.

Between one and two years bottle feeding will probably cease. In classical PKU the average daily number of 50 mg phenylalanine exchanges tolerated is between three and five and this is unlikely to change except during periods of rapid growth when protein requirements are increased. The exchanges are evenly distributed throughout the day between main meals to minimize fluctuations in plasma phenylalanine concentrations.

As the child grows the protein substitute is increased to provide amino acid requirements appropriate for age (Table 15.5). From one year an alternative protein substitute, XP Maxamaid, can be used. It contains

Table 15.11 Sample menu for infant aged 7–9 months with classical PKU

On waking	Phenylalanine-free formula e.g. XP Analog
Breakfast	2–3 teaspoons Aminogran Food Supplement + minerals 1 × 50 mg phenylalanine exchange e.g. 10 g Weetabix plus protein-free milk* Phenylalanine-free formula e.g. XP Analog Low protein bread and butter as finger food
Lunch	2–3 teaspoons Aminogran Food Supplement + minerals 1 × 50 mg phenylalanine exchange e.g. 55 g puréed potato plus puréed vegetable Cooled, boiled water or diluted fruit juice Aproten biscuit or piece of peeled apple to chew
Tea time	2–3 teaspoons Aminogran Food Supplement + minerals 1 × 50 mg phenylalanine exchange e.g. 1 Farley's rusk Phenylalanine-free formula e.g. XP Analog Puréed fruit and low protein custard
Bedtime	Breast feed or measured infant formula Phenylalanine-free formula e.g. XP Analog

Expected Daily Intake: 600–700 ml Analog XP
               (10 g Aminogran Food Supplement)
               (2.7 g Aminogran Mineral Mixture)

* Protein-free milk = 10 ml Calogen
             1 teaspoon sugar
             100 ml water

added carbohydrate, vitamins and minerals and is usually given as a drink. XP Maxamaid contributes to the energy content of the diet much more significantly than Aminogran does when providing the same quantity of amino acids. Not more than 150 g/day should be prescribed because of the possible toxic doses of Vitamin A this would provide. From eight years of age XP Maxamum, which has a higher protein to energy ratio, can be used.

School meals

For the child at school, it is best to suggest a packed lunch as not many schools can cope with such a complicated diet. The packed lunch should include 50 mg phenylalanine exchange foods and energy-giving foods which contain negligible phenylalanine. It is also very important to encourage the child to take his protein substitute at school with the meal. The school needs to understand the importance of the low phenylalanine diet; the National Society for Phenylketonuria produces some good information leaflets for teachers.

Monitoring the diet

Blood for phenylalanine measurement should be taken at a set time (ideally early morning when concentrations are likely to be at a peak following the overnight fast). Analysis by fluorimetry or High Performance Liquid Chromatography (HPLC) is preferable because of its greater accuracy, although many centres still use the Guthrie technique. Frequent blood tests are essential as plasma phenylalanine levels fluctuate so necessitating dietary changes.

After stabilization the blood tests for phenylalanine levels are taken weekly until at least four years of age. Between the ages of four and ten years the frequency of monitoring can be reduced to fortnightly and thereafter monthly, because blood phenylalanine levels are more stable as growth becomes less rapid. Parents should be contacted with the results as soon as possible by telephone and the diet adjusted accordingly. A guide to interpretation of phenylalanine levels is given in Table 15.12. High phenylalanine levels may result from:

- catabolism caused by infection, accidents or surgery
- inadequate intake of other essential amino acids and/or energy
- dietary indiscretion and food pilfering
- reduced requirement in association with reduced growth rate.

It is important to establish the cause of the changes in phenylalanine levels because it may be inappropriate to alter the diet.

Low phenylalanine levels may result from:

- a growth spurt, e.g. puberty; at times of rapid growth phenylalanine requirements will increase
- anabolic phase, following an intercurrent infection
- inadequate intake because of food refusal or misunderstandings about the diet.

Table 15.12 Adjustment of dietary phenylalanine against plasma levels

Plasma phenylalanine level μmol/l	50 mg phenylalanine exchanges
<60	Increase by 1–2
60–120	Increase by 1
120–360	No change
360–600	Decrease by ½
>600	Decrease by 1

Inadequate intake of phenylalanine, especially in infants, results in a skin rash (commonly seen around the nappy area) and growth failure. Phenylalanine intake needs to be increased immediately.

Dietary problems

Food refusal

Food refusal can be extremely difficult to manage. It is important that it is identified and dealt with in the early stages of development. Children are often very conservative in their food choices and so it is important that they are offered phenylalanine exchanges and foods that they like. If these exchanges are refused they need to be replaced later in the day. Milk is often a simple and acceptable alternative. The child must never be force fed.

Refusal of protein substitute is a common problem. Again, the child should not be forced because this could result in long term aversion. It may be beneficial to alter flavourings or offer the protein substitute at a different time during the meal. A smaller dose of protein substitute may be offered for a while and then the dose can gradually increase as the child comes to accept it. Occasionally an alternative product may be tried. If unsuccessful, a period in hospital may be necessary where trained professionals can initiate a praise and reward scheme appropriate for the child's age; this is often very successful. In the short term inadequate intakes of protein substitute can be tolerated, but with time severe nutritional deficiencies and poor growth will result.

Parents should receive adequate support to alleviate any anxiety.

Illness

During illness loss of appetite is common and combined with infection results in raised plasma phenylalanine levels. Frequent high carbohydrate drinks (e.g. glucose polymer solution, Lucozade, squash) should be encouraged. Oral rehydration solutions supplemented with glucose polymer may be indicated during gastroenteritis.

Phenylalanine exchanges can be omitted for 1–2 days, and then gradually reintroduced as the child's appetite increases. Monitoring of blood phenylalanine level is helpful in determining when phenylalanine should be reintroduced. Close monitoring of phenylalanine levels during the recovery phase to prevent persistent low levels is vital. Ideally, the protein substitute should not be discontinued. It is recognized that this may not always be possible, however a small amount taken is better than none. The full dose should be re-established as soon as possible. Medication appropriate to the intercurrent illness should be prescribed.

The child should never be forced to take either the protein substitute or exchanges during an intercurrent illness as this may lead to long term food aversion.

Adolescence

There is still some controversy amongst PKU specialist centres in the UK as to whether it is necessary to continue the low phenylalanine diet into adulthood. By adolescence the anatomical and functional development of the nervous system is nearly complete. It was previously assumed therefore that phenylalanine restriction at this age could be safely abandoned. However, numerous workers have now demonstrated that performance in neuropsychological tests of higher integrative function is impaired after diet is discontinued, especially when blood phenylalanine values exceed 1200 μmol/l [10–13]. Patients may complain of lack of concentration. Some may have brisk deep tendon reflexes and frequently a mild degree of intention tremor [8]. More severe neurological problems have also been reported [14]. The advent of magnetic resonance imaging (MRI) has revealed abnormalities of white matter composition in the periventricular regions of the brain, even in 'optimally controlled' patients [15,16]. It would therefore seem prudent to advise continuation of the low phenylalanine diet into adulthood, maintaining phenylalanine levels, where possible, of less than 700 μmol/l.

Compliance with the diet can deteriorate during adolescence because it distinguishes the adolescent with PKU from his friends [17]. In order to achieve good biochemical control, continuation of a strict dietary regimen is necessary. The majority find the protein substitutes unpalatable and the selection of low protein foods unappetizing. Adolescents may find it difficult to admit they have PKU and any social engagement involving food could cause embarrassment. It is important that adolescents maintain contact with a specialist PKU clinic which can provide them with adequate support and current research and opinions.

Pregnancy

It is essential that teenage girls are educated about the need to be on a strict low phenylalanine diet prior to conception because high maternal phenylalanine levels carry a risk to the fetus [18]. The concentration gradient across the human placenta results in the fetus being exposed to phenylalanine concentrations approximately twice those in maternal plasma [19]. The adverse effects to the infant include mental retardation, microcephaly, congenital heart disease and low birth weight [20].

It may be necessary to admit the patient to hospital to re-establish the diet if it has been discontinued for many years. This will also provide the opportunity for explanation about the diet, practising of low protein cooking with manufactured products and teaching of blood sample collection for home. The aim of dietary treatment is to maintain the pregnant woman's plasma phenylalanine levels between 120–240 μmol/l. In classical PKU during pregnancy the mother's phenylalanine intake is reduced to 3–7 exchanges per day. However tolerance increases after about 20 weeks gestation to between 30 and 35 exchanges because the fetus is growing rapidly and phenylalanine hydroxylase activity is developing in the fetal liver. Initially a daily intake of 70 g of phenylalanine-free amino acids from XP Maxamum is given [18]. Additional tyrosine is usually required from about 18 weeks gestation to provide a total intake of 8 g daily. Blood tests are taken twice a week throughout pregnancy to monitor plasma phenylalanine and tyrosine levels.

With good dietary management of the PKU mother, early indications suggest a normal outcome for the infant [18].

MAPLE SYRUP URINE DISEASE

Maple syrup urine disease (MSUD) is caused by a deficiency of branched-chain 2-ketoacid dehydrogenase enzyme complex (Fig. 15.2). This results in accumulation of the three essential branch chain amino acids leucine, isoleucine and valine and their respective ketoacids in plasma and urine. Leucine and 2-oxo isocaproate are thought to be the main toxic metabolites and responsible for irreversible neurological impairment.

MSUD can be classified clinically into three types [21].

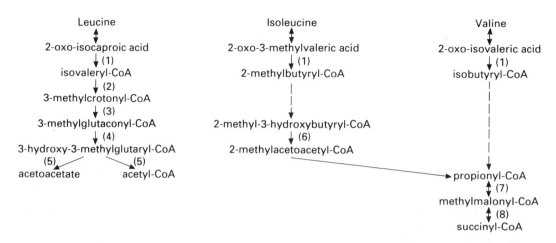

(1) Maple syrup urine disease

(2) Isovaleric acidaemia

(3) 3-methylcrotonyl-CoA carboxylase deficiency

(4) 3-methylglutaconyl-CoA hydratase deficiency

(5) 3-hydroxy-3-methylglutaryl-CoA lyase deficiency

(6) 2-methylacetoacetyl-CoA thiolase deficiency

(7) Propionic acidaemia

(8) Methylmalonic acidaemia

Fig. 15.2 Selected inborn errors of the catabolic pathways of branch chain amino acids

Classical MSUD These patients present within a few days of life; there is progressive and overwhelming illness with poor feeding, lethargy and seizures leading to coma. The main problem is toxic encephalopathy with varied signs including irritability, changes in tone and full fontanelle. Patients may have a marked metabolic acidosis. The characteristic smell of maple syrup in the urine may be present. Plasma leucine levels are grossly elevated, ranging from $1000-5000 \, \mu mol/l$ (normal reference range $65-220 \, \mu mol/l$). Untreated, patients may die and survivors are severely mentally and physically retarded.

Intermittent MSUD In this variant disorder patients are normally well between acute episodes which are usually precipitated by intercurrent infections or high dietary protein intake. Plasma branch chain amino acid levels are near normal between episodes with only a modest or no restriction of dietary leucine intake.

Thiamin responsive MSUD Thiamin is a cofactor in the branched-chain 2-ketoacid dehydrogenase reaction and occasionally patients may respond to the pharmacological doses of the vitamin. In general presentation is less severe than in non-thiamin responders. Although dietary treatment is required in addition to thiamin supplementation, the degree of dietary restriction is less severe than in the child with classical MSUD.

Dietary management of classical MSUD

Early diagnosis, combined with good long term metabolic control, is essential in minimizing neurological impairment and poor intellectual outcome in MSUD [22,23,24]. The aim of dietary treatment is to prevent accumulation of the branch chain amino acids (BCAA). Plasma branch chain amino acid levels are maintained slightly above the normal reference range to ensure an adequate rate of protein synthesis and prevention of protein deficiency. Recommendations for these are given in Table 15.13. Plasma leucine levels should, if possible, be maintained at the lower end of the recommended reference range as higher levels are associated with poorer intellectual outcome.

Plasma leucine is generally elevated much more so than isoleucine and valine. The diet is therefore based on leucine intake. The amount given is adjusted

Table 15.13 Recommendations for plasma branch chain amino acid levels in MSUD

	Aim (μmol/l)	Normal reference range (μmol/l)
Leucine	200–700	65–220
Isoleucine	100–400	26–100
Valine	100–400	90–300

according to plasma leucine levels. Leucine requirements per kg body weight decrease with increasing age.

Considerable interindividual variations of BCAA requirements are reported during the first few months of life [25]. Personal experience has shown leucine requirements to be around 100–110 mg/kg body weight/day in 2–3 month old infants, decreasing throughout the first year to around 40–50 mg/kg bodyweight/day. Most children with MSUD have leucine intakes between 400–600 mg per day.

Once a newly diagnosed infant is stabilized, there is little variation in the total leucine intake irrespective of age – except during growth spurts or occasionally after prolonged infections when there has been a reduced intake of leucine.

Leucine intake is measured by an exchange system, i.e. the weight of food which contains 50 mg leucine. Leucine is provided by a variety of low biological value protein foods such as potato, rice, cereals. The choice of foods to provide leucine is extremely limited due to the paucity of analyses of leucine content of foods, especially manufactured products. It is not possible to use the protein content of a food as an indicator of its leucine content as this is too variable and therefore unreliable (Table 15.14). Foods of a high biological value protein are usually avoided because their leucine content is so great. The leucine allowance is given throughout the day, at least three doses, to reduce fluctuations in plasma BCAA levels.

The dietary requirements of isoleucine and valine are lower than for leucine. The isoleucine and valine contents of foods are also always lower than their leucine content (Table 15.14). Normally the leucine exchange foods provide sufficient intakes of isoleucine and valine. However if plasma concentrations of isoleucine and/or valine fall too low, a supplement of these amino acids is essential to prevent them becoming the rate limiting step for protein synthesis. Isoleucine and valine are added to the diet as a solution of the pure l-amino acid, in a concentration of 100 mg of amino acid in 10 ml water. An initial

daily dose of 50–100 mg, divided into two to three doses, is given with the leucine exchanges. If isoleucine and valine levels remain low, the dose is increased according to plasma levels until isoleucine and valine levels fall within the recommended reference range.

Due to the severe restriction of leucine in the diet, the intake of natural protein is much less than that needed for normal growth requirements. It is therefore essential to give a supplement of amino acids free from the branch chain amino acids. Generous amounts of branch chain free amino acids are required because of their synthetic nature. This will also minimize disturbance of the flux of amino acids, particularly branch chain amino acids, across the blood brain barrier. The amino acid supplement intakes recommended for PKU are also used in MSUD (Table 15.5). A number of branch chain amino acid supplements of differing composition are available (Table 15.15). The supplement is given as a divided dose.

To ensure adequate protein synthesis and normal growth an adequate energy intake must be provided. Plasma BCAA levels will rise if insufficient dietary energy precipitates catabolism. Most children with MSUD eat well. However if oral intake is inadequate, nasogastric feeding is vital to prevent metabolic decompensation. Long periods of fasting are avoided, especially in infants, as plasma BCAAs increase on fasting. Dietary energy is provided by:

- foods naturally low in or free from leucine – fruits and vegetables (Table 15.16); sugar and fats (Table 15.3)
- specially manufactured low protein (low leucine) foods – bread, biscuits, pasta (Table 15.4)
- energy supplements – glucose polymers, fat emulsions.

Supplements of all vitamins and minerals are necessary because of the limited range of foods that can be taken. Free fruits and vegetables may provide sufficient amounts of vitamins A and C. The source of the vitamins and minerals varies: they may be a constituent of the branch chain free amino acid supplement (Table 15.15), or a separate supplement may be needed. Paediatric Seravit for young children or Forceval Junior Capsules, with additional calcium, for older children are commonly used. The diet and supplements together should provide the reference nutrient intake [26] for age for all vitamins and minerals. Fluoride drops are recommended because of the high sugar content of the diet.

Table 15.14 Leucine exchanges for use in MSUD

Food	Weight (g)	Energy (kcal)	(kJ)	Protein (g)*	Leucine (mg)**	Isoleucine (mg)**	Valine (mg)**
Milk							
SMA Gold	35 ml	23	96	0.5	50	27	31
Cow & Gate Premium	40 ml	26	109	0.6	54	29	32
Cows' milk	15 ml	10	42	0.5	50	27	36
Single cream	20 ml	40	167	0.5	48	26	36
Double cream	35 ml	157	656	0.6	52	30	38
Yogurt (natural/flavoured)	10	10	42	0.4	57	31	34
Custard	15 ml	18	75	0.5	57	31	42
Ice cream	15	25	105	0.4	53	28	36
Milk chocolate	5	26	109	0.4	46	27	30
Plain chocolate	15	79	330	0.7	45	27	40
Cereals							
All Bran	5	13	54	0.7	51	25	37
Cornflakes	5	18	75	0.4	54	16	20
Muesli	5	17	71	0.5	50	26	35
Oatmeal (raw)	5	19	79	0.6	47	25	34
Puffed Wheat	5	16	69	0.7	52	25	34
Ready Brek	5	19	79	0.6	48	25	34
Rice Krispies	10	37	155	0.6	48	25	34
Shredded Wheat	6	20	84	0.6	51	24	36
Sugar Puffs	12	39	163	0.7	50	25	34
Weetabix	6	21	88	0.7	49	23	31
Rice – raw	10	36	150	0.7	56	26	39
Rice – boiled	25	35	146	0.6	47	22	32
Potatoes							
Boiled	55	40	167	1.0	48	33	41
Baked (flesh only)	30	23	96	0.7	48	33	39
Baked (flesh + skin)	40	54	226	1.6	52	34	44
Roast	30	45	188	0.9	51	36	42
Chips	25	47	196	1.0	57	40	50
Crisps (plain/salted)	15	82	343	0.8	57	39	48
Sweet potato (boiled)	100	84	351	1.1	58	39	48
Vegetables							
Baked beans (canned)	15	13	54	0.8	58	31	36
Broccoli tops (boiled)	30	7	29	0.9	48	24	45
Brussel sprouts (boiled)	35	12	50	1.0	52	42	49
Cauliflower (boiled)	45	13	54	1.3	50	31	42
Lentils (boiled)	10	10	42	0.8	59	33	38
Mushrooms (raw)	30	4	17	0.5	45	27	30
Peas (boiled/fresh/frozen)	15	11	46	1.0	51	33	34
Peas (canned/processed)	10	10	42	0.7	43	27	29
Spinach (boiled)	10	2	8	0.2	48	24	31
Sweetcorn (canned)	15	18	76	0.4	55	16	21
Fruit							
Avocado	20	38	159	0.4	46	28	38
Figs (dried)	35	73	305	1.1	52	38	49

Table 15.14 (continued)

Food	Weight (g)	Energy (kcal)	Energy (kJ)	Protein (g)*	Leucine (mg)**	Isoleucine (mg)**	Valine (mg)**
Biscuits and crackers							
Plain digestive	7	33	138	0.4	50	24	31
Gingernut	12	55	230	0.7	52	29	32
Matzo	6	23	96	0.6	49	26	30
Cream cracker	7	31	130	0.7	51	28	31

* *McCance and Widdowson's 'The Composition of Foods'* 5e. Royal Society of Chemistry, Ministry of Agriculture, Fisheries and Food. London: HMSO, 1991.

** Paul AA, Southgate DAT, Russell J *First supplement to McCance and Widdowson's 'The Composition of Foods'*. London: HMSO, 1979.

Table 15.15 Branch chain free amino acid products used in MSUD

Product	Amino acids g/100 g	Energy kcals/100 g	Energy kJ/100 g	Carbohydrate g/100 g	Fat g/100 g	Vitamins and minerals	Dilution	Osmolality mOsm/kg	Comment
MSUD Analog	15.5	462	1936	54	23	full range	15%	353	Infant formula
MSUD Maxamaid	30	300	1260	51	<0.5	full range	1 to 5	782	Suitable from 2 years of age, good solubility unflavoured drink
MSUD Maxamum	47	290	1226	34	<0.5	full range	1 to 5	1181	Suitable from 8 years of age, good solubility, orange flavoured drink
MSUD Aid III	93	326	1386	4.5	nil	calcium phosphorus	5%	332	Not completely soluble therefore not suitable for continuous enteral feeding

* All products are free from leucine, isoleucine and valine but otherwise contain all essential and non-essential amino acids

All products are manufactured by Scientific Hospital Supplies and approved by the Advisory Committee Borderline Substances for prescription on FP10. Other products are manufactured but are not currently available in the United Kingdom – MSUD 1 and 2, Milupa; MSUD Diet Powder, Mead Johnson Nutritionals

Management of the newly diagnosed infant

On presentation the newly diagnosed baby with MSUD is acutely unwell, often encephalopathic and requiring intensive care. Plasma leucine level is usually greatly elevated and may be reduced with haemo or peritoneal dialysis. Nevertheless dietary treatment is also commenced as soon as possible. Nasogastric feeding is often necessary. As the plasma leucine level falls and the infant's clinical status improves, oral feeding can usually be established.

During the acute phase no dietary leucine is given until plasma leucine falls to around 800 μmol/l. Apart from dialysis, the major route of removal of leucine from the plasma pool in MSUD is into protein synthesis [27] and this is best achieved by aggressive supplementation with branch chain free amino acids, a high energy intake and frequent 2–3 hourly feeding. The infant is fed the branch chain free amino acid infant formula MSUD Analog, aiming to provide 3 g branch chain free amino acids/kg body weight/day and at least the normal energy requirement for age.

Table 15.16 Low leucine fruits and vegetables

FRUIT

Fresh, frozen or tinned in syrup
(Less than 50 mg leucine and/or less than 0.7 g protein per 100 g)

Apple	Grapefruit	Paw paw
Apricots (not dried)	Guavas	Peaches (not dried)
Banana	Lemon	Pears
Bilberries	Limes	Pineapple
Cherries	Lychees	Plums
Clementines	Mandarins	Pomegranate
Cranberries	Melon	Quince
Currants	Mulberries	Raisins
Damsons	Mango	Strawberries
Fruit Salad	Nectarines	Sultanas
Gooseberries	Olives	Tangerines
Grapes	Oranges	Water melon

Kiwi fruit, raspberries, black cherries, blackcurrant, rhubarb } Maximum of one small serving per day of any of these

VEGETABLES

Fresh, frozen or tinned
(Less than 100 mg leucine and/or less than 1 g protein per 100 g)

Artichoke	Cucumber	Pumpkin
Asparagus	Cress	Radish
Aubergine	Gherkin	Salsify
Beans (French & green)	Lettuce	Seakale
Beetroot	Marrow	Spring greens
Cabbage	Mushrooms	Swede
Carrots	Onion	Tomato
Celeriac	Parsley	Turnip
Celery	Peppers	Watercress
Chicory		

Beansprouts, courgette, leeks, okra and parsnip are higher protein vegetables, no leucine analysis is available.
A small serving of up to 30 g is allowed occasionally

Source

Royal Society of Chemistry, Ministry of Agriculture, Fisheries and Food. *McCance and Widdowson's 'The Composition of Foods'* 5e. London: HMSO, 1991.

Paul AA, Southgate DAT, Russell J *First supplement to McCance and Widdowson's 'The Composition of Foods'*. London: HMSO, 1979.

This may take a few days to achieve in the very sick infant, commencing with a more dilute MSUD Analog solution supplemented with glucose polymer to a final concentration of 10% carbohydrate.

Plasma BCAA levels need to be reported daily. If either the plasma isoleucine or valine levels fall below 100 µmol/l a supplement (50–300 mg per day) is given to maintain plasma levels between 100 and 400 µmol/l. Leucine is usually introduced as normal infant formula beginning with 50–100 mg per day (40–80 ml infant formula) divided between several feeds. The leucine intake is then increased according to plasma levels, aiming to maintain plasma leucine between 200 and 700 µmol/l.

Feeding the infant and child with classical MSUD

The diet for the infant is provided by a combination of normal infant formula as the source of leucine and MSUD Analog. The leucine-containing formula is given as a divided dose 4–5 times daily. This is followed by a feed of MSUD Analog to appetite (Table 15.17). Weaning is commenced at the usual time between four and six months, starting with low leucine foods such as puréed apple, carrot or crushed low protein biscuit. The low leucine food is given after the leucine containing formula and during or after the MSUD Analog feed. It does not matter therefore if solids are not completed as they do not affect total leucine intake. As the infant takes more solids, the amount of infant formula offered is reduced by one leucine exchange and replaced with one exchange of food, e.g. 55 g potato. The food exchange is given before the MSUD Analog. This process is continued throughout the first year until all the leucine is provided by food and is given divided between three main meals.

MSUD Aid (an amino acid supplement free from BCAA) is gradually introduced from around six months of age to condition the infant to its flavour and texture and, in some, to maintain an adequate supply of branch chain free amino acids. The MSUD Aid and vitamin and mineral supplement are mixed with water and milk shake flavouring to form a paste. A flavouring agent is essential to improve the taste of the product. Initially one teaspoon of paste is given at one meal per day before the measured leucine exchange. The MSUD Aid mixture is gradually increased in quantity and given at three meals per day and will eventually replace the MSUD Analog. The infant's acceptance of the MSUD Aid will determine how quickly the quantity offered can be increased; force feeding must be avoided. As the amount of paste taken increases it is important to give a drink of water after it because of its high osmolality. Flexibility is necessary when introducing the MSUD Aid paste; a

Table 15.17 Example of a feeding regimen for infant with MSUD aged 2 months, weight 4.5 kg

	Energy		Protein (g)	Leucine (mg)	Isoleucine (mg)	Valine (mg)
	(kcal)	(kJ)				
400 ml Cow & Gate Premium 80 ml × 5 feeds	264	1100	5.6	536	292	324
420 ml MSUD Analog 70 ml × 6 feeds	294	1226	8.2	–	–	–
Totals	558	2326	13.8	536	292	324
Per kg	124	517	3.1	119	65	72
DRV per kg for 0–3 months [26]	115–100	480–420	2.1			

combination of both Analog and MSUD Aid may be more acceptable throughout the toddler years. If MSUD Aid is not taken well as a paste, it may be added to the Analog feed, but care must be taken to ensure that the feed does not become hyperosmolar. Five grams of MSUD Aid can be safely added to 150 ml MSUD Analog.

An alternative to MSUD Aid paste is MSUD Maxamaid (branch chain free amino acid supplement with added carbohydrate and full range of vitamins and minerals) which is given as a drink. This product is not recommended for children under the age of two years because of its high osmolality (Table 15.15). However some centres have successfully used it from one year of age, both as a drink and a paste.

From around one year the diet should have progressed so that all leucine exchanges come from food, MSUD Aid paste is taken and low leucine foods are taken to appetite. Table 15.18 provides a typical example of a child's daily diet. During childhood the branch chain free amino acid supplement is increased to ensure an adequate intake of amino acids per kg body weight. MSUD Maxamum (Table 15.15) is a useful alternative branch chain free amino acid supplement which provides more protein in a smaller dose. It is recommended for use from eight years of age.

Dietary management during illness

During intercurrent infections plasma BCAAs accumulate, particularly leucine. This increase in leucine appears to be more attributable to inadequate energy intake rather than the direct catabolic effect of the actual infection [28]. At the first sign of any illness the emergency regimen is commenced to reduce and prevent the accumulation of leucine which may cause rapid neurological deterioration. The usual intake of leucine is stopped or substantially decreased. The standard emergency regimen (page 206) of two hourly glucose polymer drinks is given to reduce the effects of fasting. Supplements of branch chain free amino acids are essential to promote protein synthesis, otherwise the concentrations of the other amino acids will fall rapidly and become rate limiting for protein synthesis. The aim is to provide the child's usual intake of branch chain free amino acids and at least the normal energy requirement for age from glucose polymer, with or without additional fat. The infant is given MSUD Analog with additional glucose polymer to a total concentration of 10–12% carbohydrate.

Plasma BCAA levels are measured to monitor progress and determine when leucine can be reintroduced. Once plasma leucine is less than 800 μmol/l dietary leucine can be gradually given, increasing to the usual intake over a few days according to plasma levels. Supplements of isoleucine and valine may be necessary during the recovery period.

Monitoring the diet   The MSUD diet is monitored by clinical, biochemical and nutritional status, specifically looking for signs of protein deficiency such as skin rashes. Protein and zinc deficiency have been seen in children with MSUD (personal observation). Periodic analysis of trace element status is important (Table 1.1). The diet is assessed regularly to ensure

Table 15.18 Sample menu for child with MSUD age 4 years, weight 15 kg providing 450 mg leucine (nine exchanges per day)

Branch chain free amino acid supplement

35 g MSUD Aid III (2 g amino acids/kg)
20 g Paediatric Seravit
Flavouring e.g. Strawberry Nesquik
Add water to a paste ÷ 3
or
100 g MSUD Maxamaid (2 g amino acids/kg)
Flavouring e.g. blackcurrant juice
Add water to 450 ml
÷ 150 ml × 3 drinks

		Leucine Exchanges
Breakfast	⅓ amino acid supplement	
	3 × 50 mg leucine exchange	
	18 g Weetabix	3
	protein free milk* + sugar	
	low protein bread + margarine + honey or jam	
Lunch	⅓ amino acid supplement	
	3 × 50 mg leucine exchange	
	110 g potato	2
	30 g broccoli tops	1
	low leucine vegetables and margarine	
	low protein apple crumble	
	low protein custard	
Supper	⅓ amino acid supplement	
	3 × 50 mg leucine exchange	
	30 g peas	2
	low protein pasta + margarine + tomato ketchup	
	15 g ice cream	1
	fruit, fresh or tinned	
	Snowcrest low protein jelly	
Snacks	low protein biscuits or cake or	
	Duobar high energy supplement or fruit	
	squash, fizzy drinks, protein free milkshake*	

* Protein-free milks (Table 15.23)

all nutrients, particularly trace elements and minerals, provide the RNI for age [26]. Branch chain amino acids should be measured once a week in infants because growth is rapid, and every two weeks in 1–3 year olds. Thereafter, frequency varies between two to eight weeks depending upon the stability of the child.

Leucine intake is altered according to plasma BCAA levels. There are several reasons for high leucine levels, apart from intercurrent infections. These include inadequate energy intake with poor growth,

insufficient branch chain free amino acid supplement, or dietary indiscretion. If the plasma leucine level is around 700–800 µmol/l leucine intake is decreased by 50 mg to 100 mg daily (one to two leucine exchanges). If the plasma leucine level is less than 100–200 µmol/l leucine intake is increased by 50–100 mg (one to two exchanges). If either plasma isoleucine or valine level is less than 100 µmol/l, a supplement of 50–100 mg of the relevant amino acid is given. Any dietary alteration is reviewed with a follow-up blood test within one to two weeks.

TYROSINAEMIA TYPE I

Tyrosinaemia type I is caused by reduced activity of fumarylacetoacetate hydrolyase which catalyses the final step of tyrosine degradation (Fig. 15.3). Fumarylacetoacetate and maleylacetoacetate accumulate, and are further metabolized to succinylacetone which is found in greatly increased quantities in plasma and urine. These metabolites are considered toxic and responsible for the clinical features [29]. Tyrosinaemia type I can present at different ages with varying degrees of severity [30]:

- *acute form*, presenting in the first few months of life with progressive liver failure and early death if untreated
- *subacute form*, presenting between six months to one year with similar clinical features to the acute form, but less severe
- *chronic onset form*, presenting after one year with renal tubular dysfunction, vitamin D resistant rickets, failure to thrive and in some acute intermittent porphyria like symptoms [31].

Hepatoma can develop in all types of tyrosinaemia.

Plasma tyrosine concentration is moderately increased (2–4 times upper normal limit). In the acute form or phase of the disease plasma methionine concentration can be markedly increased. This is due to secondary inhibition of s-adenosylmethionine synthetase [29]. High plasma methionine may affect normal liver function [32].

Dietary management

Tyrosinaemia type I is treated with a low phenylalanine, low tyrosine diet to minimize formation of

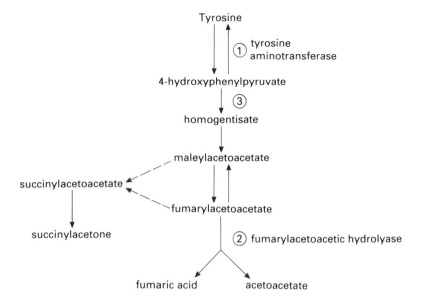

Fig. 15.3 Pathway of tyrosine degradation

toxic succinylacetone. A reduced methionine intake may also be necessary. Dietary treatment will improve renal tubular dysfunction and growth. Liver function (in particular prothrombin time) may also improve, but diet cannot prevent development of hepatoma. Dietary intake of phenylalanine and tyrosine is based on maintaining plasma tyrosine concentration within or slightly above the normal reference range, 30–120 μmol/l. The amount of natural protein tolerated varies between patients but is usually in the region of 1 g protein/kg bodyweight/day. A normal plasma tyrosine may be accompanied by a low plasma phenylalanine; care must be taken to ensure this does not become rate-limiting for protein synthesis. If plasma methionine is high the aim is to reduce this to the normal reference range. Phenylalanine and tyrosine restriction limits intake of natural protein to below minimum growth requirements and a supplement of phenylalanine and tyrosine free amino acids becomes essential. Methionine free amino acids are used if plasma methionine is high. A variety of amino acid products of varying composition are available for tyrosinaemia (Table 15.19).

The natural protein intake of phenylalanine and tyrosine is measured as 50 mg phenylalanine or 1 g protein exchanges (Table 15.1). The intake is altered according to plasma tyrosine concentrations. These are measured more frequently in infants than children because they are growing more rapidly. The natural protein intake and amino acid supplement should together provide a typical protein intake for age (10–12% energy intake) and both should be divided between feeds or meals throughout the day. When treating the newly diagnosed patient who is acutely unwell it may be desirable to decrease phenylalanine and tyrosine intake to a very low level for the first few days to help reduce production of toxic metabolites.

An adequate energy intake must be supplied for normal growth and to prevent endogenous protein catabolism causing increased tyrosine concentrations. Energy intake can be derived from protein exchanges, amino acid supplement, very low protein foods (Tables

Table 15.19 Manufactured products used in treatment of tyrosinaemia

Product	Amino acids g/100 g	Energy kcals/100 g	kJ/100 g	Carbohydrate g/100 g	Fat g/100 g	Vitamins and minerals	Dilution	Osmolality mOsm/kg	Comment
Xphen, tyr Analog (i)	15.5	462	1936	54	23	Full range	15%	353	Infant formula
Xphen, tyr, met Analog (ii)	15.5	462	1936	54	23	Full range	15%	353	Infant formula
Xphen, tyr Maxamaid (i)	30	300	1260	51	<0.5	Full range	1 to 5	782	Suitable from 2 years of age, as a drink
Xphen, tyr, met Maxamaid (ii)	30	300	1260	51	<0.5	Full range	1 to 5	782	Suitable from 2 years of age, as a drink
Phenylalanine, tyrosine free amino acid mix (i)	93	325	1381	4.5	0	Calcium and phosphorus only	5%	363	Not suitable for continuous enteral feeding as not completely soluble
Phenylalanine, tyrosine + methionine free amino acid mix (ii)	93	325	1381	4.5	0	Calcium and phosphorus only	5%	365	Not suitable for continuous enteral feeding as not completely soluble

(i)   Contains a full range of essential and non-essential amino acids except phenylalanine and tyrosine
(ii) Contains a full range of essential and non-essential amino acids except phenylalanine, tyrosine and methionine

Xphen tyr Maxamum and X tyr Maxamum are other formulations which can be produced if required.
All products are manufactured by Scientific Hospital Supplies and approved by the Advisory Committee Borderline Substances for prescription on FP10. Other products are manufactured but are not currently available in the United Kingdom.

15.2, 15.3), manufactured low protein foods (Table 15.4) and energy supplements such as glucose polymers, fat emulsions.

Vitamin and mineral supplements are essential because of the limited intake of natural protein foods. The amount prescribed needs to be individually assessed, and can be supplied from either the amino acid product, or from a vitamin and mineral supplement such as Paediatric Seravit or Forceval Junior Capsules with additional calcium. Diet and supplements together must provide the RNI [26] for all vitamins and minerals. Some patients with tyrosinaemia type I have a significant degree of cholestasis. These patients are likely to malabsorb fat soluble vitamins and an additional supplement, as Ketovite tablets and liquid, can be prescribed.

Renal tubular dysfunction leads to increased losses of phosphate and prevention of rickets usually requires both a phosphate supplement and 1-alpha-hydroxycholecalciferol (or 1,25-dihydroxycholecalciferol). There may also be increased losses of bicarbonate and potassium in the urine which necessitate supplements of these electrolytes.

During intercurrent infections the standard emergency regimen (page 206) of a protein free high energy intake is used to prevent decompensation of liver function and possible deterioration of neurological function. With dietary treatment alone many patients with the acute form of tyrosinaemia still develop progressive and fatal liver failure. In older children, deaths occur from neurological crisis and hepatoma.

Until recently liver transplantation was the only effective treatment for tyrosinaemia type I. However, Lindstet *et al.* have described the use of 2-(2-nitro-4-trifluoromethylbenzoyl)-1, 3-cyclohexanedione (NTBC) as an alternative treatment [33]. NTBC inhibits the enzyme 4-hydroxyphenylpyruvate dioxygenase, and blocks the tyrosine degradation pathway at this level (Fig. 15.2). This prevents the formation of the hepatotoxic and nephrotoxic compounds and succinylacetone (which probably plays an important role in neurotoxicity). Plasma tyrosine concentrations increased with NTBC but did not exceed $500 \mu mol/l$. Eye and skin lesions as seen in tyrosinaemia type II did not occur (see below). Dietary treatment for patients on NTBC still necessitates restriction of phenylalanine and tyrosine, but initial experience suggests a more generous intake of these as natural protein should be possible.

TYROSINAEMIA TYPE II: RICHNER-HANHART SYNDROME

In tyrosinaemia type II there is accumulation of tyrosine due to deficiency of hepatic tyrosine aminotransferase (Fig. 15.3). Crystals of tyrosine are found intracellulary and these cause inflammation. The main clinical features are corneal erosions and plaques, palm and sole erosions and hyperkeratosis. Mental retardation has been reported in some patients [29]. At presentation plasma tyrosine concentrations are usually greater than 1000 μmol/l (normal reference range 30–120 μmol/l).

Dietary management

Tyrosinaemia type II is treated with a low phenylalanine, low tyrosine diet to reduce high plasma tyrosine concentrations. The degree of dietary restriction needed is less severe than for tyrosinaemia type I. The principles of dietary management for type I tyrosinaemia can be applied to type II, but a higher intake of tyrosine and phenylalanine is normally possible. Supplementation with tyrosine and phenylalanine-free amino acids may be necessary if the total protein intake is less than minimum growth requirements. Methionine restriction is not necessary. On institution of diet, clinical features quickly resolve. The optimum level for maintenance of plasma tyrosine remains unknown. Reported cases have maintained plasma levels between 500 and 1000 μmol/l [34,35]. The resolution of eye and skin lesions has usually determined the dietary restriction and these occur readily if the plasma tyrosine level is kept below 800 μmol/l. It is not certain whether this degree of restriction will completely prevent complications of mental retardation.

During intercurrent illness, although severe metabolic decompensation does not occur, it may be prudent to use the standard emergency regimen (page 206) to prevent large increases in plasma tyrosine concentrations which have been reported to cause eye lesions during illness [35].

HOMOCYSTINURIA

Classical homocystinuria, caused by cystathionine β-synthetase deficiency, is characterized biochemically by increased plasma concentrations of homocystine and methionine. Clinical manifestations include lens dislocation, skeletal abnormalities, thromboembolism and neurological complications, probably caused by toxic effects of homocysteine [36]. Some patients are responsive to pyridoxine, the co-factor for cystathionine β-synthetase. Non-responders have traditionally been treated with low methionine diet to reduce accumulation of plasma homocystine and methionine. The aim of dietary treatment is to reduce the intake of methionine so that plasma methionine is close to the normal reference range and homocystine absent or low in blood and urine. The requirement of methionine is provided by small measured amounts of low methionine foods. Supplements of methionine free amino acids such as methionine free amino acid mix code 637 or RVHB Maxamaid or RVHB Maxamum are given to provide adequate intakes of total nitrogen. Additional cystine may also be needed because of its reduced synthesis from methionine via homocysteine. Fuller details of the practical dietary treatment are described elsewhere [37].

Compliance with the diet is usually difficult and poor because it is often started late in childhood. Nowadays, as a simpler alternative, many patients with homocystinuria are treated with oral betaine, instead of the strict low methionine diet. Betaine lowers homocysteine concentrations (although not to normal levels) by promoting the remethylation reaction of homocysteine to form methionine [38,39]. Methionine concentrations may rise to greater than pre-treatment levels in some patients although not all studies have shown this [40]. The strict low methionine diet is not necessary for patients on betaine, however a modest protein restriction may be indicated particularly if methionine levels are high, and high protein intakes should certainly be avoided. The efficacy of long term outcome of betaine treatment still remains unknown.

ORGANIC ACIDAEMIAS AND UREA CYCLE DISORDERS

LOW PROTEIN DIET FOR THE MANAGEMENT OF UREA CYCLE DISORDERS AND ORGANIC ACIDAEMIAS – PRACTICAL ASPECTS

Protein

Low protein diets must provide at least the minimum amount of protein, nitrogen and essential amino acids to meet normal growth requirements. Minimum safe levels for protein (Table 15.20) and requirements for essential amino acid intake have been set by FAO/WHO/UNU, 1985. These safe levels are based on an intake of high biological value (HBV) protein foods, milk and hens' egg, with 100% digestibility thus ensuring an adequate intake of all essential amino acids. The knowledge of the requirements of essential amino acids in children is limited. The protein source in low protein diets should ideally be mainly HBV protein, but this is not often normal practice because a greater variety of foods and a higher energy intake per gram of protein can be provided from low biological value (LBV) protein foods. Children on low protein diets who frequently consume a limited range of LBV protein foods may be at risk of one or more essential amino acids becoming rate-limiting for protein synthesis. Protein and mineral deficiencies have been reported in patients with inborn errors of metabolism on restricted protein intakes. This style of diet comprising mainly LBV protein is not uncommon in children with organic acidaemias and urea cycle disorders; therefore protein and amino acid intakes need to be monitored carefully. This should be done by clinical examination (skin and hair, looking specifically for signs of protein deficiency such as skin rashes), anthropometric measurements, biochemical assessment (quantitative amino acids, electrolytes, albumin), and regular dietary assessment. Protein tolerance will vary depending upon residual enzyme activity of the specific disorder, growth rate, age and sex. During early infancy growth is at a maximum so protein requirements per kg body weight are greatest at this time. If the child has had a period of slow growth, protein intake may need to be temporarily increased during the following period of catch-up growth.

Breast milk or a whey-based infant formula should provide the main protein source for infants. If demand breast feeding provides too much protein, intakes can be reduced by giving protein-free supplementary bottle

Table 15.20 Energy and protein requirements: Report of a Joint FAO/WHO/UNU Expert Consultation, Geneva 1985
Safe level of protein intake (milk or egg protein) for infants, children and adolescents

Age (years)	Safe level (g protein/kg/day)
0.25–0.5	1.86
0.5–0.75	1.65
0.75–1.0	1.48
1–1.5	1.26
1.5–2	1.17
2–3	1.13
3–4	1.09
4–5	1.06
5–6	1.02
6–7	1.01
7–8	1.01
8–9	1.99
9–10	1.01
Girls	
10–11	1.0
11–12	0.98
12–13	0.96
13–14	0.9
14–15	0.9
15–16	0.87
16–17	0.83
17–18	0.8
Boys	
10–11	0.99
11–12	0.98
12–13	1.0
13–14	0.97
14–15	0.96
15–16	0.92
16–17	0.9
17–18	0.86

feeds (e.g. Mead Johnson 'Protein-free' diet Powder, 80056) or a modular protein-free feed before the breast feed. The protein-free feed needs to be otherwise nutritionally complete. If a whey-based infant formula is used the amount is limited to provide the minimum safe level of protein or more if clinically indicated. Additional fluid, energy, vitamins and minerals (if necessary) are added to make it a nutritionally complete feed. An example of a low protein infant feed is shown in Table 15.21.

Weaning is commenced at the usual time between four and six months of age. The first solids given are

Table 15.21 Low protein feed for three month old male infant, weight 5 kg

	Energy		CHO	Protein	Fat	Sodium	Potassium
	kcal	kJ	g	g	g	mmol	mmol
80 g SMA Gold	423	1768	46	10	23.2	4.0	9.0
40 g Glucose Polymer e.g. Maxijul	144	600	38	–	–	<0.3	<0.2
Plus water to 750 ml Totals	567	2368	79	10	23.2	4.3 (iii)	9.2 (iii)
per 100 ml	73	316	10.5	1.3	3	0.6	1.2
per kg	113	474	–	2.0	–	0.9	1.8
DRV per kg 0–3 months (i)	115–100	480–420		2.1		2.0	3.4
Minimum protein requirement (ii)				1.86			

(i)   Dietary Reference Values [26]
(ii) FAO/WHO/UNU minimum protein requirements (Table 15.20)
(iii) Additional sodium and potassium may be necessary

NB Paediatric Seravit may need to be added if insufficient vitamins and minerals are supplied by infant formula

protein-free, so that if they are refused the total protein intake is not affected. Once these are accepted, protein containing solids are introduced from commercial baby foods or home cooked foods such as cereals, potato and pulses.

Protein intake is measured by an exchange system i.e. the weight of food which provides a specific amount of protein: 1 g protein for LBV protein (Table 15.1) or 6 g protein for HBV protein (Table 15.22).

Protein food exchanges should be weighed, at least initially. If parents are unable to cope with the concept of protein exchanges or weighing, then a set menu with handy measures for foods is used.

One gram of protein from the infant formula is replaced by 1 g of protein from solids. This process is continued throughout the first year of life or so until eventually all the protein in the diet is provided by solid food. Throughout childhood the protein intake is increased to provide at least the minimum requirement. The vitamin and mineral supplement is increased with the progressive change to solids as these foods are a poorer source than infant formula. If the child does not consume the daily protein allowance as solid food, it should be replaced with fluids; cows' milk and glucose polymer drinks are often the simplest way to do this. An example of a low protein diet is shown in Table 15.23.

If the child is consuming his protein intake mainly

Table 15.22 6 g Protein exchange list for high biological value protein foods

Food	Weight of food (g) providing 6 g protein
Egg (standard size 3 or 4)	50
Meat	
Sausage (beef or pork – not low fat)	45
Frankfurter	65
Beefburger (fried)	30
Meat – trimmed of all fat e.g. beef, chicken, pork, lamb, veal	20
Ham (canned)	30
Corned beef (canned)	25
Luncheon meat (canned)	50
Salami	30
Fish	
Fish fingers (1½ fried)	45
Fish cakes (fried)	65
Cod, plaice, haddock, lemon sole (steamed)	30
Prawns (shelled)	25
Scampi (in breadcrumbs, fried)	50
Cheese	
Cheddar, Edam, Gouda, Danish blue Stilton, White cheese	25
Full fat soft cheese e.g. Philadelphia	70

Table 15.23 Low protein diet (20 g), for 6 year old girl, weight 18 kg

	Protein (g) (using 1 g protein exchanges)
Breakfast	
20 g Cornflakes and sugar	2
Protein-free milk*	
36 g (1 slice) bread	3
Butter, jam, honey, marmalade	
100 ml pure fruit juice + 10 g glucose polymer	
Mid AM	
15 g (1) chocolate digestive biscuit	1
1 can Lucozade	
Packed lunch	
36 g (1 slice) bread	3
Butter, tomato and mayonnaise	
30 g (1 packet) crisps	2
Portion fresh fruit	
200 ml carton Ribena	
Mid afternoon	
25 g milk chocolate	2
Squash + 150 ml water + 20 g glucose polymer	
Evening meal	
25 g (1) fried fish finger	3
50 g chips	2
15 g peas	1
Carrots and butter	
30 g ice cream	1
Tinned fruit	
Bed time	
Protein free milkshake	
or Squash + 150 ml water + 20 g glucose polymer	
Daily	
8 g Paediatric Seravit	
Fluoride drops	

* Protein-free milk alternatives:
 – 15 g Duocal and water to 100 ml
 – 10 g glucose polymer or sugar
   10 ml Calogen
   + water to 100 ml
 – 10 g Coffee Mate + water to 100 ml (0.3 g protein)

from LBV protein it is important to give a variety of these to ensure an adequate intake of all essential amino acids (e.g. potato, pulses, cereals, rice, pasta). If the protein prescription is generous enough, HBV proteins are given to improve the protein quality of the diet, but these have a relatively low energy content.

Some patients, particularly those with disorders of propionate metabolism, refuse to eat or have a very limited intake of solid food. They will depend on oral or nasogastric fluids to provide most of their low protein diet. A modular feed would be designed to meet the nutritional needs of the child and the specific disorder. An example of such a low protein feed is shown in Table 15.24.

Energy

Low protein diets can often provide inadequate energy due to the restricted intake of many foods. This must be avoided as an inadequate energy intake causes poor growth and poor metabolic control with endogenous protein catabolism resulting in increased production of toxic metabolites, e.g. ammonia in urea cycle disorders. Care must be taken to give sufficient energy to ensure adequate protein synthesis and normal growth. It is also important to ensure that energy from fat provides requirements for essential fatty acids: at least 1% of total energy intake should come from linoleic acid and 0.2% from α-linolenic acid.

Dietary energy can be provided by:

- measured low protein foods
- foods naturally low in or free of protein (free foods) (Tables 15.2, 15.3)
- specially manufactured low protein foods, e.g. bread, pasta, biscuits (Table 15.4)
- energy supplements, e.g. glucose polymers, fat emulsions.

Manufactured low protein foods are not always popular with this group of patients. Children with urea cycle disorders will usually obtain sufficient energy from normal food and obviously prefer to eat these. Children with disorders of propionate metabolism usually depend upon energy supplements as their major energy source because of poor appetite.

Vitamins, minerals and trace minerals

Vitamin and mineral supplements are almost always essential as intake will be severely limited due to the protein restriction. Iron, copper, zinc, calcium and B vitamins are most likely to be deficient. An adequate intake of vitamins A and C could be provided from fruit and vegetables. The diet and supplement should

Table 15.24 Low protein tube feed for 4 year old girl, weight 14 kg

	Energy		CHO	Protein	Fat	Sodium	Potassium
	kcal	kJ	g	g	g	mmol	mmol
430 ml Cows' milk	280	1170	20	14	16	10.2	15.4
200 g Glucose polymer e.g. Maxijul	720	3000	190	–	–	<1.7	<1.0
90 ml Calogen	405	1665	–	–	45	0.8	0.4
14 g Paediatric Seravit	38	159	10	–	–	–	–
Plus water to 1200 ml							
Totals	1443	5994	220	14	61	12.7 (iii)	16.8 (iii)
Per 100 ml	120	499	18	1.2	5.1	1.0	1.2
Per kg	103	428		1.0	–		
DRV 4–6 years (i)	1460	6120		1.1		30	28
Minimum protein requirement (ii)				1.0			

(i) Dietary Reference Values [26]
(ii) FAO/WHO/UNU minimum protein requirements (Table 15.20)
(iii) Additional sodium and potassium will be needed if feed provides sole source of electrolytes

together provide the reference nutrient intakes (RNI) [26] for vitamins and minerals. The amount required will vary and needs to be assessed for the individual. Paediatric Seravit provides a comprehensive vitamin and mineral supplement. It can be added to the infant feed in the required dose, or for older children be given as a paste from a spoon. To mask the unpleasant flavour of the paste it can be flavoured with milkshake flavouring, squash, jam, honey, fruit purée; a drink is given afterwards to dilute this hyperosmolar mixture. A suitable alternative to Paediatric Seravit for older children is Forceval Junior Capsules with additional calcium provided by Sandocal (Sandoz) effervescent tablets. Periodic assessment of plasma status of vitamins, minerals and trace element status is important (Table 1.1). Fluoride supplements should be given because almost all the diets have a high sugar content.

DISORDERS OF PROPIONATE METABOLISM

The disorders of propionate metabolism, methylmalonic acidaemia (MMA) and propionic acidaemia (PA) share common biochemical and clinical features

due to accumulation of propionyl-CoA and hence propionate (Fig. 15.2).

PA is due to a defect of propionyl-CoA carboxylase which causes high plasma and urinary propionate levels and excretion of multiple organic compounds, including methylcitrate and 3-hydroxypropionate. MMA is caused by a defect of either methylmalonyl mutase or its co-factor adenosylcobalamin. Nine classes of MMA have been identified. Impairment results in accumulation of methylmalonic acid and the compounds found in propionic acidaemia. These disorders vary widely in severity depending on the degree of enzyme deficiency. Some MMA patients are completely responsive to co-factor vitamin B12, and require no dietary treatment except for an emergency regimen during intercurrent illness.

Both disorders can present in the neonatal period or early infancy with a severe metabolic acidosis manifested by poor feeding, vomiting, lethargy, hypotonia and dehydration, or in early childhood with less severe symptoms. Hyperglycinaemia and hyperammonaemia occur and are thought attributable to inhibitory effects of accumulated organic acids and CoA esters in the mitochondria [41].

The prognosis of MMA and PA is generally not good [42,43]. The mechanisms of metabolite toxicity are unclear; however propionate and its metabolites appear to be implicated. Early onset of PA is associated with poor intellectual outcome and early death, whilst late onset may be complicated by a severe disabling movement disorder [44]. Severe MMA is associated with developmental retardation and early death [42]. Other more recently recognized complications in both disorders include cardiomyopathy [45] and pancreatitis [46].

Sources of propionate

It is important to appreciate that propionate is formed from three main sources, not just from amino acid catabolism.

(1) Around 50% is derived from the catabolism of the precursor amino acids, isoleucine, valine, threonine and methionine [47].
(2) Around 20% is produced from anaerobic bacterial fermentation in the gut [47]. Oral administration of the antibiotic metronidazole will reduce gut bacteria propionate production, but the long term efficacy of this therapy is still being studied [48].
(3) Probably around 30% is derived from the oxidation of odd-numbered long chain fatty acids (C15 and C17) [49]. These odd chain fatty acids are synthesized by the normal pathway of fatty acid synthesis but propionyl CoA acts as the primer instead of acetyl CoA, hence the additional odd number of carbons in the chain [50].

Dietary management

The aims of dietary treatment are to limit production of propionate by both restriction of precursor amino acids using a low protein diet, and avoidance of fasting to limit oxidation of odd chain fatty acids.

The precursor amino acids, isoleucine, valine, threonine and methionine do not accumulate in plasma in these disorders. It is therefore not possible to use measurement of plasma levels of these amino acids to determine the intake of natural protein. Dietary protein intake can therefore only be safely restricted to the minimum required for growth (Table 15.20). Too low a protein intake can have serious effects such as poor growth, skin rashes, hair loss, vomiting and severe metabolic decompensation. Dietary protein intake is increased according to age, weight and quantitative plasma amino acid concentrations, ensuring that diet always provides at least the minimum protein requirement.

Practical aspects of low protein diets have been discussed earlier in this chapter. To improve the quality of minimum protein diets, some centres use a synthetic amino acid supplement free from the precursor amino acids (e.g. XMTVI Analog; XMTVI Maxamaid; XMTVI Maxamum; Methionine, threonine, valine free and isoleucine low amino acid mix, code 889). However, the long term value of these supplements remains uncertain. Metabolic balance can be achieved without them, they are unpleasant to taste and difficult to administer to children who already have poor appetites. One study of two patients with MMA showed that although there was an improvement in nitrogen retention when the low protein diet was supplemented with precursor-free amino acids, there was no improvement in growth or decrease in methylmalonate excretion [51].

Long fasts should be avoided to limit the production of propionate from the oxidation of odd-numbered long chain fats. A late night snack or feed and early breakfast is given to reduce overnight fasting. Continuous overnight feeding is often used in those children who have poor appetites and this has the added benefit of limiting fatty acid mobilization at night.

Impaired renal function is a common complication of MMA, manifesting as a urinary concentrating and acidification defect [52]. Supplements of sodium bicarbonate are often needed both to replace sodium losses and reduce acidosis. Increased urinary methylmalonate excretion also increases electrolyte losses.

Anorexia and feeding problems of varying severity are almost consistently present and irreversible in these children. The causative factors are unclear, but increased plasma propionate is a possibility [48]. Enteral feeding via nasogastric tube or, more recently, button gastrostomy is often essential to provide an adequate dietary intake, to prevent metabolic decompensation, and to help the parents cope with a child who is difficult to feed.

A variety of feeding problems have been observed. In general those with more severe disease have worse problems. Food and fluid refusal is often acquired during the course of the disease and is frequently a phenomenon of repeated intercurrent infections. Many children have a poor appetite for solid food and often the diet is provided solely from oral fluids. Some will only eat a few selected foods, occasionally changing the type of foods that they will eat. Some are difficult feeders; parents complain of children being slow, fussy, retching or self-inducing vomiting with foods.

Dietary management of illness

During intercurrent infections patients are at risk of developing metabolic acidosis and encephalopathy. To help prevent this the usual protein intake is stopped and the standard emergency regimen (page 206) given to reduce protein catabolism and hence propionate production. In addition, metronidazole is given to reduce gut propionate production, and carnitine (100 mg/kg/day) to increase the removal of propionyl groups as propionyl carnitine in the urine. In MMA a generous fluid intake and sodium bicarbonate are needed to prevent dehydration and reduce acidosis. Additional potassium may also be necessary.

The usual protein intake is reintroduced early (within 2–3 days) to prevent protein deficiency, which could greatly exacerbate the effects of illness. Total parenteral nutrition (TPN) is used in those patients who are unable to be reestablished on their normal diet. Surprisingly patients will tolerate a fairly generous protein intake whilst on TPN, often more than that provided from their usual oral intake.

Treatment of the newly diagnosed patient

The new patient is treated initially with a protein-free high energy feed of glucose polymer solution, with or without fat emulsion. The concentration and volume would be similar to those used for emergency regimens. The aim is to provide the normal energy requirement for age. Electrolytes (sodium and potassium) are added to the feed to provide normal requirements for age. Often more than this is required in MMA because of increased urinary losses. The feed usually needs to be administered as frequent two hourly bolus or continuous nasogastric feeds.

Protein is reintroduced once the acute metabolic derangement, including the acidosis, has been corrected and the plasma ammonia is less than or around 100 μmol/l (normal <40 μmol/l). Protein is commenced with 0.5 g protein per/kg body weight per day and increased to the final minimum protein require-

ment within a few days. Protein is added to the protein-free, high energy feed as infant formula or cows' milk. Reintroduction of protein and vitamins and minerals should not be delayed for longer than a few days because of possible deficiencies.

ISOVALERIC ACIDAEMIA

Isovaleric acidaemia (IVA) is caused by a deficiency of isovaleryl-CoA dehydrogenase which blocks the catabolism of leucine at the level of isovaleryl-CoA and causes it to accumulate (Fig. 15.2). IVA can present in neonates (acute form) or in older children (chronic intermittent form). The neonate subsequently follows the chronic intermittent course.

During remission the majority of isovaleryl-CoA is conjugated to isovalerylglycine which is non-toxic and is excreted in large amounts in urine. However, during acute episodes the natural capacity of this detoxification pathway is exceeded and isovaleryl-CoA is deacylated to produce large amounts of toxic isovaleric acid which causes overwhelming illness [53]. The outcome of IVA is variable, ranging from normal psychomotor development to severe mental retardation [54].

Dietary management

The aim of dietary treatment is to limit dietary leucine intake and minimize formation of isovaleric acid. Sufficient leucine must be given for normal growth requirements. Leucine does not accumulate in plasma so it is not possible to use measurement of this to determine protein intake.

Usually a modest protein restriction (2 g/kg in infants and young children decreasing to between 1.5 g/kg and 1 g/kg in older patients) combined with an adequate energy intake is sufficient to limit the production of isovaleric acid in the well child. Practical management of the low protein diet has been given earlier in this chapter.

Patients should also be treated with additional glycine (250 mg/kg body weight/day) or carnitine or both to reduce isovaleric acid levels, particularly during periods of metabolic decompensation [53,55]. Glycine and carnitine conjugate with isovaleric acid to form non-toxic compounds, isovalerylglycine and isovalerylcarnitine, which are rapidly excreted in the urine.

Dietary management during illness

During intercurrent infections protein catabolism will greatly increase production of isovaleric acid. The standard emergency regimen (at the end of this chapter) of a protein-free, high energy intake from glucose polymer is given to reduce isovaleric acid formation. Oral or intravenous glycine and carnitine should be included in the emergency treatment.

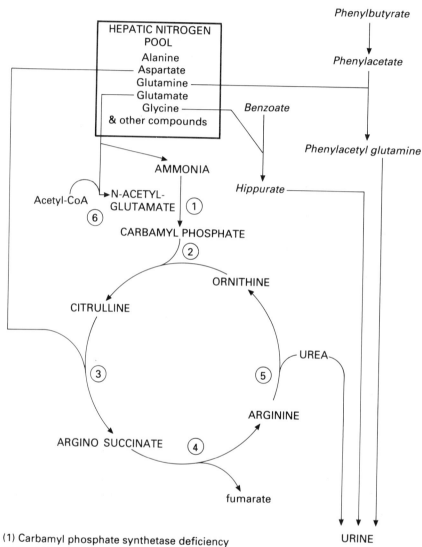

(1) Carbamyl phosphate synthetase deficiency
(2) Ornithine carbamyl transferase deficiency
(3) Citrullinaemia
(4) Arginosuccinic aciduria
(5) Arginase deficiency
(6) N-acetyl glutamate synthetase deficiency

Fig. 15.4 Hepatic nitrogen metabolism

UREA CYCLE DISORDERS

The urea cycle has two main functions – it converts waste nitrogen compounds into urea (excreted by the kidney) and it is essential for the synthesis of arginine. Inborn errors at each step of the pathway have been identified (Fig. 15.4). Arginase deficiency is distinct from the other disorders and will be discussed separately.

Deficiencies of these enzymes result in waste nitrogen accumulating as ammonia and glutamine, which are neurotoxic and may cause a severe encephalopathy. These disorders can present at any age from the neonatal period and throughout childhood. The onset of symptoms often coincides with an intercurrent infection or an increase in dietary protein intake although many of these patients self-select a low protein diet. A diet history at the time of diagnosis can usually be very revealing.

The clinical presentation varies depending on the age of onset. Loss of appetite, poor feeding and vomiting are common in all ages. In the newborn there is often respiratory distress with signs of hyperpnoea, seizures and collapse. In the later onset patients confusion, headache, disorientation, abnormal behaviour, ataxia, focal neurologial signs or coma can occur and in some there is also delayed physical growth and developmental delay [56].

The urea cycle disorders are treated by:

- restriction of dietary protein intake to decrease the need to excrete waste nitrogen
- medicines which utilize alternative pathways for the excretion of waste nitrogen
- arginine supplements.

Medicines

Sodium benzoate and phenylbutyrate increase waste nitrogen excretion by using alternative pathways to the urea cycle (Fig. 15.4) [57]. Phenylbutyrate is more effective than sodium benzoate in excreting nitrogen. Phenylbutyrate is metabolized *in vivo* to form phenyl-acetate which is conjugated with glutamine to form phenylacetylglutamine. This is then excreted so that 2 moles of nitrogen are excreted for each mole of phenylbutyrate given. Sodium benzoate is conjugated with glycine to form hippurate so that 1 mole of nitrogen is excreted for each mole of sodium benzoate given. Although phenylbutyrate is twice as effective it

is much less palatable than sodium benzoate. Both can be administered orally or intravenously (IV) and are usually prescribed in doses of up to 250 mg/kg body weight/day, divided between three or four doses. Parents are innovative in finding methods of masking the unpleasant flavour of these medicines. Some ideas are milkshake flavourings, jam, honey, yoghurt, peppermint essence and fruit purées. Some centres now have available sodium benzoate in syrup or tablet form, and phenylbutyrate as coated granules or tablets which are more readily taken.

In N-acetylglutamate synthetase (NAGS) deficiency, N-acetylglutamate, the activator of carbamylphosphate synthetase (CPS) is not formed. Patients are treated with carbamylglutamate which is an oral activator for N-acetylglutamate.

Arginine

Arginine becomes an essential or semi-essential amino acid in urea cycle disorders because its synthesis is greatly reduced [58]. In ornithine carbamyl transferase (OCT) and CPS deficiency arginine supplements of 100 mg/kg body weight/day are given to replace that which would normally be formed. Alternatively in OCT, in order to meet the arginine requirements, supplements of citrulline can be given as it is rapidly converted to arginine via the intact part of the urea cycle. Also, citrulline contains one less nitrogen atom than arginine, thereby reducing waste nitrogen production, but it is a much more expensive product than arginine.

In citrullinaemia and arginosuccinic aciduria (ASA), large doses of arginine up to 700 mg/kg/day are given to replenish ornithine supply. The carbon skeleton of ornithine is needed for the formation of citrulline and arginosuccinic acid which accumulate and are excreted in citrullinaemia and ASA respectively. Arginosuccinic acid is more effective than citrulline as it carries two waste nitrogen atoms and has a higher renal clearance. Arginine does increase the concentrations of both citrulline and arginosuccinic acid, the full consequence of which is unknown. However this appears to be less toxic than the accumulation of ammonia and glutamine.

Arginine can be administered orally or intravenously. Orally it is given as a divided dose, usually mixed with the other medicines.

Dietary management – low protein diet

Urea cycle disorders are treated with a low protein diet to reduce the accumulation of waste nitrogen. A normal energy intake for age is provided to ensure normal growth and to prevent endogenous protein catabolism with consequent metabolic decompensation.

For those with severe defects the dietary protein intake is usually reduced to the minimum safe level, but patients with milder defects will cope with a higher protein intake. Practical management of the low protein diet is given earlier in this chapter. If the child is unable to take a sufficient intake orally, nasogastric feeding must be used to prevent metabolic decompensation. Regular feeding and avoidance of prolonged fasts is recommended to help maintain good biochemical control.

Essential amino acid supplements

For some children an essential amino acid (EAA) supplement is incorporated as part of the total protein intake. This is beneficial because, by limiting the intake of non-essential amino acids, waste nitrogen is utilized to synthesize these and hence nitrogen destined for excretion as urea will be reduced.

EAA supplements are often given first when the blood biochemistry cannot be corrected by altering the medicines because the child is either on maximum doses of medicines or refusing to take more. There is no set dose of EAA supplement. The amount prescribed usually varies between 0.2 to 0.5 g/kg/day, given as a divided dose between two or three meals. EAA supplements can also be used to improve the biological value of a low protein diet which may be lacking in one or more essential amino acids. This may happen if the protein is provided from a limited range of low biological value (LBV) protein foods. Dialamine is the only EAA supplement available in the United Kingdom. It is a 30% amino acid mixture containing 25% essential amino acids and 5% non-essential amino acids. It is orange flavoured with added carbohydrate (glucose polymer and sugar) and contains a very limited range of vitamins and minerals. It can be administered either added to the infant feed, or in older children as a drink or paste, with a drink afterwards to dilute the hyperosmolar mixture.

Management of the newly diagnosed patient

Most patients when newly diagnosed will be hyperammonaemic and need to be treated with a protein-free, high energy diet and medicines. Energy is provided by glucose polymer solution and given via the oral or nasogastric route. The concentration, volume and feeding frequency would be similar to those used for emergency regimens (page 206). Maintenance electrolytes are added to the glucose polymer solution. It is important to be aware of the sodium contributed by the medicines when treating an infant. If the child is vomiting, 10% dextrose and medicines are given intravenously. Once the plasma ammonia falls to around 100 µmol/l or less, some natural protein is introduced. Often the protein intake has been low for some time prior to diagnosis so it is important to reintroduce some protein within a few days as patients, especially infants, can quickly become malnourished and protein depleted.

Protein is usually introduced at a level of either 0.5 g protein/kg/day or one quarter of the minimum safe intake (Table 15.20) divided evenly throughout the day. Protein is increased daily over a period of 3–4 days until the full allowance is reached. Occasionally it can be difficult to reintroduce protein without inducing hyperammonaemia; in these instances an EAA supplement is used and will be replaced with natural protein once the patient is more stable. Glucose polymer is given throughout the period of protein reintroduction to ensure an adequate energy intake.

Poor feeding and loss of appetite are very common in the newly diagnosed patient although this usually improves with better biochemical control. Not all patients improve at the same rate; in some appetite remains poor. It is not uncommon for a toddler still to be taking purée baby foods and refusing to chew lumps. The child must therefore be given food appropriate to his developmental stage when reintroducing the diet. Acceptance of more 'adult-type' foods can often be a slow process and is a frustrating experience for parents to cope with.

Low protein diet – monitoring

Regular measurements of plasma, ammonia and quantitative amino acids including glutamine are essential for the management of urea cycle disorders. Three to four monthly monitoring is recommended for most patients, but may need to be done more

Table 15.25 Outline of management decisions for urea cycle disorders (excluding arginase deficiency)

Ammonia µmol/l normal reference range <40	Glutamine µmol/l normal reference range 400–800	Quantitative plasma amino acids	Action
>80–100	>800	low	Increase medicines (i) Increase natural protein or essential amino acids Increase arginine in ASA and citrullinaemia (ii)
>80–100	>800	normal	Increase medicines (i) Increase arginine in ASA and citrullinaemia (ii) No change to diet
<80	400–800	low	No change to medicines (i) Increase natural protein
<80	400–800	normal	No change to medicines or diet

(i) Medicines – sodium benzoate and/or phenylbutyrate
(ii) If plasma arginine is high, arginine dose is not increased. If plasma citrulline or arginosuccinic acid is too high, arginine is not increased

frequently if the child is not well. Alterations to dietary protein, essential amino acid intakes and medicines are based on the results of these investigations (Table 15.25). High concentrations of glutamine and ammonia in plasma may not only mean that protein intake is too high, similar results will be obtained during periods of chronic catabolism so growth must also be considered when interpreting these results.

Good biochemical control may be difficult to achieve during periods of slow growth before and particularly after puberty [59]. When the adolescent stops growing there may be a period of instability because protein is no longer needed for growth; protein intake and medicines may require adjustment to restore a stable state.

Glutamine Poor appetite is common in these children [60] with high glutamine levels implicated as a cause. It is thought that glutamine causes an increased influx of tryptophan (the precursor of serotonin) into the brain and promotes serotonin synthesis. Serotonin increases a feeling of satiety [59]. If plasma glutamine is maintained within the normal range then, in some children, appetite may improve.

Management of illness

During intercurrent illness, protein catabolism may cause rapid accumulation of ammonia and glutamine. The standard emergency regimen (page 206) is used to prevent these effects of illness. Protein intake is stopped temporarily and regular drinks of glucose polymer are given. The usual doses of sodium benzoate, phenylbutyrate and arginine are administered. If necessary during acute illness the benzoate and phenylbutyrate dose can be temporarily increased to 500 mg/kg/day.

If the child does not tolerate oral fluids and medicines, 10% dextrose and medicines are given intravenously. Oral fluids can usually be recommenced within 24–48 hours, with a gradual changeover from intravenous to oral, thus ensuring an adequate energy intake. Plasma ammonia and quantitative amino acids should be measured regularly. Once the plasma ammonia is less than 80–100 µmol/l protein is gradually reintroduced over a period of two to four days. If hyperammonaemia is induced during protein reintroduction an essential amino acid supplement is used temporarily to reduce waste nitrogen.

ARGINASE DEFICIENCY

Arginase deficiency (Fig. 15.4) is a rare disorder whose presentation is distinct from the other urea cycle defects. It is characterized by a progressive spastic tetraplegia, seizures and developmental regression [56]. Hyperargininaemia and a mild hyperammonaemia occur due to defective hydrolysis of arginine. The mechanisms responsible for the neurological damage are not yet completely understood, but arginine and its guanidino metabolites are possible neurotoxins [61].

Dietary management

Arginase deficiency is treated with a low protein diet, sodium benzoate and phenylbutyrate. The aim is to maintain plasma arginine levels at less than 200 µmol/l (normal reference range 40–120 µmol/l) and a near normal plasma ammonia (normal range <40 µmol/l).

All dietary nitrogen has the potential to be converted to arginine, this source being considerably greater than the small amount of arginine which is naturally present in protein. In the past, in order to restrict the nitrogen intake, diets comprised an EAA supplement with a very limited intake of natural protein. Nowadays, by giving sodium benzoate and phenylbutyrate a more generous intake of natural protein is possible whilst still maintaining acceptable plasma arginine and ammonia levels. These medicines reduce available nitrogen destined for arginine synthesis by increasing its excretion via alternative pathways to the urea cycle (Fig. 15.4). Protein intake is restricted to the minimum protein requirement for growth, and is provided by a combination of natural protein and an EAA supplement. The precise composition of protein intake must be determined by the balance of requirements for growth and the medicines necessary for good biochemical control. The practical management of the low protein diet and EAA supplementation are provided on pages 196 and 204, respectively.

The diet is monitored by regular measurements of plasma ammonia, plasma arginine and the other amino acids quantitatively. During intercurrent illness the standard emergency regimen is used to prevent hyperargininaemia and hyperammonaemia. The usual dose of sodium benzoate and phenylbutyrate should be given orally or intravenously.

EMERGENCY REGIMENS

For some inborn errors of intermediary metabolism intercurrent infections, combined with a poor oral intake and fasting, will precipitate severe metabolic decompensation. To help prevent this, the child's usual diet is stopped and an emergency regimen (ER) is given. In some disorders the ER is combined with additional specific therapy (refer to respective disorders).

The aim of the ER is to provide an exogenous energy source, and reduce the production of potentially toxic metabolites from either protein catabolism or lipolysis. The standard ER is essentially the same for all disorders. A solution of glucose polymer is given as the main energy source. Fat emulsions are occasionally used for additional energy, but these may be less well tolerated. Fat is contraindicated in disorders of fat oxidation.

The carbohydrate concentration of the ER and fluid volumes given depend on the age of the child (Table 15.26). Too concentrated a solution of glucose polymer will be hyperosmolar, cause diarrhoea and exacerbate the effects of illness. Parents should be given a list of alternative drinks containing 10, 15 or 20 g carbohydrate per 100 ml as these may be more acceptable to the child's taste than glucose polymer alone (Table 15.27). An oral rehydration solution (ORS) supplemented with glucose polymer to provide extra energy, usually to a concentration of 10 g carbohydrate per 100 ml, is used during gastrointestinal illness. The osmolality of such feeds needs to be considered [62]; ORS with glucose polymer added to a final concentration of 10 g carbohydrate per 100 ml has an osmolality around 320 mOsm/kg water.

Table 15.26 Emergency regimens

Age (yrs)	Glucose polymer concentration %CHO	Energy/100 ml		Osmolality mOsm/kg water (i)	Daily volume	Feeding frequency
		kcal	kJ			
0–0.5	10	40	167	103	150–200 ml/kg	Initially two to three
0.5–1	10	40	167	103	120–150 ml/kg	hourly, night and
1–2	15	60	250	174	95 ml/kg	day
2–6	20	80	334	245	1200–1500 ml	
6–10	20	80	334	245	1500–2000 ml	
>10	25	100	418	342	2000 ml	

(i) Data provided by Scientific Hospital Supplies Group UK Ltd

Table 15.27 Emergency regimen drinks providing 15 g carbohydrate

Drink	Volume ml	Glucose polymer added per 100 ml
Orange squash	15 ⎫ add water to 100 ml	10
Ribena	10 ⎭	10
Fruit juice	100	5
Coca Cola	100	5
Lemonade	100	10
Lucozade	80	–

To reduce the period of fasting and optimize energy intake, the ER is fed at frequent intervals two hourly night and day.

The ER is normally commenced at home at the first signs of illness and is given via the oral or enteral route. It is useful to teach the parents of patients who refuse to drink when they are unwell how to feed their child nasogastrically at home. If the child persistently vomits the ER or is obviously not recovering, then a hospital admission for stabilization with intravenous (IV) therapy is usually necessary. A concentrated solution of 10% dextrose is given by peripheral drip or more concentrated dextrose can be administered through a central line. When oral fluids are reintroduced there is a gradual changeover from IV to oral feeding, thus ensuring an overall adequate energy intake.

The basic ER of glucose polymer must not be continued for long periods of time because it does not provide adequate nutrition. Poor growth and nutritional deficiencies will occur in patients on low protein diets, who have repeated infections and are frequently on the ER. If so, it may be necessary to increase protein intake temporarily when the child is well to compensate for inadequate intakes of protein whilst on the ER.

During the recovery phase when the usual diet is being reintroduced ER drinks or feeds are still given. Frequency of night feeds can be reduced to 3–4 hourly.

For patients on low protein diets, the protein is increased daily, providing one quarter, one half, then three quarters of the usual intake resuming the normal allowance by the fourth day. For infants or children on low protein feeds the protein intake is increased in quarterly increments, as described above. Additional glucose polymer is added to the formula feed to the same concentration as that in the ER.

Instructions for parents

Treatment of intercurrent infections can be an anxious and difficult time for parents. To make this easier, parents are taught a three staged plan telling them what to do and when [63]. This type of approach can also help reduce episodes of metabolic decompensation and hospital admissions.

(1) If the parents are unsure whether their child is showing the first signs of illness (pallor, lethargy, irritability) then an ER drink is given as a precaution. The child's clinical state is then reviewed within 1–4 hours.
(2) • If on reassessment the child has improved, the normal diet is resumed;
   • if however the child has deteriorated or shown no signs of improvement the full ER is commenced for a period of 24–48 hours. The parents are instructed how to reintroduce the usual diet.
(3) If the child is not tolerating the ER (i.e. refusing ER drinks, vomiting or becoming encephalopathic) then the child is admitted to hospital.

The parents are taught to recognize signs of encephalopathy such as disorientation, poor responsiveness, accompanied by a glazed look.

REFERENCES

1 Folling A Uber Ausscheidung von Phenylbrenztraubensaure in den Harn Stoffwechselanomalie in Verbindung mit Imbezillitat. *Z Physiol Chem*, 1934, **227** 169–187.
2 Woo S *et al*. Regional mapping of the human phenylalanine hydroxylase gene and the PKU locus on chromosome 12. *Proc National Academy of Science USA*, 1985, **82** 6221–6225.
3 Jervis GA Phenylpyruvic oligophrenia: introductory study of 50 cases of mental deficiency associated with excretion of phenylpyruvic acid. *Arch Neurol Psychiatr (Chic)*, 1937, **38** 944–963.
4 Paine RS The variability and manifestations of untreated patients with phenylketonuria (phenylpyruvic aciduria). *Paediatrics*, 1957, **20** 290–302.
5 Guthrie R, Susi A A simple phenylalanine method for detecting phenylketonuria in large populations of newborn infants. *Paediatrics*, 1963, **32** 338–343.
6 Smith I The hyperphenylalaninamias. In: Lloyd JK, Scriver CR (eds.) *Genetic and Metabolic Disease*. London: Butterworth, 1985.
7 Smith I Disorders of tetrahydrobiopterin metabolism.

In: Fernandes J, Saudubray JM, Tada K (eds.) *Inborn Metabolic Disease: Diagnosis and Treatment*. Berlin: Springer-Verlag, 1990.

8 Smith I Recommendations on the dietary management of phenylketonuria. *Arch Dis Childh*, 1993, **68** 426–427.

9 Pratt OE Transport inhibition in the pathology of phenylketonuria and other inherited metabolic diseases. *J Inher Metab Dis*, 1982, **2** 75–81.

10 Guttler F, Lou H Dietary problems of phenylketonuria: effect on CNS transmitters and their possible role in behaviour and neuropsychological function. *J Inher Metab Dis*, 1986, **9**(Suppl 2) 169–177.

11 Brunner RL, Jordan MK, Berry HK Early treated phenylketonuria: neuropsychological consequences. *J Pediatr*, 1983, **102** 831–835.

12 Krause W *et al.* Biochemical and neuropsychological effects of elevated plasma phenylalanine in patients with treated phenylketonuria. *J Clin Invest*, 1985, **75** 40–48.

13 Lou HC *et al.* Decreased vigilance and neurotransmitter synthesis after discontinuation of dietary treatment for phenylketonuria in adolescents. *Eur J Paediatr*, 1985, **144** 17–20.

14 Thompson AJ *et al.* Neurological deterioration in young adults with phenylketonuria. *Lancet*, 1990, **336** 602–605.

15 Lou HC *et al.* An occipito-temporal syndrome in adolescents with optimally controlled hyperphenylalaninaemia. *J Inher Metab Dis*, 1992, **15** 687–695.

16 Thompson AJ *et al.* Magnetic resonance imaging changes in early treated patients with phenylketonuria. *Lancet*, 1991, **337** 1224.

17 Schmidt H *et al.* Continuation vs discontinuation of low phenylalanine diet in PKU adolescents. *Eur J Pediatr*, 1987, **146**(Suppl) A17–A18.

18 Smith I, Glossup J, Beasley M Fetal damage due to maternal phenylketonuria: effects of dietary treatment and maternal phenylanine concentrations around the time of conception (an interim report from the UK phenylketonuria register). *J Inher Metab Dis*, 1990, **13** 651–657.

19 Brenton DP, Haseler ME Maternal phenylketonuria. In: Fernandes J, Saudubray JM, Tada K (eds.) *Inborn Metabolic Disease: Diagnosis and Treatment*. Berlin: Springer-Verlag, 1990.

20 Lenke RR, Levy HL Maternal phenylketonuria and hyperphenylalaninaemia. *N Engl J Med*, 1980, **303** 1202–1208.

21 Daner D, Elsas L Disorders of branched chain amino acid and keto acid metabolism. In: Scriver CR *et al.* (eds.) *The Inherited Metabolic Basis of Inherited Disease*, 6e. New York: McGraw-Hill, 1989.

22 Hilliges C, Awiszus D, Wendel U Intellectual performance of children with maple syrup urine disease. *Eur J Paed*, 1993, **152** 144–147.

23 Nord A, Doornick W, Greene C Developmental profile of patients with maple syrup urine disease. *J Inher Metab Dis*, 1991, **14** 881–889.

24 Treacy E *et al.* Maple syrup urine disease: interrelations between branched-chain amino, oxo and hydroxy acids; implications for treatment; associations with CNS dysmyelination. *J Inher Metab Dis*, 1992, **15** 121–135.

25 Wendel U Disorders of branched-chain amino acid metabolism. In: Fernandes J *et al.* (eds.) *Inborn Metabolic Diseases, Diagnosis and Treatment*. Berlin: Springer-Verlag, 1990.

26 Department of Health Report on Social Subjects No 41. *Dietary Reference Values for Food, Energy and Nutrients for the United Kingdom*. London: HMSO, 1991.

27 Thompson G *et al.* Protein and leucine metabolism in maple syrup urine disease. *Am J Physiol*, 1990, **258** 654–660.

28 Thompson G, Francis D, Halliday D Acute illness in maple syrup urine disease: dynamics of protein metabolism and implications for management. *J Paediatr*, 1991, **119** 35–41.

29 Goldsmith L, Laberge C Tyrosinaemia and related disorders. In: Scriver CR *et al.* (eds.) *The Metabolic Basis of Inherited Disease*, 6e. New York: McGraw-Hill, 1989.

30 Halvorsen S, Kvittingen E, Flatmark A Outcome of therapy of hereditary tyrosinaemia. *Acta Paediatr Jpn*, 1988, **30** 425–428.

31 Mitchell G *et al.* Neurologic crisis in hereditary tyrosinaemia. *N Engl J Med*, 1990, **322** 432–437.

32 Michaels K, Matalon R, Wong K Dietary treatment of tyrosinaemia type I. *J Am Diet Assoc*, 1978, **73** 507–514.

33 Lindstedt S *et al.* Treatment of hereditary tyrosinaemia type I by inhibition of 4-hydroxyphenylpyruvate dioxygenase. *Lancet*, 1992, **340** 813–817.

34 Halvorsen S Tyrosinemia. In: Fernandes J, Saudubray J, Tada K (eds.) *Inborn Metabolic Disease: Diagnosis and Treatment*. Berlin: Springer-Verlag, 1990.

35 Barr D, Kirk J, Laing S Outcome in tyrosinaemia type II. *Arch Dis Childh*, 1991, **66** 1249–1250.

36 Mudd SH, Levy HL, Skovby F Disorders of transsulfuration. In: Scriver CR *et al.* (eds.) The Metabolic Basis of Inherited Disease, 6e. New York: McGraw-Hill, 1989.

37 Francis D Disorders of amino acid metabolism. In: *Diets for Sick Children*, 4e. Oxford: Blackwell Scientific Publications, 1987.

38 Smolin L, Benevenga N, Berlow S The use of betaine for the treatment of homocystinuria. *J Pediatr*, 1981, **99** 467–472.

39 Wilken D *et al.* Homocystinuria – the effects of betaine in the treatment of patients not responsive to pyridoxine. *New Eng J Med*, 1983, **309** 448–453.

40 Surtees R, Bowron A, Leonard J The effect of betaine therapy on plasma and cerebrospinal fluid one carbon metabolites in children with cystathionine β-synthetase deficiency. (In press).

41 Rosenberg L, Fenton W Disorders of propionate and methylmalonate metabolism. In: Scriver CR *et al.* (eds.) *Inherited Metabolic Basis of Disease*, 6e. New York:

McGraw-Hill, 1989.

42 Matsui S, Mahoney M, Rosenberg L The natural history of the inherited methylmalonic acidaemias. *N Engl J Med*, 1987, **38**(15) 857–861.

43 Leonard J *et al*. The management and long term outcome of organic acidaemias. *J Inher Metab Dis*, 1984, **7**(Suppl) 13–87.

44 Surtees R, Matthews E, Leonard J Neurologic outcome of propionic acidaemia. *Pediatr Neurol*, 1992, **8**(5) 333–337.

45 Massoud A, Leonard J Cardiomyopathy in propionic acidaemia. *Eur J Pediatr*, 1993, **152** 441–445.

46 Kahler S *et al*. Pancreatitis in patients with organic acidaemias. (In press).

47 Thompson G *et al*. Sources of propionate in inborn errors of propionate. *Metabolism*, 1990, **39** 1133–1137.

48 Thompson G *et al*. The use of metronidazole in management of methylmalonic and propionic acidaemias. *Eur J Pediatr*, 1990, **149** 792–796.

49 Sbai D *et al*. Possible contributions of odd-chain fatty acid oxidation to propionate production in methylmalonic and propionic acidaemia. *Paedatr Res*, 1992, **31** 188A.

50 Wendel U Abnormality of odd-numbered, long-chain fatty acids in erythrocyte membrane lipids from patients with disorders of propionate metabolism. *Pediatr Res*, 1989, **25**(2) 147–150.

51 Ney D *et al*. An evaluation of protein requirements in methylmalonic acidaemia. *J Inher Metab Dis*, 1985, **8** 132–142.

52 D'Angio C, Dillon M, Leonard J Renal tubular dysfunction in methylmalonic acidaemia. *Eur J Pediatr*, 1991, **150** 259–263.

53 Sweetman L Branched chain organic acidurias. In: Scriver CR *et al*. (eds.) *The Metabolic Basis of Inherited Disease*, 6e. New York: McGraw-Hill, 1989.

54 Berry G, Yudkoff M, Segal S Isovaleric acidaemia: medical and neurodevelopmental effects of long-term therapy. *J Paediatr*, 1988, **113** 58–63.

55 Naglak M *et al*. The treatment of isovaleric acidaemia with glycine supplement. *Pediatr Res*, 1988, **24**(1) 9–13.

56 Brusilow S, Harwich A Urea cycle enzymes. In: Scriver CR *et al*. (eds.) *The Metabolic Basis of Inherited Disease*, 6e. New York: McGraw-Hill, 1989.

57 Brusilow S, Tinker J, Batshaw ML Amino acid acylation: a mechanism of nitrogen excretion in inborn errors of urea synthesis. *Science*, 1980, **207** 659–661.

58 Brusilow S Arginine, an indispensable amino acid for patients with inborn errors of urea synthesis. *J Clin Invest*, 1984, **74** 2144–2148.

59 Bachman C Ornithine carbamyl transferase deficiency: findings, models and problems. *J Inher Metab Dis*, 1992, **15** 578–591.

60 Hyman S *et al*. Behaviour management of feeding disturbances in urea cycle and organic acid disorders. *J Paediatr*, 1987, **III**(4) 558–562.

61 Lambert M *et al*. Hyperargininaemia; intellectual and motor improvement related to changes in biochemical data. *J Pediatr*, 1991, **118**(3) 420–424.

62 Verber I, Bain M Glucose polymer regimens and hypernatraemia. *Arch Dis Childh*, 1990, **65** 627–628.

63 Dixon M, Leonard J Intercurrent illness in inborn errors of intermediary metabolism. *Arch Dis Childh*, 1992, **67** 1387–1391.

FURTHER READING

Bachman C Urea cycle disorders. In: Fernandes J, Saudubray J, Tada K (eds.) *Inborn Metabolic Diseases, Diagnosis and Treatment*. Berlin: Springer-Verlag, 1990.

Brusilow S Inborn errors of urea synthesis. In: *Genetic and Metabolic Disease in Paediatrics*. London: Butterworths, 1985.

Maestri N, McGowan K, Brusilow S Plasma glutamine concentration; a guide in the management of urea cycle disorders. *J Paediatr*, 1992, **121**(2) 259–261.

USEFUL ADDRESSES

National Society for Phenylketonuria (NSPKU)
7 Southfield Close, Willen, Milton Keynes MK15 9LL.

Research Trust for Metabolic Diseases in Children
Golden Gates Lodge, Weston Road, Crewe CW1 1XN.

CHAPTER 16

Disorders of Carbohydrate Metabolism

GLYCOGEN STORAGE DISEASE TYPE I

Glucose-6-phosphatase has a central role in glucose production, catalysing the final common pathway for endogenous glucose synthesis from glycogenolysis and gluconeogenesis (Fig. 16.1). The enzyme glucose-6-phosphatase is normally expressed in liver, kidney and intestine. Glycogen storage disease type I (GSDI) is caused by either deficiency of glucose-6-phosphatase itself (type Ia) or a defect of any one of its associated transport proteins (types Ib, c or d) [1]. The clinical manifestations include growth retardation and hepatomegaly (due mainly to fatty infiltration of the liver). Increased glycolytic flux leads to lactic acidosis and hyperlipidaemia, with triglycerides being more markedly elevated than cholesterol [2]. Additionally in type Ib, there is neutropenia and impaired neutrophil function which increases susceptibility to bacterial infections [2]. A chronic inflammatory bowel disease similar histopathologically to Crohn's disease is also seen [3].

Dietary management

The aim of dietary treatment is to promote normal growth by maintaining a normal blood glucose level. This will also improve the secondary metabolic abnormalities, but it is recognized that these cannot be completely normalized [4]. Infants and children are administered a frequent supply of exogenous glucose both day and night at least until they have stopped growing. Glucose requirements are calculated from basal glucose production rates [5]. It is important to be aware that these requirements for glucose decrease with age (Table 16.1). Dietary energy is provided as follows: 60–70% by carbohydrate (CHO), 20–25% from fat and 10–15% from protein. Fat intake is decreased to compensate for increased carbohydrate intake.

Provision of carbohydrate to GSDI patients has altered over the years. Traditionally frequent CHO feeding was given day and night. In 1976, Greene *et al.* reported the intensive regimen of regular drinks of glucose polymer by day and continuous nasogastric feeding at night [6]. In 1984 Chen *et al.* introduced uncooked cornstarch to the diet to provide a source of slow-release glucose [7].

Some centres restrict fructose and galactose in the diet because these sugars are not converted to glucose via the gluconeogenic pathway but, instead, increase lactate production [8]. However a mildly elevated blood lactate level of up to 4.0 mmol/l is considered acceptable because lactate provides an alternative source of energy to the brain and therefore has a protective effect against fuel depletion [9]. Consequently many feel that the restriction of these sugars is not essential and that regular provision of glucose is the more important dietary manoeuvre.

Replacement of saturated fat with polyunsaturated fat is recommended by some in an attempt to improve the hyperlipidaemia [10], but this is less important than supplying a frequent CHO intake. Despite persistent hyperlipidaemia, no evidence of premature arteriosclerosis has yet been observed [11,12].

Nasogastric feeding

Continuous nasogastric feeding is used to provide glucose overnight. Careful management of this is necessary because it can render patients much more sensitive to hypoglycaemia. Indeed one reported case of unplanned cessation in delivery of glucose was fatal [13]. It is therefore important that a paediatric enteral feeding pump, which accurately controls flow rate and alarms if there is a fault in the system, is used.

Table 16.1 Glucose requirements in GSD type I

| Age | Glucose: mg per kg per minute | Glucose: grams per kg per hour | |
		Day	Night
Infants	8–9	0.5	0.5
Toddlers and children	5–7	0.3–0.4	0.3–0.4
Adolescents and adults	2–4 at night		0.2–0.25

Table 16.2 Infant feeding regimen GSD type I
5 kg infant: aim 0.5 g carbohydrate per kg per hour

| | Fluid ml | Energy | | CHO g | Protein g | Fat g |
		kcal	kJ			
SMA Gold	840	546	2282	60	12.6	30
Amount per kg	170	110	456	12.0	2.5	
Amount per kg per hour				0.5		

Daily feed distribution:

Day: Oral feeds 70 ml
8.30 AM, 10 AM, 12 noon, 2 PM, 4 PM, 6 PM = 420 ml
Night: Continuous nasogastric feeds 35 ml
every hour from 8 PM finishing at 8 AM = 420 ml
Bolus nasogastric feeds – 20 ml at 8 PM and 8 AM
(extra to calculated fluid requirement)

It is likely that the child will not have fed for two hours prior to commencing nasogastric night feeds so at the start a small oral or bolus feed is given. This also compensates for the slow delivery of glucose via the enteral feeding pump. The child must also be fed within 15 minutes of discontinuation of the night feed to avoid hypoglycaemia. Parents need thorough teaching and must be adept and confident with the enteral feeding system prior to home use.

Diet for infants

For the first few months of life glucose requirements (0.5 g CHO/kg/hour) are provided by infant formula, fed at volumes of 150 to 200 ml/kg. Additional glucose polymer is not usually necessary. Regular two hourly feeds during the day and continuous nasogastric feeding by night are needed to maintain a normal blood glucose level. At the beginning and end of the night feed, an oral or bolus feed providing sufficient glucose to last for 30 minutes is given. An example of an infant's feed regimen is shown in Table 16.2.

Weaning is commenced at the normal time between 4–6 months of age, and a regular intake of starchy foods is recommended, e.g. baby rice, rusk, potato. As the intake of starchy food increases it can replace the infant feed at main meals as the source of glucose. As relatively small quantities of food provide the glucose requirements a complicated CHO food exchange system is not necessary. It is usually sufficient just to teach parents which foods provide CHO and to include these at main meals. However for those infants and children who have poor appetites or are fussy eaters a list of foods which provide appropriate amounts of CHO can prove extremely useful.

As more energy is derived from solids, the infant should take smaller volumes of feeds. To ensure adequate intake of CHO, glucose polymer is added to the infant feed to give a final concentration of 10–15% CHO. From nine months onwards, some of the infant feeds can be replaced by CHO drinks such as baby juices with added glucose polymer, fruit juices or glucose polymer solution. However, it is important that the daily intake of infant formula should not fall to less than 600 ml because it continues to provide a major source of nutrients in the older baby's diet. Care must be taken to avoid giving drinks which are too concentrated in CHO content because of high osmolality precipating diarrhoea. Intermittent diarrhoea or loose stools does occur in some patients, but the cause is not completely understood [14,15]. A maximum concentration of 12–15% CHO is recommended in older infants. An example of a weaning diet is shown in Table 16.3.

Diet for children

During the daytime a source of glucose continues to be given at two hourly intervals either from a meal or snack containing CHO, or CHO drink. Parents are given a list of different drinks to supply the appropriate amount of CHO. Starchy foods such as bread, rice, pasta and cereals are encouraged in preference to sugary foods because these provide a slower release of glucose. The diet should provide the child's normal requirement for all nutrients. This point is emphasized

Table 16.3 Example of a diet for a 10 month old infant with GSD type I
Weight 8 kg, providing 0.5 g carbohydrate per kg per hour

Time	Food or drink	Total CHO g	Grams CHO per kg per hr*	Protein g	Energy kcal	kJ
8.15 AM	1 Weetabix	10.0	0.9	1.7	50	209
	100 ml SMA Gold	7.2		1.5	65	272
10.00 AM	15 ml concentrated baby juice diluted to 100 ml	9.0	0.5	–	36	150
12.00 AM midday	Minced beef, vegetable	–		6.0	60	250
	Small potato	10.0	1.6	1.0	40	167
	100 g yoghurt	15.0		5.0	80	334
2.00 PM	90 ml SMA Gold + glucose polymer to 10% CHO	9.0	0.5	1.3	68	284
4.00 PM	1 slice bread + butter	12.0		2.2	70	292
	Ham filling		1.3	4.0	30	125
	Small banana	10.0		0.5	40	167
6.00 PM	90 ml SMA Gold + glucose polymer to 10% CHO	9.0	0.5	1.3	68	284
8.00 PM to 8.00 AM finish	30 ml hourly for 12 hours SMA Gold + glucose polymer to 13% CHO	47.0	0.5	5.4	317	1325
8.00 PM and 8.00 AM	15 ml bolus SMA Gold + glucose polymer to 13% CHO	3.9		1.0	26	109
Totals		142		30.0	950	3968
% Energy intake		60%		13%		

* The portion size of carbohydrate foods (appropriate for age) will make the carbohydrate content of main meals in excess of the specified requirement of 0.5 g per kg per hour

as some parents have a tendency to be overzealous in providing CHO, which can lead to either inadequate intake of essential nutrients for growth, or obesity. Fluoride supplements are recommended because of high intake of sugars, and also the possible prolonged use of bottle feeding beyond young infancy. From one year of age the night feed is often changed to a solution of glucose polymer provided that the requirements for other nutrients are supplied by the daytime diet. As the child gets older the glucose polymer solution is made more concentrated; 15% CHO in 1–2 year olds and 20% CHO thereafter. Occasionally a paediatric enteral feed is administered at night in preference to glucose polymer alone, particularly when growth and nutrient intakes are inadequate.

Glucose requirements decrease with age. It is important to ensure that only the required amount of glucose is administered at night and as two hourly daytime drinks. Large quantities of exogenous glucose will exacerbate swings in blood glucose and make patients more sensitive to rebound hypoglycaemia [16]. Equally important is the need to supply adequate glucose as insufficient amounts will lead to high plasma lactate levels and growth retardation. Achieving optimum biochemical control is difficult. For some patients it may be beneficial to measure blood glucose levels at home by using blood glucose monitoring strips, however this is not perceived to be essential.

Cornstarch therapy

Uncooked cornstarch (UCCS) as cornflour is slowly digested, primarily by pancreatic amylase to release glucose. When compared with glucose polymer feeding, less glucose is required and a smoother blood glucose profile is produced [17]. UCCS is administered in doses of 1.5 to 2 g/kg body weight/day and on average will maintain a normal blood glucose for between 4–10 hours, obviating the need for two hourly feeding. UCCS can be introduced around two years of age. In younger children it may not be adequately digested to maintain a normal blood glucose because pancreatic amylase activity only reaches adult levels between two and four years, although its activity is reported to be induced by oral starch [10]. Success has been reported with UCCS in children under two years of age using smaller more frequent doses [18,19]. Cornflour is given raw; cooking or heating disrupts the starch granules by hydrolysis and thus makes it less effective. To increase palatability of UCCS it can be mixed with different drinks such as milk, squash, carbonated drinks or with cold foods such as ice cream, yoghurt, fruit purée or thin cold custard. Some studies have reported that mixing UCCS with sugary drinks makes it less effective [7,17,20].

When initiating UCCS treatment, a fasting cornflour load test under controlled conditions in hospital is important to assess the child's metabolic response by serial measurement of blood glucose and lactate. These biochemical results are used to determine the frequency and quantity of UCCS feedings. Prior to this UCCS will have been introduced at home to test its palatability and acceptance. The dose of UCCS is gradually increased to 2 g/kg at one meal over a few weeks. Some patients may experience side effects such as diarrhoea, abdominal distention and flatulence, but these are usually transient. Two hourly feeding will continue during this introductory period of UCCS.

UCCS is administered in doses of 1.75–2 g/kg/day at 4–6 hourly intervals with main meals, decreasing to a lower dose of 1.5 g/kg/day in adolescents who have stopped growing. A lower dose may be given late afternoon if there is a relatively short interval between this time, the evening meal and commencement of

Table 16.4 Example of a diet for a seven year old child with GSD type I Weight 25 kg; aim 0.3 g carbohydrate per kg per hour overnight

Time	Food or drink	
7.30 AM	**Breakfast** including: CHO foods e.g. breakfast cereal, bread, chapatti, pitta bread 50 g cornflour mixed with 100 ml water	2 g per kg
12.30 PM	**School dinner** including: CHO foods e.g. potato, rice, pulses, biscuits (crackers or semi-sweet), fruit 50 g cornflour mixed with yoghurt	2 g per kg
5.30 PM	**Evening meal** including: CHO foods e.g. potato, pasta, bread, fruit, yoghurt 25 g cornflour mixed with 50 ml milk	1 g per kg
8.00 PM to 7.00 AM	20% glucose polymer 40 ml hourly	Provides 0.3 g CHO per kg per hour overnight
8.00 PM and 7.00 AM	20 ml bolus of 20% glucose polymer	

night feeds. An example of a diet incorporating UCCS is given in Table 16.4. In children nocturnal enteral feeding is usually continued until they have stopped growing. Some may prefer to use UCCS at night, but the main disadvantage of this for young children is the need to take it at around six hourly intervals, thereby interrupting sleep. A comparison of long term management of both forms of treatment reported no significant differences in physical growth and biochemical parameters [21]. Cornflour and glucose polymer are approved by the Advisory Committee Borderline Substances for prescription on FP10.

Hypoglycaemia

It is inevitable that hypoglycaemia will occasionally occur. Parents need to recognize early warning signs such as sweating, irritability or drowsiness. They should respond to these by immediately giving a CHO drink and, on recovery, some starchy foods. Hypostop (page 106) is another extremely useful alternative for treatment of hypoglycaemia.

Illness

During intercurrent infections, the frequent supply of glucose must be maintained. Often a change in dietary regimen is needed, with replacement of meals and snacks with glucose polymer drinks, because of poor appetite. If the child has diarrhoea and is vomiting, an oral rehydration solution supplemented with glucose polymer is given. Nasogastric feeding during the daytime may be necessary. If the child does not tolerate the intensive glucose polymer regimen then a hospital admission for intravenous therapy becomes essential.

GSD type Ib

The dietary treatment of patients with type Ib is the same as for GSDI. However the additional problems seen in type Ib may necessitate further dietary manipulation. Mouth ulcers are a feature of type Ib and can make oral feeding difficult and painful. Meals and snacks may need to be temporarily replaced with nutritionally complete fluid supplements and if necessary these can be given via the enteral route. An elemental feed is sometimes used if the bowel is inflamed and bleeding.

GLYCOGEN STORAGE DISEASE TYPE III

Glycogen storage disease type III (GSDIII) is characterized by deficiency of the glycogen debranching enzyme (amylo-1,6-glucosidase), in various tissues including liver and muscle (Fig. 16.1). On fasting glycogen is only degraded to the 1,6 branch points. Consequently the production of glucose from glycogenolysis is greatly limited. However the gluconeogenic pathway is functional for endogenous glucose production and prevents the development of profound hypoglycaemia during fasting, although hypoglycaemia can still occur.

The debranching enzyme can be absent in liver (type IIIb) or liver and muscle (type IIIa) resulting in clinical features of varying severity. Hypoglycaemia and poor growth are common during childhood when cerebral demands are greatest but these become less severe with increasing age. Hepatomegaly occurs due to both glycogen and fat accumulation. Additional in type IIIa patients also suffer from myopathy and cardiomyopathy [2].

Dietary management

The dietary treatment of children with GSDIII will vary depending upon the severity of the disorder and the diet needs to be individually tailored to the child's specific requirements. A high protein diet is recommended because of increased demand for gluconeogenesis and loss of muscle amino acids which are substrates for gluconeogenesis.

Some children require a more intensive dietary regimen of frequent feeding similar to GSD type I (page 211) if fasting tolerance and/or growth is inadequate. At night continuous nasogastric feeding or uncooked cornstarch (UCCS) can be used [22,23]. During the daytime, there is greater emphasis on increased protein intake compared with GSDI. UCCS is often used in addition during the daytime. For other children a high protein, high starch diet of regular daytime meals and a late protein-rich bedtime snack is sufficient dietary treatment.

In young patients with debrancher enzyme myopathy a high protein diet combined with a high protein night feed has been beneficial in improving muscle strength [24].

The diet should provide 20–25% energy intake from protein, 50–55% from carbohydrate and 20–25% from fat. Fat intake is decreased to compensate for increased protein and carbohydrate intakes, thus preventing possible obesity. Starchy foods are given in preference to sugary food as on digestion they release glucose more slowly. Practical guidelines are given for a high protein, high starch, low fat diet in Table 16.5.

Children who have a good appetite and enjoy milk may possibly achieve sufficient protein intake from high protein foods, but protein supplements are usually necessary. Despite use of these it can be difficult, particularly in young children, to provide such a high protein intake; a lower protein intake with a higher carbohydrate intake is an acceptable alternative.

A variety of high protein supplements are available. Often the choice of supplement is dictated by what the child will happily take. Pure protein powders, such as Maxipro HBV and Vitapro, are versatile and can be fairly easily incorporated into food or drinks. Protein powders are often preferable to some of the prescribable high protein drink or dessert supplements because these often have too high an energy content. Table 16.6 provides a list of high protein, lower energy supplements suitable for children.

For infants, protein powders can be added to infant formula milks to provide around 3 g protein per

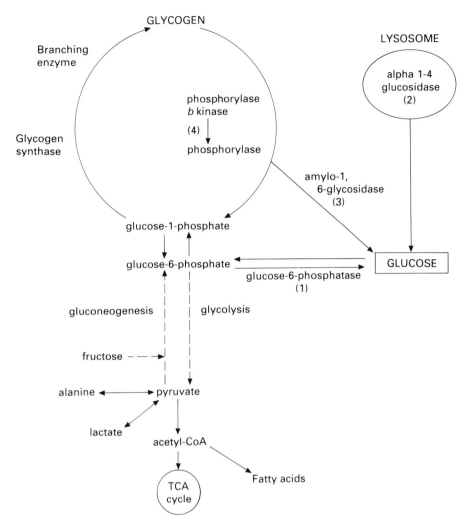

(1) Glycogen storage disease type I
(2) Glycogen storage disease type II
(3) Glycogen storage disease type III
(4) Phosphorylase system deficiencies

Fig. 16.1 Pathway of liver glycogen metabolism

100 ml, or a combination of glucose polymer and protein powder added to infant milks may be preferred. From six months onwards follow on formulas such as Progress or Farley's Follow-on Milk, which provide around 2.0 g protein per 100 ml, can be used.

Adolescents and adults must be made aware that alcohol is a potent inhibitor of gluconeogenesis and even quite moderate amounts may reduce glucose production. Alcohol intake should be limited and must always be taken in combination with food [25].

GLYCOGEN STORAGE DISEASE TYPE II

GSD type II is caused by deficiency of acid maltase (alpha 1–4 glucosidase) (Fig. 16.1). It is a generalized

Table 16.5 High protein, high starch, low fat diet for glycogen storage disease type III

High protein low fat foods

One serving of high protein food at three main meals and bedtime snack. Generous intakes of milk or high protein drinks (Table 16.6) should be given

Milk	Semi-skimmed or skimmed milk, milk puddings e.g. rice, custard, semolina
Meat	Lean red meat (<10% fat content), trim off all visible fat
Poultry	White meat in preference to dark meat
Fish	White fish instead of oily
Cheese	Low fat cheese e.g. cottage, Edam type, half fat Cheddar
Yoghurt	Low fat yoghurt
Pulses	Beans, lentils, peas, sweetcorn
Eggs	Egg white in preference to yolk

Carbohydrate foods (starch and sugar)

Starch foods At least one serving at three main meals and include at bedtime snack:

e.g. bread, chapatti, pitta, cereal, potato, rice, pasta, fruit, plain biscuits or crackers, tea cake, muffins, scones

Sugar These foods are allowed but should be kept to a minimum e.g. table sugar, sweets, cakes, ice cream, preserves

Fats

High fat foods should be used sparingly e.g. butter, margarine, vegetable oil, animal fats, cream (double, whipping, single), imitation cream, mayonnaise, salad dressings

Avoid fried or roasted foods. Spread butter or margarine thinly on bread

Snack foods

Most children choose high fat or sugary snack foods e.g. crisps, nuts, sweets, chocolate

Low fat, high protein, high carbohydrate snack foods should be used instead e.g. yoghurt, fromage frais, sandwich with protein filling, crackers and cheese, glass of milk

Table 16.6 High protein drinks

	Protein (g/100 ml)	Energy/100 ml		Comments
		kcal	kJ	
Build Up + skimmed milk (i)	6.4	77	323	Milk based Various flavours
Fortimel	10	100	420	Milk based Various flavours
Protein Forte	10	100	420	Milk based Various flavours
Skimmed Milk + Vitapro (ii)	6.3	45	272	Milk based
Provide	3.6	60	250	Fruit juice Various flavours

(i) 13 g Build-Up plus 100 ml skimmed milk
(ii) 4 g Vitapro plus 100 ml skimmed milk

form [26,27]. Fat and carbohydrate intakes are decreased so that each provides 35–40% of energy intake to compensate for increased protein intake.

Dietary protein intake is increased in a similar manner to GSD III (page 214). High protein low fat foods are encouraged and high protein supplements, such as drinks or pure protein powders, are invaluable in increasing protein intake.

THE PHOSPHORYLASE SYSTEM

Deficiencies of the phosphorylase system (Fig. 16.1) of which phosphorylase *b* kinase is most prevalent have similar symptomatology to but are much milder than GSD III [2]. In these disorders glycogen degradation is reduced but gluconeogenesis is functional for endogenous glucose production. Children present with hepatomegaly and growth retardation but catch-up growth usually occurs before puberty [28]. Hypoglycaemia is generally mild and usually only occurs after prolonged fasting or infection [10]. Most adults will be entirely asymptomatic with a normal life expectancy.

Many patients do not require specific dietary treatment. Nevertheless, general dietary advice on provision of increased intakes of protein and starch and avoidance of prolonged fasts particularly during illness would be appropriate. To reduce the period of overnight fasting a late night bedtime snack rich in protein

lysosomal storage disorder in which deficiency of lysosomal acid maltase leads to accumulation of glycogen. The infantile form (Pompe's disease) is associated with poor prognosis and early death. The childhood form is less severe and progresses more slowly. There is generalized muscle weakness, which can eventually lead to cardiorespiratory insufficiency and cause death between the second and fourth decade [2].

A high protein diet providing 25% dietary energy from protein is reported to improve muscle strength and to delay the downward course of the childhood

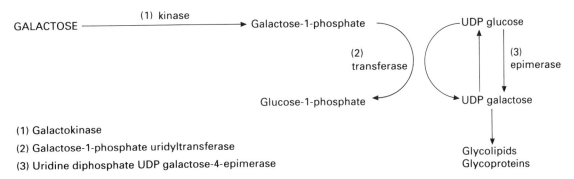

Fig. 16.2 Pathways of galactose metabolism

and starch should be given. However for some patients more aggressive treatment with uncooked cornstarch (page 213) may be necessary both to prevent low blood glucose levels and improve growth. Since alcohol is a potent inhibitor of gluconeogenesis, it is recommended that these patients only drink in moderation and preferably in combination with food [25].

INBORN ERRORS OF GALACTOSE METABOLISM

There are three inborn errors of galactose metabolism, deficiencies of the enzymes galactokinase, uridine diphosphate galactose-4-epimerase and galactose-1-phosphate uridyl transferase which result in the inability to metabolize the monosaccharide galactose (Fig. 16.2).

Galactosaemia

Of the defects in this pathway, classical galactosaemia is by far the most common disorder with an incidence of 1 in 44 000 in the United Kingdom [29]. It is caused by a deficiency of the enzyme galactose-1-phosphate uridyl transferase which catalyses the reaction that converts galactose-1-phosphate (gal-1-p) to glucose-1-phosphate and uridine diphosphate galactose (UDPgalactose) (Fig. 16.2). The latter is the substrate for the incorporation of galactose into complex glycoproteins and glycolipids. Absence of transferase causes the accumulation of gal-1-p, galactitol and galactonic acid.

As galactose is a constituent of breast milk and most infant formulas, the majority of infants present in the

first week of life. The most common features are jaundice, failure to thrive, hepatomegaly, vomiting and cataracts. It is thought that the accumulation of gal-1-p is responsible for the acute symptoms and galactitol for the formation of cataracts.

Dietary management

The main treatment of this disorder is exclusion of dietary galactose (Table 16.7). The diet needs to be continued for life and without any relaxation. However complete elimination of galactose is virtually impossible because of traces of galactose and galactolipids, particularly in plant foods. Despite the early introduction of diet and continuation of good dietary control, long term complications of galactosaemia are increasingly recognized. These include learning difficulties, speech abnormalities, growth retardation and ovarian dysfunction in females [30,31]. The mechanisms of damage are not clear and several have been suggested. These include chronic intoxication by galactose metabolites from both endogenous and exogenous sources or a deficiency of UDPgalactose which is essential as the donor of galactose into complex glycoproteins and glycolipids.

On minimal galactose diet the symptoms rapidly regress. The red cell gal-1-p level initially falls rapidly and then more slowly to an 'acceptable' low, but it is not possible to reduce this to zero which would be the value for a normal individual. Treated patients usually have a gal-1-p level below the 'acceptable' figure of 0.57 μmol per gram haemoglobin, but levels often fluctuate. It is not completely clear what is responsible for this variation. Gal-1-p is often used as a marker for dietary compliance, but its limitations should be

Table 16.7 Minimal galactose and lactose diet

	Foods allowed freely	Foods forbidden
Milk and milk products	Infant soya formula, liquid soya milk (Table 16.9)	Human, cows', sheeps' and goats' milk Evaporated, skimmed and filled milk Cows' milk based infant and follow-on formula Cream, cheese (cows', goats' and sheeps') Yoghurt, ice-cream, non-milk fat ice creams, milk puddings and desserts
Fats and oils	Milk free margarine e.g. Tomor, Granose Edible oils e.g. vegetable, sunflower, corn, rapeseed, nut Lard, dripping	Butter, margarine containing milk protein (whey and casein)
Meat, fish and eggs	Fresh meat, poultry, fish and shellfish Bacon, ham Egg, offal	Tinned meat, ham and cured meat and fish products Sausages*, burgers*, fish fingers*, fish in batter*
Cereals, flour and pasta	Wheat, rye, barley, oats, rice, corn, maize, pasta Flour, cornflour, rice flour, soya flour (if permitted) Custard powder, sago, tapioca, semolina	Egg noodles, macaroni cheese, tinned pasta with cheese Milk pudding e.g. rice pudding, instant custard mix, Instant Whip
Breakfast cereals	Most are milk free e.g. Cornflakes, Weetabix, Rice Krispies, Shreddies, Sugar Puffs	Coco Pops, Special K, muesli* Baby cereals*
Bread	White, wholemeal Some prepacked bread may contain milk protein	Milk bread, Procea
Cakes and biscuits	If known to be milk-free	Many contain milk and milk products
Fruit	All varieties, fruit juices	Fruit juices with whey protein
Vegetables	All varieties without butter or milk products Potatoes, plain crisps Pulses (if permitted)	Instant mashed potato containing milk/butter Potato salad*, vegetable salad* Flavoured crisps*
Seasonings, gravies, soups	Herbs and pure spices, mustard salt, pepper Marmite, Bovril, Oxo, Bisto Tomato ketchup, pickles, chutney Consommé	Gravy mixes* Mayonnaise*, salad cream* Monosodium glutamate* Cream soups, tinned and packet soups*
Sugars, sweets, miscellanous	Sugar, jam, honey, jelly, syrup, boiled sweets, jelly sweets, water ice-lollies, mints, non-dairy milk chocolate Carob chocolate Baking powder, yeast	Artificial sweeteners containing lactose e.g. Sweet 'n' Low Milk and plain chocolate, fudge
Drinks	Tea, coffee Milk shake fruit flavouring, fruit drinks, squashes, fizzy drinks, fruit juice Cocoa if permitted, carob	Malted drinks e.g. Horlicks Drinking Chocolate

NB Check all medicines particularly tablets to ensure they are lactose and galactose-free

* denotes some brands of manufactured foods may be suitable

recognized. Caution should be applied when interpreting red blood cell gal-1-p levels.

Sources of galactose

The main source of galactose in the diet is the disaccharide lactose (milk sugar). Lactose is hydrolysed in the gut to form galactose and glucose. Galactose is then transported across the epithelial cells and enters the portal vein to undergo further metabolism in the liver (Fig. 16.2).

The source of lactose in the diet is milk. Therefore to exclude galactose all milk, milk products and manufactured foods containing milk need to be avoided. Another potential source of galactose is from the oligosaccharides, raffinose, stachyose and verbacose which are found predominantly in pulses and legumes. However it is thought unlikely that galactose is absorbed from these sources as the small intestine does not contain the alpha-galactosidase enzyme that is required to split galactose from the oligosaccharide [32]. Instead they are fermented to produce volatile fatty acids in the large intestine. It has been suggested that in the presence of diarrhoea the small intestine can be colonized with bacteria capable of releasing α-linked galactosides [33]. With this knowledge most UK centres initially recommend that galactosides are excluded for the first year or two of life, but opinions differ. Foods containing galactosides that would be restricted are drawn mainly from a list compiled by a group of paediatric dietitians in 1978, reported at a Galactosaemic Workshop in 1982 [34] (Table 16.8). However even this list was compiled from tenuous sources. An extensive search of the literature can substantiate only some of these reported foods as containing galactosides [35].

More recent work by Gross and Acosta [36] indicates that plants, including fruit and vegetables, may contain significant sources of galactose in the form of free galactose, plant cell wall galactans and beta-1,4-linked galactosyl residues in chloroplast membranes of green plant tissue (galactolipids). These galactans and galactolipids might be hydrolysed by beta-galactosidase, present in the small intestine, to liberate galactose. More investigation has been recommended by the authors before the diets of galactosaemic children are restricted further.

Traditionally, foods which are rich in nucleoproteins were also excluded from the diet because of them being a possible source of galactose; again this is far from proven. These foods were also listed at the 1982 Galactosaemic Workshop [6] (Table 16.8).

Milk substitutes

Breast feeding and cows' milk based infant formulas are contraindicated for the galactosaemic infant because they contain lactose. Infant soya formulas (Table 16.9) are the feeds of choice; they are lactose free and oligosaccharides are removed during manufacture. Only in those with severe liver disease would a protein hydrolysate formula containing MCT, such as Pregestimil, be used. It should be noted that some of the accepted milk substitutes used in galactosaemia do contain small amounts of lactose, and therefore galactose, as it is virtually impossible to completely remove this during manufacture.

Milk is normally the main source of calcium in children's diets. For the galactosaemic child an infant

Table 16.8 Dietary sources of galactosides and nucleoproteins

Galactosides	Peas, beans, lentils, legumes, chick peas, dahls, grams, spinach
	Texturized vegetable protein
	Soya (other than soya protein isolates), soya beans, soya flour
	Cocoa, chocolate
	Nuts
Nucleoproteins	Offal – liver, kidney, brain, sweetbreads, heart
	Eggs

Table 16.9 Milk substitutes for use in galactosaemia

Infant formula	Protein source	Calcium mmol per 100 ml
InfaSoy	soya-protein isolate	1.3
Wysoy	soya-protein isolate	1.7
Prosobee	soya-protein isolate	1.6
OsterSoy	soya-protein isolate	1.4
Isomil	soya-protein isolate	1.7
Galactomin 17 (i)	sodium and calcium caseinate	1.4
Pregestimil (i) (ii)	casein hydrolysate	1.5

All infant formulas are approved by the Advisory Committee Borderline Substances for prescription on FP10. InfaSoy and Pregestimil are not specifically listed for disorders of galactose metabolism

(i) Galactomin 17 contains up to 6.5 mg galactose per 100 ml and Pregestimil contains 8.7 mg galactose per 100 ml

(ii) Contains medium chain triglyceride

soya milk can continue to be used to provide calcium, but as the content is relatively low an additional medicinal supplement may still be needed. From one year a commercial liquid soya milk can be used (if soya beans are permitted). A variety of liquid soya milks are available, some of which are devoid of calcium. Those which contain calcium provide on average 3.5 mmol/100 ml, for example Sainsbury's UHT soya milk (calcium enriched), Tesco's calcium enriched soya milk, Vande Moortele's Provamel calcium enriched soya milk. As children often develop a dislike for the taste of soya milks, medicinal calcium supplements are required. Care must be taken to ensure that these are galactose free. It is important to check the diet regularly to ensure that the reference nutrient intake [37] for calcium is always being achieved, particularly during adolescence, when requirements are high.

Milk products and milk derivatives

Milk is processed to make several different foods: cheese, yoghurt, butter, cream. These products need to be avoided in a minimal galactose diet. Often, they are added to manufactured foods such as biscuits, desserts, pasta which therefore need to be excluded. Even when milk is processed and separated into component parts both the protein fractions, casein, and in particular whey, still contain lactose. Therefore these milk derivatives (protein or fat based) must be excluded from the diet to ensure it is lactose free (Table 16.10).

Difficulties frequently arise with manufactured foods because milk derivatives often occur in a form which is not instantly recognizable as milk, e.g. casein, hydrolysed protein. It is imperative that parents are taught to interpret food labels for the presence of

Table 16.10 Milk derivatives and non-milk derivatives

Milk derivatives

Skimmed milk powder, milk solids, milk protein, separate milk solids

Whey, hydrolysed whey protein, margarine or shortening containing whey, whey syrup sweetener, hydrolysed whey sugar

Casein, caseinates, hydrolysed casein, sodium caseinate

Butter, cream, animal fat (may be butter), buttermilk, butterfat, artificial cream

Cheese, cheese powder, non-fat milk solids

Lactose

Non-milk derivatives

Lactic acid E270, sodium lactate E325, potassium lactate E325 or calcium lactate E327

Cocoa butter, non-dairy cream

---

these products. Unfortunately reading the label will not always provide a conclusive answer as UK labelling does not require the listing of all compound ingredients (if the compound ingredient forms less than 25% of the final product its individual constituents need not be declared [38]). This makes it very difficult to guarantee from the ingredient label that the food is milk free. Also, it is not a legal requirement for all foods to have ingredient labels e.g. those found in a baker's or butcher's shop. These may need to be avoided because of limited information concerning their composition. Conversely confusion may also occur with words which might alert parents to thinking milk is an ingredient when this is not the case (Table 16.10).

Lactose is sometimes used as a filler or carrier and is found in medicines especially tablets, artificial sweeteners and flavourings, e.g. monosodium glutamate (E621). Obtaining this information pertaining to manufactured foods is particularly difficult as these are usually compound ingredients. Often the decision has to be made whether to avoid these completely or to allow them, knowing that the quantity of galactose is likely to be insignificant.

Galactosides and nucleoproteins in processed foods

Galactosides and nucleoproteins (Table 16.8) are usually avoided for the first year or two of life. Many commercial baby foods contain egg, soya protein, soya flour and pulses. Excluding these in addition to milk severely limits the range of suitable commercial baby foods.

Alcohol

In adolescents with galactosaemia, avoidance of alcohol is often recommended because alcohol inhibits galactose metabolism [39]. However, if the pathway is blocked the restriction of alcohol has little logic. UK practice varies and most centres do allow alcohol in moderation.

Heterozygote mothers – dietary treatment

There is considerable uncertainty about the management of pregnancy in heterozygote mothers. There is no clear evidence that the outcome of pregnancy is better for those who have been on a strict low galactose diet and those who have not [40]. Usually, intakes of the major sources of lactose, i.e. milk and milk products is restricted, whilst ensuring the mother has an adequate supply of calcium.

Galactokinase deficiency (Fig. 16.2)

The clinical manifestations of galactokinase deficiency are much less severe than in classical galactosaemia. Cataracts are the main feature and there is no liver disease or developmental delay. The dietary treatment is the same as for galactosaemia i.e. galactose avoidance. Gitzelmann [32] has suggested that the degree of galactose avoidance can be less strict but recognizes that no systematic study has been done.

UDPgalactose 4 – epimerase deficiency (Fig. 16.2)

Two forms of epimerase deficiency exist; only the severe form which is extremely rare requires dietary

treatment. Epimerase forms UDPgalactose from UDPglucose. A complete absence of galactose from the diet and lack of UDPgalactose formation would result in an inability to form complex glycoproteins and glycolipids. Only two cases are reported in the literature [41,42]. The dietary treatment differed slightly; both were maintained on a minimal galactose diet but in addition one patient was supplemented with 1.5 g galactose per day. This was deemed necessary to provide substrate for the production of galactocerebrosides and other glycoproteins and glycolipids. Although the other patient had no supplements sufficient galactose may well have been obtained from unrecognized dietary sources. The optimal dietary therapy of patients with epimerase deficiency is not known. Complete exclusion of galactose appears deleterious. Either the diet can be relaxed slightly or a small supplement of dietary galactose can be given to supply sufficient substrate for synthesis of glycoproteins and glycolipids [43].

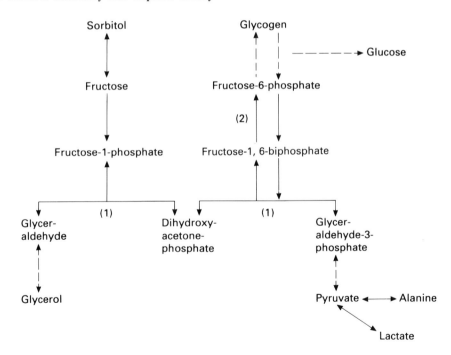

(1) Fructose-1-phosphate aldolase B (Hereditary fructose intolerance)

(2) Fructose-1, 6-bisphosphatase

Fig. 16.3 Fructose metabolism

HEREDITARY FRUCTOSE INTOLERANCE

Hereditary fructose intolerance (HFI) is caused by a greatly reduced activity of the enzyme fructose-1-phosphate aldolase B in the liver, kidney and small intestine. This enzyme is an essential step in the metabolism of fructose (Fig. 16.3).

Symptoms will only develop when the child is given fructose. In the UK exposure to fructose is uncommon prior to weaning as breast milk and infant formula are fructose free. During the introduction of solid food sources of fructose become abundant from fruits, vegetables and commercial baby foods. Whilst the clinical picture and dietary history should enable a diagnosis of fructosaemia to be made in older patients, the diagnosis can be more difficult in young patients. However, even in older patients symptoms may be minimal because they develop an aversion to sweet tasting foods and self-select a low fructose diet. Nevertheless, these children may still be given fructose from unexpected sources such as medicines.

In the infant and young child the main clinical symptoms include poor feeding, vomiting, abdominal distention and failure to thrive. Hypoglycaemia may develop after exposure to fructose. Continued exposure to fructose causes severe liver failure, proximal renal tubular dysfunction and specific metabolic disturbances [44]. None of these problems are specific and the key to diagnosis is a very accurate clinical and dietary history.

The main treatment of HFI is strict exclusion of fructose, sucrose and sorbitol from the diet. This results in a rapid improvement of symptoms. The long term prognosis is good although hepatomegaly and fatty changes in the liver may persist [45]. The diet needs to be continued for life without relaxation as even small amounts of fructose have been shown to be harmful [46]. Abdominal pain and vomiting can occur if a child on the diet is accidentally exposed to fructose.

Sources of fructose

Fructose in the diet comes from fructose, sucrose and sorbitol. Fructose is absorbed by a carrier mediated process across the small intestine and then enters the liver to undergo further metabolism (Fig. 16.3). The disaccharide sucrose is cleaved in the small intestine by sucrase-isomaltase to form a molecule of both glucose and fructose. Sorbitol, a sugar alcohol, diffuses slowly across the intestinal absorptive surface with

only 10% to 30% being absorbed. In the liver it is rapidly converted via sorbitol dehydrogenase to fructose. Another potential source of fructose is from complex oligosaccharides such as raffinose and stachyose; however it is thought unlikely that these are hydrolysed to any significant extent in the small intestine and therefore little of the fructose is absorbed. Fructose polymers such as inulin are widespread in various plants e.g. artichokes [47]. Again these are not absorbed; instead they undergo bacterial fermentation in the colon.

In recent years there has been an increase in the use of commercially prepared sugar alcohols as artificial sweeteners which are potential sources of fructose. Isomalt is a mixture of two disaccharide alcohols, glucose-sorbitol and glucose-mannitol. During digestion in the small intestine it is hydrolysed to 50% glucose, 25% sorbitol and 25% mannitol. Lycasin is a glucose syrup in which all glucose units with free aldehyde groups have been reduced by hydrogenation to sorbitol. The product consists of sorbitol, hydrogenated oligo- and higher polysaccharides. Oligofructose is obtained from inulin through enzymatic hydrolysis, producing a mixture of chains of fructose molecules of varying chain length (2 to 20 molecules). Commercial syrups of oligofructose contain small amounts of fructose and sucrose. As yet these oligofructose syrups are not used in the United Kingdom.

Minimal fructose, sucrose, sorbitol diet

The aim of dietary treatment of HFI is complete elimination of fructose, sucrose and sorbitol, but it is not possible to exclude these sugars completely (Table 16.11). In practice the intake of fructose from all sources is 1–2 g per day. The normal average daily intake of fructose (including contribution from sucrose) in unaffected infants has been reported as 20 g per day [48]. Obviously intakes in older children on normal diets would be much greater and could easily be of the order of 100 g per day.

Fructose is the natural sugar present in fruit, vegetables and honey. Sucrose is also found in fruit and vegetables but a much greater source is from sugar cane or beet. These are refined to produce table sugar which is used extensively in food manufacture as a sweetener and bulking agent. Sugar is a major ingredient in cakes, biscuits, desserts and soft drinks. Many other commerical foods (e.g. stock cubes, tinned meats, bottled sauces, savoury snack biscuits) contain

Table 16.11 Minimal, fructose, sucrose and sorbitol diet (<2 g per day)

Foods allowed freely	Foods to avoid
Sugars and sweeteners Glucose, glucose polymers, glucose syrup, dextrose, lactose, starch, maltose, maltodextrin, malt extract Saccharin, aspartame Glucose tablets – Dextrosol Lucozade Sport Glucose Energy tablets – original only	Sugar (cane or beet) – white, brown, castor, icing Fruit sugar, fructose, laevulose, Sorbitol, Lycasin, Isomalt, Hydrogenated glucose syrup Honey, syrup, treacle, caramel, molasses, corn syrup Jam, marmalade, lemon curd Sweets, chocolate, toffee Dessert sauces, jelly, ice lollies
Fruits Avocado, rhubarb (occasionally)	All other fruit and fruit products
Vegetables (cooked) (boil and discard water)	
Group 1 (<0.5 g fructose per 100 g) Broccoli (fresh), celery, globe artichokes, mushrooms (fried), old potato, plain potato crisps, spinach, watercress. Pulses – beans: haricot, mung, red kidney – peas: chick, dried split, mangetout – lentils	Beetroot, brussel sprouts, carrots, gherkins, green beans, onion, parsnip, pepper, spring onion, sweetcorn, tomato Pulses – beans: green, runner, baked in tomato sauce Tinned vegetables with added sugar, mayonnaise or salad cream Coleslaw Flavoured crisps
Group 2 (0.5–1 g fructose per 100 g) Asparagus, beansprouts, broccoli (frozen), cabbage, cauliflower, courgette, cucumber, Jerusalem artichoke, leeks, lettuce, marrow, new potato, pumpkin, radish, spring greens, swede, turnip Pulses – beans: broad, soya – peas: marrow fat, processed	
Dairy products Infant formula milk Cows' milk – whole, semi-skimmed, skimmed Unsweetened evaporated milk Coffee-Mate, Coffee Compliment, dried milk powder	Liquid soya milk Flavoured milk, condensed milk, milkshake powders and syrups Aerosol cream Fruit and flavoured yoghurt Fromage frais

Table 16.11 (continued)

Foods allowed freely	Foods to avoid
Cream Cheese, plain cottage cheese Natural yoghurt	Cheese with added ingredients e.g. pineapple, nuts
Eggs Allowed	
Meat, fish and poultry All fresh meat, fish and poultry If processed read label to check for added sucrose, fructose or honey	Processed meats which have added sucrose e.g. meat pastes, frankfurters, salami, paté, sausages Tendersweet meats e.g. ham Honey cured meats Ready-made meals containing vegetables
Cereals Arrowroot, cornflour, custard powder, sago, semolina, tapioca, oats, barley Flour, rice, pasta (white in preference to brown) Puffed wheat, porridge, Readybrek or Shredded Wheat (one serve per day of either) White bread (pre-packed), Bakers' bread – check if sugar is added to dough mixture Cream crackers, Matzo crackers, water biscuits, Ryvita, plain rice cakes	Bran, wheatgerm Pasta tinned in tomato sauce Most manufactured breakfast cereals Wholemeal bread, sweetened breads, e.g. malt bread, soda bread, currant bread Cakes, biscuits, pastries Savoury snack biscuits
Fats and oils Butter, margarine, lard, suet Vegetable oils	
Drinks Tea, coffee, cocoa Lucozade (not fruit flavour), Ferguzade, Glucose Syrup Beverage, Soda water, mineral water Squashes and fizzy drinks sweetened with only saccharin or aspartame, (free from sugar, fruit flavourings or comminuted fruits) Milupa Baby Drinks (glucose and herb extracts)	Instant tea mixes, coffee essence Drinking chocolate, malted milk drinks Fruit juices, vegetable juices Fizzy drinks, fruit squash Diabetic squash containing sorbitol or fructose
Miscellaneous Pure herbs, mustard and spices	Gravy browning, stock cubes

Table 16.11 (continued)

Foods allowed freely	Foods to avoid
Salt, pepper, vinegar	Pickles, chutney, tomato purée
Marmite, Bovril	Mayonnaise, salad cream
Food colouring, gelatine	Bottled sauces and dressings
Baking Powder	e.g. tomato ketchup,
Sesame seeds	horseradish sauce
Pumpkin and sunflower seeds	Packet and tinned soups
maximum of 10 g per day	All other nuts, peanut butter,
	marzipan

NB 1 Always read the label of manufactured foods to check for sources of fructose
2 Check with the chemist that prescribed medicines (syrups or tablets) do not contain sucrose or sorbitol

Analysis of fructose and sucrose content of foods

1 *Cereals and Cereal Products – The Third Supplement to McCance and Widdowson's 'The Composition of Foods'* 4e. 1988.
2 *Milk and Milk Products and Eggs – The Fourth Supplement to McCance and Widdowson's 'The Composition of Foods'* 4e. 1989.
3 *Vegetables, Herbs and Spices – The Fifth Supplement to McCance and Widdowson's 'The Composition of Foods'* 4e. 1991.
4 *Fruit and Nuts – The First Supplement to McCance and Widdowson's 'The Composition of Foods'* 5e. 1992.

Publishers of above: Holland B, Unwin ID, Buss DH, The Royal Society of Chemistry and Ministry of Agriculture, Fisheries and Food, HMSO.

sugar but are much less obvious sources. Indeed, very few manufactured foods are suitable for inclusion in the diet. Flavourings can be another potential trace source of sucrose and fructose as these sugars are sometimes used as carriers for flavouring compounds.

Only vegetables which contain predominantly starch can be included in the diet (Table 16.11). Permitted vegetables have been divided into two groups (with a fructose content of 0.5 g per 100 g and 0.5–1.0 g per 100 g) to give a wider choice. However, fructose from vegetables should not exceed 1.0–1.5 g per day as small amounts of fructose from cereals will increase the total intake to the 2 g maximum. It is important to note the difference in fructose content between raw and cooked vegetables. Cooking causes a loss of free sugars, consequently cooked vegetables have a lower fructose content and are recommended in preference to raw. New potatoes have a higher fructose content than old (0.65 g/100 g versus 0.25 g/100 g). Sucrose content of stored potatoes, has previously been reported to both decrease and increase on storage [49,50]; however no further analysis is available to resolve this issue. Wholemeal flour contains more

fructose than white because the germ and bran contains sucrose. Similarly other wholegrain foods (e.g. brown rice, wholemeal pasta) contain more sucrose than the refined varieties. No accurate analysis for the fructose content of bread is available; however it would appear prudent to choose white in preference to wholemeal. Bread has previously been restricted in the diets of children with HFI. Nowadays this restriction is probably unnecessary because most flour improvers for bread making do not contain sugar. If the bread does contain sugar it has to be declared on the ingredient label. Caution should be applied where richer doughs are used (e.g. in soft rolls) because often the flour improver does contain sugar in these instances. Bread bought from craft bakers may also contain sugar, and bakers are under no legal obligation to declare this information to the consumer.

Sorbitol is used as an artificial sweetener and bulk sweetener, particularly in diabetic foods and drinks; these foods must be avoided. Isomalt and lycasin are used as alternative sweeteners, predominantly being used in confectionery. Isomalt may also be found in baked goods, breakfast cereals, desserts, snack foods and jam. These need to be avoided because of their sorbitol content. Sucrose and sorbitol are often used in medicines (particularly syrups) as bulking agents or to improve the flavour. Parents need to be made aware of this and know to check with a pharmacist about the sucrose content of prescribed medicines.

Intravenous fructose and sorbitol are potential lethal sources of fructose; these are rarely used in the United Kingdom, but are more commonly used in Europe [51].

Starch, glucose and lactose can be included in the diet. Glucose can be used as an alternative sweetener to sucrose and can also provide a useful source of energy. The relative sweetness of glucose is only half that of sucrose, so additional sweetening may be needed in baked goods. Some intense sweeteners, e.g. Sweetex, can be successfully added to cooked food; others, e.g. aspartame, decompose on heating and are therefore not suitable for baking. However, extra sweetening may not be necessary or desirable as children with HFI dislike and avoid sweet tasting foods. Glucose is not prescribable on FP10 for treatment of HFI.

Nutritional problems

Children with HFI are at risk of vitamin C and possible folic acid deficiency due to the exclusion of the major dietary sources of these vitamins i.e. fruits and vegetables. A suitable medicinal supplement (e.g. Vitamin C Powder from Boots the Chemist plc) should be prescribed to meet the RNI [37]. Lack of dietary fibre may also be a problem. This could be overcome by including pulses and oats, which contain only very small amounts of fructose, in the diet.

FRUCTOSE-1,6-BISPHOSPHATASE DEFICIENCY

In the fasting state, glycogen initially provides the major fuel source for glucose production. As the duration of fast extends and glycogen stores are depleted, glucose is synthesized via gluconeogenesis from lactate, glycerol and the gluconeogenic amino acids such as alanine. A deficiency of fructose-1,6-bisphosphatase (Fig. 16.3) blocks the gluconeogenic pathway and, as a result, during fasting patients develop hypoglycaemia and a marked lactic acidosis with ketosis.

Fructose-1,6-bisphosphatase deficiency may present in the newborn period or, in older children, during intercurrent infections associated with prolonged fasting [44]. Once diagnosed, these life threatening acute episodes can be prevented with careful treatment. The prognosis is good, with normal growth and development.

Dietary treatment

The aims of the dietary management of fructose-1,6-bisphosphatase deficiency are to:

- prevent hypoglycaemia
- reduce the need for gluconeogenesis
- provide good glycogen reserves.

This can be achieved by avoidance of prolonged fasts and provision of regular meals, with a high intake of carbohydrate from starch. Patients should be carefully assessed for fasting tolerance, which should improve with age. The majority of children will be well controlled without the need for fructose restriction when they are well. Nevertheless, it is inadvisable for them to have a very high intake of fructose as this may cause hypoglycaemia and lactic acidosis. During illness fructose must be completely avoided.

Diet when well

The young infant is fed at four hourly intervals during the day and night. Even when weaning is well established, a late night and early morning feed is still given to reduce the duration of overnight fasting.

The older child is given regular meals containing a high carbohydrate intake from starch to provide a constant supply of 'slow-release' glucose. Fasting overnight is not normally a problem provided a starchy bedtime snack and early breakfast is given. A modest decrease in fat intake is necessary to compensate for the increased carbohydrate intake to prevent an excessive intake of energy. A high intake of fructose as sucrose in cakes and confectionery is discouraged.

Alcohol inhibits gluconeogenesis and if taken in excess in healthy adolescents can precipitate hypoglycaemia. Alcohol should therefore be taken in moderation and only with food.

Diet during illness

Poor appetite and fasting is common in the sick child. In the child with fructose-1,6-bisphosphatase deficiency it is critical to prevent such prolonged fasts; during intercurrent illnesses an exogenous source of glucose must be supplied. The standard emergency regimen (page 206) must be given during times of illness to reduce the risk of hypoglycaemia and lactic acidosis. Fructose, sucrose and sorbitol must be excluded because these will exacerbate the metabolic derangement. Fat should be avoided during decompensation as glycerol may exacerbate the illness. Emergency regimen drinks are restricted to those which are glucose based; glucose polymer and low calorie squash (sorbitol free) or Lucozade (original variety). Medications must be free of fructose, sucrose and sorbitol. Some patients may decompensate rapidly, becoming very ill with marked acidosis. The impact can be reduced by giving sodium bicarbonate up to 4 mmol/kg body weight/day. If there are signs of metabolic acidosis the patient's condition must be assessed in hospital. Once the child improves, normal diet can be resumed, with a gradual reintroduction of fructose and sucrose-containing foods. During the recovery period extra drinks should continue to be given, particularly at night.

REFERENCES

1 Burchell A, Waddell I Identification, purification and genetic deficiencies of the glucose-6-phosphatase system transport proteins. *Eur J Pediatr*, 1993, **152**(Suppl 1) 14–17.

2 Hers H, Van Hoof F, de Barsy T Glycogen storage diseases. In: Scriver CR *et al.* (eds.) *The Metabolic Basis of Inherited Disease*, 6e. New York: McGraw-Hill, 1989.

3 Roe T *et al.* Inflammatory bowel disease in glycogen storage disease type IB. *J Paediatr*, 1986, **109**(1) 55–59.

4 Stanley CA, Mills J, Baker L Intragastric feeding in Type I glycogen storage disease: Factors affecting the control of lacticacidaemia. *Pediatr Res*, 1981, **15** 1504–1508.

5 Bier D *et al.* Measurement of true glucose production rates in infancy and childhood with 6,6-diodeuteroglucose. *Diabetes*, 1977, **26**(11) 1016–1023.

6 Green H *et al.* Continuous nocturnal nasogastric feeding for management of Type I GSD. *New Eng J Med*, 1976, **294** 423–425.

7 Chen Y, Cornblath M, Sidbury J Cornstarch therapy in Type I glycogen storage disease. *New Eng J Med*, 1984, **310** 171–175.

8 Fernandes J The effect of disaccharides on the hyperlacticacidaemia of glucose-6-phosphatase-deficient children. *Acta Paediatr Scand*, 1974, **63** 695–698.

9 Fernandes J, Berger R, Smit P Lactate as a cerebral metabolic fuel for glucose-6-phosphatase deficient children. *Pediatr Res*, 1984, **18**(4) 335–339.

10 Fernandes J The glycogen storage diseases. In: Fernandes J, Saudubray JM, Tada K (eds.) *Inborn Metabolic Diseases, Diagnosis and Treatment*. Berlin: Springer-Verlag, 1990.

11 Fernandes J, Alaapovic P, Wit J Gastric drip feeding in patients with glycogen storage disease Type I: its effects on growth and plasma lipids and apoliproproteins. *Pediatr Res*, 1989, **25**(4) 327–331.

12 Schmitz G, Hohage H, Ullrich K Glucose-6-phosphate; a key compound in glycogenosis I and favism leading to hyper- or hypolipidaemia. *Eur J Pediatr*, 1993, **152** (Suppl 1) 77–84.

13 Leonard J, Dunger D Hypoglycaemia complicating feeding regimens for glycogen storage disease. *Lancet*, 1978, **11** 1203–1204.

14 Fine R, Kogut M, Donnell G Intestinal absorption in type I glycogen storage disease. *J Pediatr*, 1969, **75** 632–635.

15 Milla P *et al.* Disordered intestinal function in glycogen storage disease. *J Inher Metab Dis*, 1978, **1** 155–157.

16 Collins J *et al.* Glucose production rates in Type I glycogen storage disease. *J Inher Metab Dis*, 1990, **13** 195–206.

17 Smit G *et al.* The dietary treatment of children with Type I glycogen storage disease with slow release carbohydrate. *Pediatr Res*, 1984, **18**(9) 879–881.

18 Hayde M, Widhalm K Effects of cornstarch treatment in very young children with Type I glycogen storage disease. *Eur J Pediatr*, 1990, **149** 630–633.

19 Ogata T *et al.* Effect of cornstarch formula in an infant with Type I glycogen storage disease. *Acta Paediatr Jpn*, 1988, **30** 547–552.

20 Sidbury J, Chen Y, Roe L The role of raw starches in the treatment of type I Glycogenosis. *Arch Intern Med*, 1986, **146** 370–373.

21 Chen YT *et al.* Type I glycogen storage disease: nine years of management with cornstarch. *Eur J Pediatr*, 1993, **152**(Suppl 1) 56–59.

22 Gremse D, Bucuvalas J, Balisteri W Efficacy of cornstarch therapy in Type III glycogen storage disease. *Am J Clin Nutr*, 1990, **52** 672–674.

23 Borowitz S, Greene H Cornstarch therapy in a patient with Type III glycogen storage disease. *J Paediatr Gastroenterol Nutr*, 1987, **6**(4) 631–639.

24 Slonim A, Coleman R, Moses W Myopathy and growth failure in debrancher enzyme deficiency: improvement with high protein nocturnal enteral therapy. *J Paediatr*, 1984, **105**(6) 906–911.

25 Collins JE *et al.* The effect of ethanol on glucose production in phosphorylase b kinase deficiency. *J Inher Metab Dis*, 1989, **12** 312–322.

26 Slonim E *et al.* Improvement of muscle function in acid maltase deficiency by high protein therapy. *Neurology*, 1983, **33** 34–38.

27 Umpleby M *et al.* Protein turnover in acid maltase deficiency before and after treatment with a high protein diet. *J Neurosurgery Psychiatry*, 1987, **50** 587–592.

28 Smit GPA *et al.* The long term outcome of patients with glycogen storage diseases. *J Inher Metab Dis*, 1990, **13** 411–418.

29 Honeyman M *et al.* Galactosaemia: Results of the British Paediatric Surveillance Unit Study 1988–90. *Arch Dis Childh*, 1993, **69** 339–341.

30 Waggoner DD, Buist NR, Donnell GN Long-term prognosis in galactosaemia: results of a survey of 350 cases. *J Inher Metab Dis*, 1990, **13** 802–818.

31 Schweitzer S *et al.* Long-term outcome in 134 patients with Galactosaemia. *Eur J Pediatr*, 1993, **152** 36–43.

32 Gitzelmann R, Auricchio S The handling of soya alpha-galactosides by a normal and a galactosaemic child. *Paediatrics* 1965, **36** 231.

33 Gitzelmann R Disorders of galactose metabolism. In: Fernandes J, Saudubray JM, Tada K (eds.) *Inborn Metabolic Diseases*. Berlin: Springer-Verlag, 1990.

34 Clothier CM, Davidson DC Galactosaemia workshop. *Hum Nutr: Appl Nutr*, 1983, **37a** 483–490.

35 Southgate DAT *et al.* Free sugars in foods. *J Hum Nutr*, 1978, **32** 335–347.

36 Gross KC, Acosta PB Fruits and vegetables are a source of galactose. *J Inher Metab Dis*, 1991, **14** 253–258.

37 Department of Health Report on Health and Social Subjects No 41. *Dietary Reference Values for Food Energy*

and Nutrients for the United Kingdom. London: HMSO, 1991.

38 *The Food Labelling Regulations*, No 1305. London: HMSO, 1984.

39 Brandt NJ How long should galactosaemia be treated? In: *Inherited Disorders of Carbohydrate Metabolism*. Lancaster: MTP Press, 1980.

40 Irons M *et al.* Accumulation of galactose-1-phosphate in the galactosaemic fetus despite maternal milk avoidance. *J Paediatr*, 1985, **107** 261–263.

41 Holton JB *et al.* Galactosaemia: a new severe variant due to uridine diphosphate galactose-4-epimerase deficiency. *Arch Dis Child*, 1981, **56** 885–887.

42 Sardharwalla IB *et al.* A patient with a severe type of epimerase deficiency galactosaemia. *Abstracts of the 25th SSIEM Annual Symposium*, 1987:91.

43 Segal S Disorders of galactose metabolism. In: Scriver CR *et al.* (eds.) *The Metabolic Basis of Inherited Disease*, 6e. New York: McGraw-Hill, 1989.

44 Gitzelmann R, Steinmann B, Van den Berghe G Disorders of fructose metabolism. In: Scriver CR *et al.* (eds.) *The Metabolic Basis of Inherited Disease*, 6e. New York: McGraw-Hill, 1989.

45 Odièvre M *et al.* Hereditary fructose intolerance in childhood diagnosis, management and course in 55 patients. *Am J Dis Childh*, 1978, **132** 605–608.

46 Oberhaensli R *et al.* Study of Hereditary fructose intolerance by the use of magnetic resonance spectroscopy. *Lancet*, 1987, (24 October) 931–934.

47 Rumessen J *et al.* Fructans of Jerusalem artichokes: intestinal transport, absorption, fermentation and influence on blood glucose, insulin and C-peptide responses in healthy subjects. *Am J Clin Nutr*, 1990, **52** 675–681.

48 Mills A, Tyler H *Food and Nutrient Intakes of British Infants aged 6 to 12 Months*. London: Ministry of Agriculture, Fisheries and Foods, HMSO, 1992.

49 Francis D Galactosaemia, fructosaemia and favism – dietary management. In: *Diets for Sick Children*, 4e. Oxford: Blackwell Scientific Publications, 1987.

50 Bell L, Sherwood W Current practices and improved recommendations for treating hereditary fructose intolerance. *J Am Diet Assoc*, 1987, **87**(6) 721–731.

51 Collins J Metabolic disease, time for fructose solutions to go. *Lancet*, 1993, **341** 600.

FURTHER READING

Coleman R *et al.* Glycogen debranching enzyme deficiency: long term study of serium enzyme activities and clinical features. *J Inher Metab Dis*, 1992, **15** 869–881.

Moses S Pathophysiology and dietary treatment of the glycogen storage diseases. *J Paediatr Gastroenterol Nutr*, 1990, **11**(2) 155–174.

USEFUL ADDRESSES

Association for Glycogen Storage Disease (UK)
9 Lindop Road, Hale, Altrincham, Cheshire WA15 9DZ.

Galactosaemia Support Group
31 Cotysmore Road, Sutton Coldfield, West Midlands.

CHAPTER 17

Disorders of Fatty Acid Oxidation

Fatty acids are metabolized by many tissues, including cardiac and skeletal muscle. They form a major source of energy, particularly during prolonged fasting and infections.

Fat stored in adipose tissue as triglycerides is hydrolysed releasing free fatty acids into the blood stream. These are transported to the tissues bound with albumin. Long chain fatty acids enter the mitochondria via a carnitine dependent pathway, whereas medium chain fatty acids do not require carnitine. The fatty acids then undergo progressive beta-oxidation, a cycle of four steps; on each turn of the cycle one molecule of acetyl-CoA is produced and the fatty acids are shortened by two carbon atoms. Acetyl-CoA is then metabolized in the tricarboxylic acid cycle. In the liver it may be converted to form ketones (Fig. 17.1).

Several defects of the beta-oxidation pathway have now been described. The clinical features are thought to be the result of both the inability to oxidize fatty acids and the accumulation of toxic intermediates. Many of the disorders of fatty acid oxidation present with an acute encephalopathy often accompanied by hypoglycaemia. As a result of the defect in fatty acid oxidation the production of ketones is reduced, hence 'hypoketotic hypoglycaemia'. In some there is associated chronic muscle weakness and cardiomyopathy.

Treatment of these disorders is mainly by diet. The two major principles are to control the mobilization of fatty acids and to limit the intake of long chain fat, in some cases replacing long chain fat with medium chain fat. With the exception of medium chain acyl-CoA dehydrogenase deficiency, disorders of fatty acid oxidation are rare and experience of dietary treatment is therefore limited.

Acyl-CoA dehydrogenases

The first step of beta-oxidation is catalysed by an acyl-CoA dehydrogenase. There are three separate enzymes which metabolize fatty acids of different chain length although there is some overlapping of substrate specificity:

Fatty acid chain length
long chain acyl-CoA
    dehydrogenase – C12 to C18
medium chain acyl-CoA
    dehydrogenase – C6 to C12
short chain acyl-CoA
    dehydrogenase – C4 to C6

Medium chain acyl-CoA dehydrogenase

Medium chain acyl-CoA dehydrogenase (MCAD) deficiency is the most common of the fatty acid oxidation defects with an estimated incidence of approximately 1:6000 births. MCAD most commonly presents in infancy or early childhood (mean age 13.5 months) [1]. Acute decompensation, characterized by encephalopathy and hypoketotic hypoglycaemia, is triggered by metabolic stress such as fasting or gastrointestinal or respiratory infections and if not recognized and treated will progress ultimately to coma.

Dietary management

The medium chain acyl-CoA dehydrogenase acts specifically on C6 to C12 fatty acids. C6 to C10 fatty acids are present only in trace amounts in a normal diet. C12 is found in the diet, but can be oxidized by the long chain enzyme. In the well child, the diet can

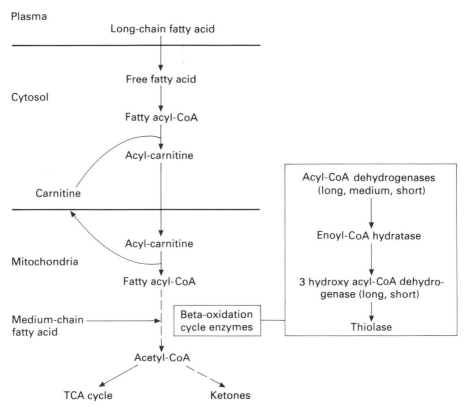

Fig. 17.1 Pathway of mitochondrial fatty acid oxidation.
Long chain fatty acids are transported into the mitochondria and sequentially degraded via β-oxidation to 2-carbon acetyl-CoA which is used for ketone synthesis (in liver) or oxidised in the tricarboxylic acid cycle. Medium chain fatty acids enter directly into β-oxidation.

be completely normal, but it is important to avoid prolonged fasts and to ensure that the child has regular meals containing starch to provide 'slow-release glucose'. Missed meals should be replaced by a sugary or glucose polymer drink. Fatty acid oxidation rates increase as the period of fasting is extended and this includes night time. Therefore it is essential to provide a late night snack and breakfast to prevent decompensation. Infants should continue a late night feed at least during the first year and children should not fast for more than 10–12 hours. Older children may tolerate longer fasts. Restriction of dietary fat is not necessary provided the child is well. Long chain fats can be oxidized by long or short acyl-CoA de-hydrogenases or alternate pathways. Medium chain triglycerides (MCT) occur in only a few foods and are not present in significant quantities to cause a prob-lem. Coconut is the only exception (9 g MCT per 100 g), however small amounts are acceptable. Some

specialized infant formulas (e.g. Pregestimil, MCT Pepdite) contain a high percentage of MCT and must not be given.

The following guidelines should be followed when treating a child with MCAD:

- prolonged fasts should be avoided
- meals containing starch must be taken regularly
- a late night snack should be given
- breakfast must not be missed
- missed meals should be replaced with a sugary drink
- MCT products must be avoided.

Diet during illness

In contrast to the diet when well, a much stricter dietary regimen is needed during illness. It is critical to inhibit the mobilization of fatty acids which would result in the production of toxic fatty acid intermediates and precipitate overwhelming illness. If the child is not eating well and missing meals the standard emergency regimen should be used (page 200). Long chain fat should be excluded from the diet during the acute period and MCT is strictly contraindicated. As the child improves the normal diet can be resumed, but extra emergency regimen drinks should be given particularly during the night until the child is fully recovered and eating well.

Hypoglycaemia is a relatively late complication so that monitoring blood glucose can give a false sense of security. These patients may develop a marked encephalopathy before becoming hypoglycaemic and treatment must be started before this [2].

Long chain acyl-CoA dehydrogenase deficiency

Long chain acyl-CoA dehydrogenase deficiency (LCAD) is much rarer than MCAD but is substantially more severe. Lack of LCAD reduces the oxidation of fatty acids for either energy production in the tricarboxylic acid cycle or hepatic ketone synthesis. The clinical picture is one of collapse, coma and fasting hypoglycaemia, often presenting in the neonatal period or early weeks of life. There is also muscle weakness and cardiomyopathy. This is not only due to impaired energy production, but may reflect a toxic effect of accumulated fatty acids and long chain acyl-CoA intermediates in the mitochondria.

Dietary management

The long chain acyl-CoA dehydrogenase enzyme acts specifically on C12 to C18 fatty acids. Both dietary fat and adipose tissue contain predominantly C16 and C18 fatty acids. In LCAD deficiency fatty acid oxidation from both sources needs to be limited. The diet should contain minimal long chain fat and be high in carbohydrate with frequent feeding. Medium chain fat can be included in the diet provided a medium chain defect has been excluded. Frequent feeding is necessary to reduce fatty acid mobilization. The interval between feeding is based on the response to fasting which is assessed by measuring the plasma concentration of free fatty acids and glucose under carefully controlled conditions. During the day, three hourly feeding may be needed and, at night, continuous nasogastric feeding if fasting tolerance is low. Since fatty acid oxidation rates decrease with age,

those patients who have initially been stabilized on a strict diet may be able to have more fat and feed less frequently once they are older. Patients with milder defects can have a more relaxed diet.

Energy distribution in the diet for LCAD should be provided as follows:

- 70% energy from carbohydrate (CHO)
- 10–15% energy from protein
- 1–2% energy from essential fatty acids (EFA)
- 10–20% energy from medium chain fat.

The diet can contain 3–5 g long chain fat, including essential fatty acids (EFA). Frequent feeding is essential.

Infants

Infants need a minimal long chain fat (<3 g), high carbohydrate feed (Table 17.1) with frequent feeding. In the newly diagnosed infant 24 hour continuous nasogastric feeding is often necessary to achieve an adequate intake and to prevent further metabolic decompensation. At present a modular feed is the only way of providing this, therefore great care must be taken to ensure all nutrients meet the reference nutrient intake for age particularly the requirement for EFA. At least 1% of total energy intake should come from linoleic acid and 0.2% from alpha-linolenic acid [3]. Soya or walnut oil provides the optimum ratio of linoleic to alpha-linolenic acids and allows a minimum amount of long chain triglyceride (LCT) to be given. The oil can be given medicinally from a spoon. When commencing the modular feed, skimmed milk powder is used as the protein base with glucose polymer added to a total concentration of 10% CHO. A lower CHO concentration may be necessary if the child has diarrhoea, as has been encountered in the newly diagnosed patient (personal observation). MCT emulsion, because of its high osmolar load and rapid absorption, should be introduced gradually by 1 or 2 g increments per day to prevent any gastrointestinal side effects such as diarrhoea, vomiting or abdominal distention. The vitamin and mineral mixture should be gradually added from day one, increasing to the full dose within a few days. Monogen, a minimal long chain fat nutritionally complete infant formula, is currently being evaluated for use in LCAD.

Weaning is commenced at the normal age of 4–6 months. Solids should have a minimal fat content and be high in starch. As solid food intake increases the

Table 17.1 Minimal fat feed for an infant with LCAD: age three months, weight 4 kg

Ingredients	Energy		CHO (g)	Protein (g)	Fat (g)		Na mmol	K mmol	Vit A μg	Vit D μg
	kcal	kJ			LCT	MCT				
30 g Skimmed milk powder*	107	447	16	11	0.4	–	7.5	13.2	110	0.4
65 g Glucose polymer e.g. Maxijul	234	975	62	–	–	–	1.1	0.2	–	–
20 ml Liquigen	80	334	–	–	–	10	0.2	–	–	–
7 g Paediatric Seravit	21	89	5.2	–	–	–	–	–	–	–
plus water to 600 ml										
3 Mothers' and Children's vitamin drops	–	–	–	–	–	–	–	–	120	4.5
2 ml Walnut or soya oil	18	75	–	–	2	–	–	–	–	–
0.1 ml Folic acid (Lexpec)	–	–	–	–	–	–	–	–	–	–
Totals	460	1920	78.6	11	2.4	10	8.6	13.4	525	8.8
Per 100 ml	77	320	13.1	1.8	0.4	1.7	1.4	2.2	–	–
Per kg	115	480		2.8			2.1	3.3	–	–
DRV per kg 0–3 months	115–100	480–420		2.1			2.0	3.1	350	8.5
% total energy	–		68	10	5	17	–	–	–	

* e.g. Marvel fortified with Vitamins A and D

Table 17.2 Minimal long chain fat (<3 g daily)–weaning diet: sample menu

Breakfast **7.30 AM**	Commercial baby cereal (<0.1 g fat per 100 g) Purée fruit and sugar Minimal fat feed
10 AM	Baby juice
Lunch **12.30 PM**	Purée white fish, turkey (light meat, no skin), lentils Purée potato Purée vegetables Commercial baby savoury foods can be used (<1.5 g fat per 100 g) Minimal fat feed
3 PM	Baby juice
Supper **5 PM**	Skimmed milk pudding (custard, ground rice or cornflour) Purée fruit and sugar Very low fat yoghurt or fromage frais (<0.2 g fat per 100 g) Commercial baby dessert (<0.2 g fat per 100 g) Minimal fat feed
Overnight Feed **7 PM to 7 AM**	Minimal fat feed

volume of feed can be decreased, but frequent feeding must continue. Carbohydrate can be supplied from either the feed, starchy food, or juice during the daytime, and continuous nasogastric feeds overnight. Table 17.2 provides a suggested menu plan.

Children

The older child should continue on a minimal fat, high carbohydrate diet with frequent feeding (Table 17.3). From one year of age, providing growth is satisfactory, the night feed can be changed from infant feed to a glucose polymer solution. The amount of glucose given overnight should at least equal basal glucose production rates (page 210), but more generous amounts could be given to further minimize lipolysis.

It is best to give the necessary high carbohydrate intake from starchy foods (e.g. rice, pasta, potato, bread) as these will give a better metabolic profile by providing 'slow-release glucose'. However, it is recognized that not all children can manage such a bulky diet and supplementary drinks may be needed, particularly between meals, to provide adequate glucose.

MCT oil can be incorporated into the diet to increase palatability and provide an alternative energy source. Also, some MCT can be stored in adipose tissue and used as an energy source [4]. MCT oil has a low smoke point compared with other cooking oils and care must be taken to ensure it does not burn. The optimum cooking temperature for MCT is 160°C. If MCT is overheated it develops a bitter taste and unpleasant odour.

Supplements of fat soluble vitamins (A, D, E) will be needed. Additional iron, zinc and B12 are also required, the amount required depending upon the

Table 17.3 Minimal long chain fat diet

	Foods allowed	Foods not allowed
Milk	Skimmed milk, condensed skimmed milk, Nestlé Build-up Very low fat yoghurt or fromage frais (<0.2 g/100 g) Low fat cottage cheese, Quark (skimmed milk soft cheese)	Whole milk, cream, dried whole milk Full fat yoghurt, ice cream Cheese
Egg	Egg whites	Egg yolks
Fish	White fish e.g. haddock, sole plaice, cod, whiting Crab, lobster, prawns, shrimps	Oily fish e.g. sardines, mackerel, kipper
Poultry	Turkey, light meat (no skin) chicken*, light meat (no skin)	Chicken and turkey skin and dark meat, basted poultry, duck
Meat	*	Fatty meat, sausages, salami, paté, meat paste
Pulses	Peas, beans, lentils	
Fats	Medium chain triglyceride oil, as permitted	Butter, margarine, low fat spread, vegetable oils, lard, dripping, suet, shortening
Cereals	Spaghetti, macaroni, pasta Rice Flour (white) Custard powder, semolina, sago, tapioca, cornflour Breakfast cereals*	Oats, soya flour, bran, pastry, pies Ordinary milk puddings, instant pudding mixes Some breakfast cereals: All Bran, Muesli, Ready Brek
Bread	*	
Cakes, Biscuits, Puddings	Only those made from suitable low fat ingredients Meringue, jelly, sorbet	Cakes, buns, biscuits, crackers, shop bought desserts
Fruit	Most varieties–fresh, frozen, tinned, dried	Avocado pears, olives
Vegetables	All vegetables and salad	Chips, crisps, roast potato, tinned potato salad, salad with dressing
Sauces	Tomato ketchup, pickles, Marmite, Oxo, Bovril	Salad cream, mayonnaise, oil and vinegar dressing
Drinks	Fizzy drinks, squash, fruit juice, milkshake flavourings, tea, coffee	Instant chocolate drinks, Bournvita, Horlicks, Ovaltine, cocoa
Confectionery	Boiled sweets, fruit gums, pastilles, water ices, jelly	Chocolate, toffee, fudge
Miscellaneous	Sugar, honey, jam, golden syrup, treacle, marmalade Herbs, spices, salt, pepper, vinegar, essences	Lemon curd Nuts, peanut butter

degree of fat restriction. Paediatric Seravit is a suitable comprehensive vitamin and mineral mix; for the older child Forceval Junior capsules provide a good alternative.

Frequent feeding must be maintained to reduce the effects of fasting. Regular meals and snacks or drinks are given. In children over the age of two years uncooked cornstarch (cornflour) is a useful way of providing 'slow-release glucose' and can reduce the need for such frequent feeding. Younger children may

not produce sufficient pancreatic amylase to digest cornflour. Cornflour can give good metabolic control (i.e. maintenance of blood glucose levels and prevention of a rise in free fatty acids) for around six hours in young children and even longer in older patients. However this must be assessed for each individual. A hospital admission is recommended when initiating this treatment so that fasting tolerance can be accurately measured under controlled conditions. It is usual to give a dose of 2 g cornflour/kg body

Table 17.3 (continued)

---

* Restricted list
These foods do contain fat but may be permitted in measured amounts depending upon the amount of fat allowed. In a minimal fat diet i.e. <5 g the restricted meats are avoided completely with bread and cereals given in measured amounts.

Lean Meats (cooked)	Fat content (g/100 g) (i)	Cereals	Fat content (g/25 g) (i)
Chicken (light meat)	5.0	Cornflakes	0.4
Ham (canned)	5.0	Puffed wheat	0.3
Gammon (lean only)	5.5	Rice Krispies	0.5
Beef rump steak (lean only)	6.0	Sugar Puffs	0.2
Beef topside (lean only)	4.4	Weetabix	0.8
Veal fillet (raw)	2.7		
		Bread, white	0.4
		Bread, wholemeal	0.7

(i) *McCance and Widdowson's The Composition of Foods* 5e. London: Royal Society of Chemistry, Ministry of Agriculture, Fisheries and Food, 1991

weight which is administered raw. To improve the palatability, cornflour can be mixed with skimmed milk, low fat yoghurt, fruit juice, squash or water. Cornflour can be given during the daytime with main meals reducing the need for between-meal snacks or drinks. Eventually it may be able to replace overnight nasogastric feeding.

Diet during illness

Throughout intercurrent infections the standard emergency regimen should be used. LCT is strongly contraindicated. It is important to stress the early use of the emergency regimen to inhibit the mobilization of fatty acids as decompensation may be rapid. As in MCAD, blood glucose monitoring is not always helpful as often patients are acutely unwell before they become hypoglycaemic.

3-hydroxy acyl-CoA dehydrogenase deficiency (3-OH-ACD)

The third step of beta-oxidation involves the 3-hydroxy acyl-CoA dehydrogenases. Two enzymes exist: one specific to long and medium-chain fats, the other to short chain fats. There is some overlapping substrate specificity, but the precise chain length specificity has yet to be defined. The clinical presentation of the long chain 3-hydroxy enzyme deficiency is similar to severe LCAD deficiency, with episodes of fasting-induced coma, hypoketotic hypoglycaemia, muscle and cardiac weakness.

Long chain 3-hydroxy acyl-CoA dehydrogenase deficiency

The dietary treatment of long chain 3-hydroxy acyl-CoA dehydrogenase deficiency when well and unwell is similar to that of LCAD with one exception: medium chain fat should be used cautiously. The diet should contain minimal long chain fat, be high in carbohydrate with frequent feeding and be individually tailored to the child's specific requirements. Because the long chain 3-hydroxy enzyme oxidizes both long and medium chain fats, the tolerance to medium chain fats in the diet may also be limited. However, MCT can be added into the diet slowly, but its introduction should be carefully monitored. If MCT is poorly tolerated, extra energy will need to be supplied from carbohydrate and minimal fat protein foods.

Multiple acyl-CoA dehydrogenase deficiency

Multiple acyl-CoA dehydrogenase deficiency (MAD) is caused by defects in either the electron transfer flavoprotein (ETF) or the ETF-ubiquinone oxidoreductase which carry electrons to the respiratory chain from the six flavin-dependent acyl-CoA dehydrogenases [5]. Defects in this pathway will therefore affect the oxidation of fatty acids (long, medium, short) as well as the oxidation of branch chain organic acids and lysine and tryptophan. MAD deficiency can present as either a severe neonatal form which is usually fatal, or a milder later onset form. The latter presents with episodes of hypoglycaemia, coma, vomiting and muscle weakness.

Dietary management

As MAD deficiency blocks the oxidation pathways of fat and some amino acids a modest restriction of dietary protein and fat intake may be beneficial in the mild form. The degree of restriction necessary would need to be assessed individually. To reduce the effects of fasting it is important to give regular meals and a high carbohydrate intake from starch. Overnight fasting might be a problem. It may be sufficient just to give a late night bedtime snack; however some may require a more frequent feeding regimen. If necessary uncooked cornflour can be used in older children to provide a supply of 'slow-release glucose' and reduce the need for frequent feeding (refer to LCAD for use of cornflour). Medium chain triglycerides are contraindicated in MAD deficency. The following dietary guidelines should be followed:

- 65–70% energy from carbohydrate
- 8–10% energy from protein
- 20–25% energy from fat
- frequent feeding – to tolerance.

During illness the standard emergency regimen should be used to prevent endogenous protein catabolism and lipolysis (page 206). Long chain fats should be excluded during the acute period and MCT is contraindicated. The usual diet can be reintroduced during the recovery period, but extra emergency regimen drinks should be given throughout this time.

3-hydroxy-3-methylglutaric aciduria

Children with 3-hydroxy-3-methylglutaric aciduria (HMGCoA lyase deficiency) effectively have defects in two metabolic pathways: the final steps of leucine catabolism and the last step of hepatic ketone synthesis. The latter prevents acetyl-CoA from fatty acid oxidation being converted to form ketone bodies. Patients normally present either in the early neonatal period or later between three and eleven months of age with episodes of illness characterized by vomiting, lethargy, hypotonia, hypoglycaemia, and a metabolic acidosis (with a notable absence of ketones) which may progress to coma [6].

Dietary management

The dietary treatment is a restriction of both dietary protein and fat, as the accumulated toxic metabolites are derived from both leucine catabolism and the ketone body synthesis pathway. However fat restriction has been shown to be more effective in reducing the abnormal metabolite production [7] and only a modest protein restriction is necessary. To reduce the effects of fasting it is important to give regular meals and a high carbohydrate intake from starch.

Dietary guidelines are to provide:

- 8–10% energy from protein
- 25% energy from fat
- 65% energy from carbohydrate.

Long fasts should be avoided by:

- eating a late night snack
- not missing breakfast
- replacing missed meals with a sugary drink.

During intercurrent infections the standard emergency regimen is used to reduce protein catabolism and lipolysis hence limiting the production of toxic metabolites from both defective pathways. During the recovery phase the usual intake of protein and fat can be reintroduced over a period of a few days.

REFERENCES

1 Touma EH, Charpentier C Medium chain acyl-CoA dehydrogenase deficiency. *Arch Dis Childh*, 1992, **67** 142–145.
2 Dixon M, Leonard J Intercurrent illness in inborn errors of intermediary metabolism. *Arch Dis Childh*, 1992, **67** 1387–1391.
3 Department of Health Report on Health and Social Subjects No 41. *Dietary Reference Values for Food Energy and Nutrients for the United Kingdom*. London: HMSO, 1991.
4 Sarda P *et al.* Storage of medium chain triglycerides in adipose tissue of orally fed infants. *Am J Clin Nutr*, 1987, **45** 399–405.
5 Stanley C Disorders of fatty acid oxidation. In: Fernandes J, Saudubray JM, Tada K (eds.) *Inborn Metabolic Diseases:*

Diagnosis and Treatment. Berlin: Springer-Verlag, 1989.

6 Sweetman L Branched chain organic acidurias. In: Scriver CR *et al.* (eds.) *The Metabolic Basis of Inherited Disease*, 6e. New York: McGraw-Hill, 1989.

7 Walter J, Clayton P, Leonard J Case Report, 3-Hydroxy-3-methylglutarly-CoA lyase deficiency. *J Inher Metab Dis*, 1986, **9** 286–288.

FURTHER READING

Roe C, Coates M Acyl-CoA dehydrogenase deficiencies. In: Scriver CR *et al.* (eds.) *The Metabolic Basis of Inherited Disease*, 6e. New York: McGraw-Hill, 1989.

Stanley C New genetic defects in mitochondrial fatty acid oxidation and carnitine deficiency. *Adv Pediatr*, **34** 59–88.

SECTION 6

Lipids

CHAPTER 18

Lipid Disorders

There are three main types of lipid in the body: triglycerides, cholesterol and phospholipids. They are transported in the serum bound to specific proteins called apolipoproteins to form the four major lipoprotein families (Table 18.1). Each of these lipoproteins contain a different amount of cholesterol and triglyceride and have different functions:

- *chylomicrons* carry dietary triglycerides from the intestine to peripheral tissues
- *very low density lipoproteins (VLDL)* are synthesized by the liver and carry excess triglycerides produced by the liver to other tissues
- *low density lipoproteins (LDL)* are formed from VLDL and transport cholesterol from the liver to the peripheral tissues
- *high density lipoproteins (HDL)* transport excess cholesterol from the cells to the liver for excretion in the bile.

Disorders of lipid metabolism which are managed by dietary intervention can be classified into those in which serum lipoproteins are deficient or absent (hypolipoproteinaemia) or those in which they are increased (hyperlipoproteinaemia) (Tables 18.2 and 18.3). The nature of the lipid disorder should be determined by measurement of serum lipoprotein fractions as well as total serum cholesterol and triglycerides.

Hyperlipoproteinaemia, secondary to diabetes, nephrotic syndrome or glygogen storage disease, is treated by management of the underlying disease and specific dietary measures are not usually necessary. The dietary management of the primary disorders which are genetically inherited are reviewed. A brief description of the biochemical defect of each disorder is given; more detailed information on the biochemistry can be found in the references at the end of the chapter.

THE HYPOLIPOPROTEINAEMIAS

All the primary hypolipoproteinaemias (Table 18.2) are rare and only abetalipoproteinaemia and occasionally hypobetalipoproteinaemia require dietary management.

ABETALIPOPROTEINAEMIA

This disorder is characterized by malabsorption of fat resulting in steatorrhoea and poor weight gain. It usually presents at birth or in early infancy. The defect is thought to involve the synthesis of apolipoprotein B or intracellular assembly of apolipoprotein B with the lipid. There is a failure of the intestinal

mucosa to synthesize chylomicrons which results in the complete absence of chylomicrons, VLDL and LDL in the serum [1]. It is inherited as an autosomal recessive trait. Other features of this condition are acanthocytosis of the red blood cells, ataxic neuropathy and pigmentary retinopathy. The neurological features may become apparent during the first decade and are slowly progessive [2]. The fat malabsorption results in deficiencies of fat soluble vitamins, including vitamin K. Levels of the essential fatty acid (EFA) linoleic acid are low in blood and tissue, but clinical deficiency has not been reported. Although there is a complete absence of chylomicrons about 50% of dietary fat is absorbed. It is thought that long chain triglycerides

Table 18.1 Composition of lipoproteins

Lipoprotein class	Principal lipids	Major apolipoproteins
Chylomicrons	Dietary triglycerides	A,B,C
VLDL	Endogenous triglycerides	B,C,E
LDL	Cholesterol ester and cholesterol	B
HDL	Cholesterol ester and phospholipid	A

Table 18.2 Classification and treatment of hypolipoproteinaemias

Primary disorder	Lipoprotein class	Treatment
Abetalipoproteinaemia	Chylomicrons LDL	Very low fat diet Vitamin A, E, K supplements MCT not recommended
Hypobetalipoproteinaemia	LDL	None usually indicated Low fat diet if steatorrhoea is a problem

MCT Medium chain triglycerides

(LCT) are transported via the portal vein, which is normally used by medium chain fatty acids. Treatment results in catch up growth and further growth and development are normal.

Dietary management

The steatorrhoea will respond to a low fat diet. The neurological features can be prevented, halted or reversed by large doses of vitamin E [3]. The management, therefore, involves a low fat diet with a high carbohydrate intake to provide adequate energy, and fat soluble vitamin supplements.

Fat restriction   The degree of fat restriction is determined by individual tolerance which increases with age and intake can vary from 5 g a day in infants to 20 g a day in an older child. Although clinical evidence of essential fatty acid deficiency has not been reported, some of the fat should be given as polyunsaturated fatty acids to provide essential fatty acids. The WHO/FAO (1980) recommends a minimum of 3% energy from EFA in normal infants and adults [4]. A more recent report recommends that neonakes require 1% energy intake from linoleic acid and 0.2% energy from alpha-linolenic acid (pp. 148, 230).

Table 18.3 Classification and treatment of hyperlipoproteinaemias

Primary disorder	Lipoprotein class	Treatment
Familial hyperchylomicronaemia (type I)	Chylomicrons	Low fat diet (20–30 g/day) MCT can be used to provide extra energy and to improve palatabilty
Familial hypercholesterolaemia (type IIa)	LDL	Reduce fat intake to 30% of energy. Polyunsaturated and monounsaturated fat can be used in moderation Usually requires a combination of diet and drugs
Familial combined hyperlipidaemia (type IIb)	LDL VLDL	As above
Familial type III hyperlipidaemia (broad beta disease)	IDL	Restriction of energy intake if obese Clofibrate effective
Familial hypertriglyceridaemia (type IV)	VLDL	Decrease CHO intake
Familial hyperlipoproteinaemia (type V)	Chylomicrons	Reduction in fat and CHO intake

IDL   Intermediate density lipoprotein
CHO Carbohydrate

In infants a low fat feed can be made by using Maxipro, Vitapro or skimmed milk powder as the protein base, a glucose polymer as an energy source and requires supplementation with vitamins, minerals and trace elements (Table 18.4). Fat in the form of a LCT emulsion (Calogen) can then be added to tolerance. Fat-free weaning foods such as baby rice, potato, fruit and vegetables can be introduced at the normal weaning age (Table 17.2).

Medium chain triglycerides (MCT) The use of MCT is not recommended as they will compete for binding sites in the portal system with LCT and may exacerbate malabsorption [5] and promote fatty changes and micronodular cirrhosis in the liver [6].

Energy In infants and young children it will be necessary to use glucose polymers to achieve sufficient energy intake for growth. Older children may be able to meet their requirements from refined carbohydrates, fruit squash, sweets, jam, or unrefined carbohydrates such as bread, potatoes, pasta and rice. Low fat cakes and biscuits can also be made.

Protein Adequate protein can be provided by the use of skimmed milk, low fat yoghurts, cottage cheese, white fish, cereals, pulses, and most beans.

Vitamin supplements The following are recommended [3]:

- vitamin A 7000 µg/day are required to maintain normal plasma concentration
- vitamin D normal requirements
- vitamin E 100 mg/kg/day
- vitamin K 5–10 mg/day.

THE HYPERLIPOPROTEINAEMIAS

The main types of primary hyperlipoproteinaemia are summarized in Table 18.3 and the typing system advocated by the World Health Organization is used. The two most commonly encountered in childhood are familial hyperchylomicronaemia (type I) and familial hypercholesterolaemia (type IIa). These two are discussed in detail. The other disorders, familial combined hyperlipidaemia (type IIb), familial type III hyperlipidaemia, familial hypertriglyceridaemia (type IV) and familial hyperlipoproteinaemia (type V) are rarely expressed in childhood.

Table 18.4 Minimal fat feed for infants for use in abetalipoproteinaemia

Per 100 ml	Energy		Protein (g)	CHO (g)	Fat (g)	Sodium (mmol)	Potassium (mmol)
	kJ	kcal					
2 g Maxipro	33	8	1.6	Trace	Trace	0.1	0.2
15 g Glucose Polymer	225	60	0	14	0	Trace	Trace
Water to 100 ml							
Total	258	68	1.6	14	Trace	0.1	0.2

1 Fat can be added to tolerance using an LCT emulsion (e.g. Calogen), and the glucose polymer can be decreased accordingly
2 Minerals and trace elements can be added as metabolic mineral mixture, see manufacturers data for dose
3 Vitamins can be given as 5 ml Ketovite Liquid and three Ketovite tablets a day
4 Alternatively vitamins and minerals can be added as Paediatric Seravit and electrolytes added to suit individual requirements

Care should be taken to ensure that the minimum recommendations for all nutrients, including essential fatty acids, are met and that the electrolyte content of the feed is calculated

FAMILIAL HYPERCHYLOMICRONAENIA (type I)

The manifestation of the clinical features of this rare disorder varies greatly and often the child is asymptomatic. The asymptomatic child may be diagnosed by a chance finding of turbid plasma when a blood sample is taken for some other reason, or the finding of hepatomegaly or lipaemia retinalis in an older child. Alternatively, the child may present with attacks of acute abdominal pain due to pancreatitis and/or eruptive xanthomata and hepatosplenomegaly. The defect is a deficiency of lipoprotein lipase which hydrolyses dietary triglycerides, or the apoprotein C which activates it [7]. It is inherited as an autosomal recessive trait. There is a failure to clear chylomicrons at the normal rate which leads to an accumulation in the serum and there is a gross elevation of triglycerides (35–115 mmol/l, normal fasting level 0.5–2.2 mmol/l), and moderate elevation of cholesterol. There is no current evidence that the high triglyceride levels are associated with an increased risk of atherosclerosis in later life. Growth and development are normal and clinical deficiency of linoleic acid has not been reported.

Dietary management

The aim of the dietary treatment is to relieve the symptoms. Restriction of fat to 5 g a day will result in optically clear fasting serum and lowering of serum triglycerides. However it is difficult to maintain this restriction long term, and fat intake is determined by tolerance. Triglycerides will remain high but as the condition is not associated with premature atherosclerosis there is no need for severe dietary restriction.

Acute episodes

During attacks of acute abdominal pain, a fat free diet should be given (<5 g LCT a day) (Table 17.3). This will produce a rapid decrease in serum triglyceride levels within 5–7 days. A suitable feed for an infant is shown in Table 18.4. Older children should have frequent high carbohydrate drinks and very low fat foods as tolerated.

Long term management

Fat Fat intake can be gradually increased to tolerance which is usually around 20–30 g a day, although there is individual variation. Tolerance does not seem to increase with age. The fat should be equally distributed between meals. The serum triglyceride level will increase, but the restriction should be sufficient to avoid attacks of acute pancreatitis or the development of xanthomata. In infants a LCT emulsion (Calogen) can then be added to the low fat feed (Table 18.4) to tolerance.

Medium chain triglycerides MCT emulsion (Liquigen) can also be used to provide additional energy. Several MCT based formulas are available (Table 6.16):

- *Portagen* – whole protein formula providing 3.2 g of fat/100 ml, with 88% of the total fat as MCT
- *Monogen* – complete whole protein, low fat infant formula providing 2 g of fat/100 ml, with 93% of the total fat as MCT (Table 12.4)
- *Caprilon* – complete, whole protein infant formula providing 3.6 g of fat/100 ml with 75% of the total fat as MCT. This feed should be available in 1994; further information can be obtained from the manufacturer (Table 8.1).

The amount of LCT in some of these feeds may be too high for the acute phase. Feeds containing MCT should always be introduced slowly and care should be taken to ensure that the feed provides sufficient essential fatty acids [4].

In older children MCT oils and emulsions can also be used to provide extra energy and to improve the palatability of the diet. It should always be introduced slowly. MCT oils and emulsions can be used in cooking and baking.

Energy Energy requirements can be met by the use of MCT, refined carbohydrates, and glucose polymers if necessary.

Vitamins and minerals In infants on modular feeds, supplementation of the feeds is essential. MCT-based complete infant formula feeds should provide adequate intakes provided sufficient volume is taken. Older children should have a supplement of fat-soluble vitamins.

FAMILIAL HYPERCHOLESTEROLAEMIA (type IIa)

This is the most common primary lipoprotein disorder of childhood and is characterized by raised serum cholesterol levels and results in an increased risk of ischaemic heart disease. It is transmitted by an autosomal dominant gene and therefore occurs in two forms – the heterozygous and the homozygous. The heterozygous form is the more common and occurs in 1 in 500 of the population. Total serum cholesterol levels are usually around 7.3–13.0 mmol/l (normal level is <6.2 mmol/l). It is generally asymptomatic in childhood, but heart disease will occur in early to middle adult life. In the rare homozygous form serum cholesterol levels are between 20–25 mmol/l. Skin and tendon xanthomata are present in early childhood and ischaemic heart disease is evident in later childhood leading to death in early adolescence. The defect is in the production of LDL receptors in the hepatic and extrahepatic cells which catabolize LDL cholesterol. In the heterozygous form individuals have half the number of receptors and in the homozygous form there are essentially no LDL receptors.

Screening of children for hypercholesterolaemia is not routinely undertaken, but serum lipid and lipoproteins should be measured in children of adults with hypercholesterolaemia or where there is a family history of early coronary heart disease. There are diagnostic difficulties in children under one year as blood cholesterol levels vary widely whilst the infant is receiving predominantly milk feeds [8]. Diagnosis and treatment is therefore best deferred until after one year of age, when the child is taking a varied toddler diet.

Dietary management

The aim of dietary treatment is to lower total serum and LDL cholesterol by restricting dietary fat intake and help to decrease the risk of cardiovascular disease in later life. LDL and HDL cholesterol levels are usually measured. LDL cholesterol is a derived value, usually between 75 and 85% of the total cholesterol. British, European and American expert panels [9,10,11] agree a total serum concentration of 5.2 mmol/l or less as the ideal for the general population; however, a level of less than 6.2 mmol/l is generally regarded as acceptable for this group of children.

Once the diagnosis has been confirmed dietary modification can be started straight away as changes in dietary habits may be more easily achieved if started in early childhood. The degree of fat restriction in toddlers needs to be assessed individually and diet and growth should be closely monitored. There is no evidence of a deleterious effect of a low fat diet on growth and development.

Dietary recommendations

Many factors affect plasma lipid and lipoprotein levels including total fat intake, type of fat taken, non starch polysaccharide intake and obesity [12]. Each of these should be considered when planning the diet for the child with familial hypercholesterolaemia.

Energy intake This should be based on age, weight and activity levels [13].

Total fat intake This should be decreased to approximately 30–35% of energy intake. The type of fat in the diet also needs to be considered. Saturated fatty acids have a hypercholesterolaemic effect and should be limited to 10% of the total energy intake. Monounsaturated fatty acids have been shown to have a hypocholesterolaemic effect when substituted for saturated fatty acids in the diet. As polyunsaturated fatty acids lower HDL and LDL cholesterol, and there is concern over their long term safety, it is generally recommended that intake should not exceed 10% of total energy intake.

Fat intake can be reduced by decreasing the intake of fried foods and other high fat foods. Skimmed or semi skimmed milk and low fat cheese and yoghurt should be used instead of the full fat varieties. Lean meat should be limited to one serving a day, and fish, poultry, pulses and beans used in preference. Eggs can be included as part of the fat allowance. An allowance of some high fat foods should be included to help improve compliance. Polyunsaturated and monounsaturated fats and oils can be substituted for saturated fat but should be used in moderation.

Dietary cholesterol Emphasis on restriction of cholesterol intake is not necessary as most cholesterol is synthesized endogenously and dietary intake has little influence on serum levels. However, excessively high intakes may increase serum cholesterol levels.

Non-starch polysaccharides (NSP) Soluble NSP, which is found in oats, oat bran, legumes and pectin, will help to reduce serum cholesterol levels [14]. An intake of around 120 g oat bran per day or 100–130 g of dried beans per day is needed to have a long term effect [14]. Although this is more than most children will eat on a regular basis, families should be encouraged to include a variety of foods high in soluble NSP in their diet. Care needs to be taken, especially with very young children, that an excessive intake of NSP in combination with a low fat diet, does not affect energy intake. The recommendation to increase soluble NSP intake should form part of the advice on healthy eating to this group of children, but an over emphasis may detract from the most important of the advice, that is decreasing total fat intake.

Fat-soluble vitamins Fat-soluble vitamins (e.g. Abidec 0.6 ml/day) should be given to children under five years.

Effectiveness and compliance

A low fat diet can lower serum cholesterol levels by around 10–15%; for individuals with pre-treatment levels greater than 8.0 mmol/l, diet alone will usually be inadequate management. The maintenance of a strict diet over a number of years is very difficult. In a study conducted by West and Lloyd in 1974 [15], only about 20% of children had satisfactory control on diet alone after three years, though compliance with diet seems to be better when treatment is started in early childhood rather than in adolescence [16]. Regular and intensive family education sessions may also help to improve motivation and compliance [17]. The long term management of most of these children will usually require a combination of diet and drug therapy. In the homozygous form a reduction in serum cholesterol levels of greater than 40% is rarely achieved with a regimen of diet and drug treatment and radical therapy such as plasmapheresis may be required [2].

Drug therapy

Dietary intervention should always be the first line of treatment and should be continued for approximately

six months before considering drugs. Children with the homozygous form and children with pre-treatment levels greater than 8.0 mmol/l will not respond adequately to dietary treatment alone. In the majority of children, effective long term management will probably require the use of diet and drugs. The choice of drug therapy in children is cholestyramine or colestipol (Questran and Colestid) which are anion exchange resins that bind bile salts in the gut preventing their reabsorption. Thus the total cholesterol pool is decreased with a resultant increase in the breakdown of LDL cholesterol for conversion into bile acids. Reduction in serum cholesterol levels is proportional to the size of the dose, the number of doses and timing in relation to meals [18]. The starting dose in children is generally a half to one sachet a day, which is then gradually increased in response to the cholesterol levels and compliance. It can be taken as one single dose with the evening meal, or once the dose exceeds two packets it is best taken in two divided doses [18]. It should be increased slowly to minimize the side effects which may include nausea and steatorrhoea. Questran and Colestid are available as powders and can be mixed with fruit juice to help improve palatability [19]. Long term administration of these drugs may result in malabsorption of fat-soluble vitamins and folate [20] and serum levels should be monitored annually in children on long term treatment with these drugs. New drugs have been developed which act by inhibiting cellular cholesterol production. Simvastation is licensed for use in adults and has proven to be an effective hypocholesterolaemic agent. It is not yet licensed for use in children.

Follow-up

As this condition is inherited by the child by an autosomal dominant gene, in the heterozygous form one of the parents is affected and in the homozygous form both parents are affected. It is beneficial to see the parent(s) and child in a combined clinic if possible to ensure uniformity of advice. The parents should be encouraged to incorporate the dietary changes into the meal plans for the whole family. Dietary advice and monitoring should be undertaken frequently to help improve compliance and to ensure nutritional adequacy of the diet. Support is also available from the Familial Hypercholesterolaemic Association (see Useful address).

REFERENCES

1 Herbert PN *et al.* The disorders of lipoprotein and lipid metabolism. In: Stanbury JB *et al.* (eds.) *The Metabolic Basis of Inherited Disease*, 5e. New York: McGraw-Hill, 1983.

2 Lloyd JK, Muller DPR Disorders of lipid metabolism. In: McLaren DS *et al.* (eds.) *Textbook of Paediatric Nutrition*, 3e. Edinburgh: Churchill Livingstone, 1991.

3 Muller DPR, Lloyd JK, Wolf OH Vitamin E and neurological function. *Lancet*, 1985, **1** 225–228.

4 FAO/WHO *Dietary Fats and Oils in Human Nutrition*. Rome: FAO of the United Nations, 1980: 21–37.

5 Lloyd JK, Muller DPR Management of abetalipoproteinaemia in childhood. In: Peters H (ed.) *Protides of the Biological Fluids, 19th Colloquium*. Oxford: Pergamon Press, 1972.

6 Partin JS *et al.* Liver ultrastructure in abetalipoproteinaemia and evolution of micronodular cirrhosis. *Gastroenterology*, 1974, **67** 107–118.

7 Durrington PN Hyperlipoproteinaemia. In *Hyperlipidaemia, Diagnosis and Management*. London: Butterworth, 1989.

8 Darmady JM, Fosbrooke AS, Lloyd JK Diagnosis and management of familial hypercholesterolaemia in the first year of life. A prospective study of serum cholesterol concentration. *Brit Med J*, 1972, **2** 685–688.

9 The British Cardiac Society Working Group on Coronary Prevention. Conclusions and recomendations. *Brit Heart J*, 1987, **57** 188–189.

10 Study Group European Atherosclerosis Society The recognition and management of Hyperlipidaemia in adults: a policy statement of the European Atherosclerosis Society. *Eur Heart J*, 1988, **9** 571–600.

11 National Cholesterol Education Programme Expert Panel. Report on detection, evaluation and treatment of high blood cholesterol in adults. *Arch Intern Med*, 1988, **148** 36–39.

12 Kris-Etherton PM *et al.* The effect of diet on plasma lipids, lipoproteins, and coronary heart disease. *J Am Diet Assoc*, 1988, **88** 1373–1400.

13 Department of Health Report on Health and Social Subjects No 41 *Dietary Reference Values for Food Energy and Nutrients for the United Kingdom*. London: HMSO, 1991.

14 Anderson JW, Gustafson NJ Hypocholesterolaemic effects of oat and bean products. *Am J Clin Nutr*, 1988, **48** 749–753.

15 West RJ, Lloyd JK Adherence to treatment in children with familial hypercholesterolaemia. *Paed Res*, 1974, **8** 911 (abstract).

16 Koletzko B, Kupke I, Wendal U Treatment of hypercholesterolaemia in children and adolescents. *Acta Paed*, 1992, **81** 682–685.

17 McMurray MP *et al.* Family-orientated nutrition intervention for a lipid clinic population. *J Am Diet Assoc*, 1991, **91** 57–65.

18 Stein EA Management of hypercholesterolaemia. Approach to diet and drug therapy. *Am J Med*, 1989, **87**(Suppl 4A) 20S–27S.

19 Shaefer MS *et al.* Acceptability of cholestyramine or colestipol combinations with six vehicles. *Clin Pharm*, **6** 51–54.

20 Schwarz KB *et al.* Fat soluble vitamin concentrations in hypercholesterolaemic children treated with colestipol. *Paed*, 1980, **65** 243–250.

FURTHER READING

Durrington PN *Hyperlipidaemia, Diagnosis and Management*. London: Butterworth, 1989.

Stanbury JB *et al.* (eds.) *The Metabolic Basis of Inherited Disease*, 5e. New York: McGraw-Hill, 1983.

USEFUL ADDRESS

Familial Hypercholesterolaemic Association
PO Box 133, High Wycombe, Bucks, HP13 6LF.

SECTION 7

Peroxisomal Disorders

CHAPTER 19

Refsum's Disease

Heredopathia atactica polyneuritiformis (Refsum's disease) is a rare inborn error of lipid metabolism inherited as an autosomal recessive trait. The chief characteristics are retinitis pigmentosa, peripheral neuropathy, and cerebellar ataxia. Other manifestations can include nerve deafness, anosmia, ichthyosis, cardiac abnormalities and skeletal abnormalities. There is no developmental or mental retardation.

Patients accumulate phytanic acid (3,7,11,15 tetramethyl hexadecanoic acid) in plasma and body tissues, and it is this which distinguishes Refsum's disease from many other neurological disorders. This unusual 20-carbon branched chain fatty acid is normally rapidly degraded in the human body. The major mechanism involves an initial alpha-hydroxylation step followed by decarboxylation before the beta-oxidation analogous to that found in the oxidation of straight chain fatty acids. Patients with Refsum's disease have an isolated deficiency of the enzyme phytanic acid alpha-hydroxylase needed to effect the initial step in this sequence of reactions. The onset of symptoms is usually slow and diagnosis is not usually made until the second to fifth decade of life, although some patients have been diagnosed in early childhood [1,2].

Phytanic acid is exogenous in origin, and treatment is aimed at reducing plasma and tissue levels by means of a diet low in phytanic acid and free phytol which must be followed for life. Reduction of plasma phytanic acid levels significantly improves peripheral nerve function, ichthyosis and cardiac arhythmias; it cannot, however, reverse the damage done to the sensory nerves although further deterioration can be arrested. It is thought that in the case of young children early diagnosis and treatment could delay or prevent the development of these irreversible lesions.

Steinberg and Gibberd *et al.* provide an overall review of Refsum's disease [2,3].

PEROXISOMAL DISORDERS

Patients with global peroxisomal defects can also show raised plasma levels of phytanic acid. These conditions, e.g. infantile Refsum's, Zelwegger syndrome and neonatal adrenoleukodystrophy, must be distinguished from 'true' Refsum's disease (HAP). While patients with HAP appear to have an isolated phytanic acid alpha-hydroxylase deficiency, infantile Refsum's disease is associated with many more defective metabolic functions including that of very long chain fatty acids, especially C:26. These metabolic defects result in severe clinical symptoms, including mental and physical retardation, which present in infancy [4–7].

A low phytanic acid diet may be requested for children with infantile Refsum's disease and some improvement in behaviour has been claimed [8].

Reference values for plasma phytanic acid

Normal	$0–33\ \mu mol/l$
	(usually <10)
Heterozygote for HAP	$0–130\ \mu mol/l$
Peroxisomal disease	$0–320\ \mu mol/l$
HAP after one year treatment	$16–1000\ \mu mol/l$
HAP untreated	$990–6400\ \mu mol/l$

DIET FOR TREATMENT OF REFSUM'S DISEASE (HAP)

The aims of dietary treatment are:

- to avoid dietary sources of phytanic acid and free phytol
- to encourage suitable weight gain and guard against weight loss (phytanic acid moves between body fat

stores and plasma; when weight loss occurs plasma levels will rise causing exacerbation of symptoms)
- to ensure an adequate intake of all nutrients.

Dietary sources of phytanic acid

Phytanic acid derives from phytol, which is a part of the chlorophyll molecule. It is found in the fats of ruminant animals (cows, sheep, goats) and also of fish. The average Western diet will provide between 50 mg and 100 mg per day [9].

Free phytol in food is absorbed and metabolized to phytanic acid by humans and, therefore, would present an additional source in the diet. Most phytol in food however is bound to chlorophyll which is poorly absorbed by humans [10]. The free phytol content of a typical Western diet has been found to be less than 10% of the preformed phytanic acid [9]. The phytanic acid and free phytol content of some foods have been reported from various sources [9,11–17]. Varying values have been obtained for similar foods. This reflects the difficulty of the estimation and the variation to be expected when allowing for changes in the diet of the animals, food processing methods (especially oils) and the composition of commercial food ingredients.

Little information is available on the phytol content of individual foods [2,9,18]. Again, published values show variation, reflecting perhaps the changes in food processing or the presence of other branched chain substances. Initially, many fruits and vegetables were excluded from the diet as a potential source of phytol: this meant that vitamin supplements were necessary and the diet was extremely restricted and unpalatable. In 1988 it was shown that fruit and vegetables could be introduced into the diet without any deterioration in clinical condition [18] and these are now permitted.

Patients with Refsum's disease have a residual capacity to metabolize phytanic acid by an alternative pathway, possibly involving ω-oxidation. Opinions as to the efficacy of this vary between 10 and 30 mg per day for adults [2]. Accordingly, diets were devised to provide less than 10 mg phytanic acid per day based on published food analyses. Recent analysis of foods has demonstrated the variability of these values and foods are now simply placed in one of three groups. Actual values will be found in the literature [9,11–17].

Table 19.1 lists foods as presenting low risk, moderate risk, and high risk for phytanic acid content based on recent analysis. Patients are advised to:

- habitually choose low risk foods
- avoid high risk foods altogether
- limit their intake of moderate risk foods to one single choice per day, and preferably not every day.

Treatment on diagnosis

A child presenting with classical Refsum's disease may be anorexic and vomiting , making it very difficult to establish feeding. If plasma phytanic acid levels are very high, plasma exchange may be performed. It is still of vital importance, however, to feed the child since any weight loss mobilizes body fat stores, releasing further phytanic acid into the blood and exacerbating symptoms. If the child is not able to take adequate nutrition orally, then total or supplementary nasogastric feeding should be instituted as a matter of urgency.

Most commercial enteral feeding products are free from animal fats (and hence phytanic acid) and are, therefore, suitable for use. Products available are listed in Table 19.2 together with the origin of the vegetable oils used. The choice of feed should be made commensurate with the age and requirements of the child.

If the child is able to eat, the diet should be devised to provide enough energy for growth appropriate for age and chosen from low risk foods (Table 19.1).

Suitable nutritional supplements will almost certainly need to be prescribed to promote weight gain at the beginning of treatment. Their use can be discontinued at the discretion of the dietitian when the child is eating suitable foods in adequate amounts and is clinically stable.

Supplements

Those whose lipid source is solely vegetable oils are suitable for a low phytanic acid diet; those containing fats from animal sources are not suitable since these are likely to be from cows' milk or hydrogenated fish oils, both of which contain phytanic acid.

It has been suggested that oils which are high in linoleic acid are preferable since this has a faster metabolic turnover and would prevent further release of body stores of phytanic acid [11,12]. Sunflower and safflower oils have therefore been favoured. The recent concern with $\omega6:\omega3$ ratio of essential fatty acids (EFA) perhaps points to the use of rape seed and

Table 19.1 Sources of phytanic acid in food

Low risk (no phytanic acid, allowed freely)	Moderate risk (up to 10 mg per serving)	High risk (more than 10 mg per serving)
Cereals and cereal products		
Wheat, rice, maize, oats, sago, tapioca		Biscuits with animal fat e.g. McVitie's Rich Tea
Crispbreads, bran cereals		
Biscuits containing only vegetable and hydrogenated vegetable oils, e.g. Sainsbury Rich Tea		
Dairy products		
Flora 'alternative to Cheddar Cheese', very low fat cottage cheese <1% fat	Half fat cottage cheese	Butter
		Margarines containing butter or animal fats
Fat free fromage frais		All cheeses including goats', sheep, cheese spreads, processed cheese
Skimmed milk, and powder	Semi-skimmed milk	
Very low fat yoghurt <1% fat	Low fat yoghurt	
		Full fat milk. Sheep, goat milks, Evaporated milk
Soya milks		Sheep and goat milk yoghurts, cream, Elmlea
Soya based yoghurts e.g. Berrydales		Infant formulas containing animal fats
Non-dairy ice cream e.g. Walls' Vanilla Blue Ribbon, containing only vegetable fats		Dairy ice cream
Eggs		
Fats and oils		
Margarines and spreads containing only vegetable oils and hydrogenated vegetable oils, e.g. Flora, Tomor, Tesco soya		Margarines and spreads containing animal fats e.g. Stork Special blend, Krona
Oils: corn, sunflower, safflower, soya, olive, rapeseed, arachis		Butter
Lard		Beef suet
Fish		
	Coley, cod (no skin), smoked haddock, tuna, crab, prawns	Plaice. All fatty fish e.g. herring, mackerel, sardines, salmon fresh and canned
		Fish oils e.g. Maxepa, Cod-Liver oil
		Fish in sauces (boil in bag)
Meat		
Pork, pig liver, pig kidney	Rabbit	Beef and offal
Ham, bacon		Lamb and offal
Chicken, chicken liver, turkey, duck		Goat (not analysed)
Safeway pork and turkey sausages		Beefburgers, Sausages (not analysed)
		All meat products (not analysed)
Vegetarian meat substitutes		
Soya based TVP products e.g. Protoveg soya chunks, Sosmix		
Tofu		
Quorn mycoprotein		
Vegetables		
Root vegetables, potatoes, crisps cooked in all vegetable oil e.g. Golden Wonder, Sainsbury lower fat		Beef, cheese, prawn flavour crisps (not analysed)
Dried beans and pulses		
Green vegetables		
Fruit		
All fresh and canned fruit	Dried fruit (possible phytol content)	

Table 19.1 *Continued*

Low risk (no phytanic acid, allowed freely)	Moderate risk (up to 10 mg per serving)	High risk (more than 10 mg per serving)
Nuts		
Almonds, peanuts, coconut, Brazil, peanut butter	Walnuts	
Tahini (sesame)	Skins of nuts (possible phytol)	
Miscellaneous		
Beverages – coffee, cocoa, drinking chocolate	Tea in large amounts (phytol content)	
Supplements – See Table 19.2		
Chicken Oxo, Bisto, Marmite		Beef Oxo
Clear Vegetable soups		Cream soups
Confectionery		
Sugar based sweets containing no fat, e.g. boiled sweets, fruit gums, jellies, turkish delight, marshmallows		Milk chocolate e.g. Mars Bars, Dairymilk
Plain chocolate with no butter fat, e.g. Waitrose continental plain chocolate, Plamil plain chocolate with soya		Plain chocolate with butter e.g. Terry's, Sainsbury plain
Carob e.g. Plamil raw sugar confection		

soya oils. Table 19.2 lists suitable supplements and the vegetable oil used where this is known.

Fresubin (Fresenius) has been used successfully for adults and is suitable for children above six years of age although it may be used with care in younger children. It is prescribable for patients with Refsum's disease.

Maintenance diet and long term management

Dietary treatment (sometimes together with plasma exchange) will usually lower plasma phytanic acid within a matter of weeks. The child will then be put on a diet low in phytanic acid and phytol which must be followed for life. Initially, the child is restricted to low risk foods only (Table 19.1). As the condition improves, one food from the moderate risk group may be allowed occasionally at the discretion of the physician. High risk foods must be avoided altogether. Attention to satisfactory growth (or weight maintenance in older children) is essential, since any weight loss mobilizes stored phytanic acid. With rigorous adherence to diet these stores can be gradually eliminated.

Special care is needed during infection or other intercurrent illness to maintain nutritional status and liquid supplements may need to be used at these times.

Table 19.2 Tube and sip feed products free from animal fats

Product	Fat source/oil
Fresubin	Sunflower
Ensure	Corn
Osmolite	Coconut, corn, soya
Paediasure	Sunflower, soya, MCT
Fortisip ⎫ Nutrison ⎬ Nutrison paediatric ⎭	Canola, corn, palm, coconut
Isocal	Soya, MCT

In general the diet, if chosen from a variety of permitted foods, should be adequate in all nutrients. The exclusion of many saturated fats from animal sources shifts the diet of these patients towards a much higher polyunsaturated to saturated fat ratio than that of the general population. This means that the dietitian should check that there is an adequate intake of antioxidant nutrients, especially vitamin E. Although most oils do contain vitamin E, it is prudent to recommend the use of fat spreads which have extra vitamin E added e.g. Flora (Van den Berg Ltd).

The inclusion of convenience and manufactured foods in the diet of patients with Refsum's disease requires extreme vigilance in reading the ingredients list on food labels. The guidance of the dietitian can be very helpful here. Many commercial fats used in desserts and baked goods contain fish oils which are a rich source of phytanic acid.

Patients are advised to look for and AVOID the following: butter, cream, animal fats, full cream milk, cheese, butter oil, ghee, beef, lamb, suet, milk fat, fish, fish products, fish oils.

Foods labelled as suitable for vegans are quickly and easily identified as safe. Most large retail food shops now issue lists of vegan foods on request. These are updated at regular intervals.

DIETARY TREATMENT OF INFANTILE REFSUM'S DISEASE

Infantile Refsum's disease is a global peroxisomal disease which, unlike classic Refsum's, presents in infancy with more widespread biochemical deficiencies including raised plasma phytanic acid and abnormal levels of very long chain fatty acids. There are also physical and mental abnormalities [2,5,6,7,19,20]. Despite the more complex nature of this condition some paediatricians will prescribe a low phytanic acid diet. Some improvement has been claimed in lowering plasma phytanate but not for other parameters [6].

Infant feeding

If the mother is breast feeding this should be encouraged since human breast milk does not contain phytanic acid. Infant formulas should contain no animal fats (milk, beef etc.) since the amount of phytanic acid in these is variable and could be significant. Soya based milks are acceptable.

Suitable infant feeds free from animal fats are given in Table 19.3. The formulation of feeds is liable to change and, therefore, the composition should always be checked before use.

Nuts and seed oils (especially peanuts/arachis oil) have been shown to contain hexacosanoic acid ($C26:0$). The use of feeds containing medium chain triglyceride (MCT) oils, and which are also free of phytanic acid, might be of some benefit to infantile Refsum's patients although this is, at present, untested in practice.

Table 19.3 Infant formulas free from animal fats

Product	Fat source/oil
InfaSoy / Galatomin 17 / Galactomin 19	Palm, coconut, canola, sunflower
Pepti-Junior	50% MCT
Farley's First Milk / Farley's Second Milk / OsterSoy	Groundnut, palm, palm kernel
Wysoy / SMA Gold / SMA White / Progress	Palm, coconut, soya, lecthin
SMA low birthweight	10% MCT
ProSobee / Pregestimil	Soy, coconut palm, sunflower
Portagen	MCT, corn, soy
Nutramigen	MCT, corn
	Corn, soy
Prejomin	Vegetable fat, lecthin
Pepdite 2+	Maize, coconut
MCT Pepdite 0–2 / MCT Pepdite 2+	Coconut, sunflower
Neocate	Safflower, coconut, soya

Solid food

The choice of weaning foods should be based on those shown in Table 19.1. Only low risk foods should be used. Proprietary baby foods should be checked for the presence of 'milk solids', milk fat, butter, cream, cheese, beef and beef fat, lamb and fish. These ingredients should be avoided.

Products labelled as suitable for vegans will again be suitable.

Since children with infantile Refsum's syndrome also have abnormal metabolism of very long chain fatty acids (VLCFA) especially C26, as in adrenoleukodystrophy (ALD), they might benefit from the dietary treatment applied in ALD.

REFERENCES

1 Dickson N *et al.* A child with Refsum's disease, successful treatment with diet and plasma exchange. *Develop Med Child Neurol*, 1989, **31**(Feb) 92–97.
2 Steinberg D Refsum disease. In: Scriver CR *et al.* (eds.)

Metabolic Basis of Inherited Disease, 6e. New York: McGraw-Hill, 1989.

3 Gibberd FB *et al.* Heredopathia atactica polyneuritiformis: Refsum's disease. *Acta Neurol Scand*, 1985, **72** 1–17.

4 Stokke O, Skjeldal O, Hoie K Disorders related to the metabolism of phytanic acid. *Scand J Clin Lab Invest*, 1986, **46**(Suppl 184) 3–10.

5 Poulos A, Sharp P, Whiting G Infantile Refsum's disease (phytanic acid storage disease): a variant of Zellwegger's syndrome? *Clinical Genetics*, 1984, **26** 579–586.

6 Poulos A *et al.* Accumulation and defective β-oxidation of very long chain fatty acids in Zellwegger's syndrome, adrenoleukodystrophy, and Refsum's disease variants. *Clin Gen*, 1986, **29** 397–408.

7 Poll-The BT, Saudebray JM *et al.* Infantile Refsum's disease: an inherited peroxisomal disorder. Comparison with Zellwegger's syndrome and neonatal adrenoleukodystrophy. *Europ J Pediatr*, 1987, **146** 477–483.

8 Robertson EF *et al.* Treatment of infantile phytanic acid storage disease: clinical, biochemical and ultrastructural findings in two children treated for two years. *Europ J Pediatr*, 1988, **147** 133–142.

9 Steinberg D *et al.* Refsum's disease, a recently characterised lipidosis involving the nervous system. *Ann Intern Med*, 1967, **66** 365–395.

10 Baxter J Absorption of chlorophyll phytol in normal man and in patients with Refsum's disease. *J Lipid Res*, 1968, **9** 636–641.

11 Masters-Thomas A *et al.* Heredopathia atactica polyneuritiformis, (Refsum's disease). 1 Clinical features and dietary management. *J Hum Nutr*, 1980, **34** 245–250.

12 Masters-Thomas A *et al.* Heredopathia atactica polyneuritiformis (Refsum's disease). 2 Estimation of phytanic acid in foods. *J Hum Nutr*, 1980, **34** 251–254.

13 Steinberg D Phytanic acid storage disease (Refsum's disease). In: Stanbury JB (ed.) *Metabolic Basis of Inherited Disease*, 5e. New York: McGraw-Hill, 1983.

14 Ackman RG, Harrington M Fishery products as components of diets restricted in phytanic acid for patients with Refsum's syndrome. *J Canad Diet Assoc*, 1975, **36** 50–53.

15 Ackman RG, Hooper SN Isoprenoid fatty acids in the human diet: distinct geographical features in butterfat and importance in margarines based on marine oils. *Can Inst Food Tec J*, 1973, **6** 159–165.

16 Lough AK The phytanic acid content of the lipids of bovine tissues and milk. *Lipids*, 1977, **12** 115–119.

17 Brown PJ *et al.* Diet and Refsum's disease. The determination of phytanic acid and phytol in certain foods and the application of this knowledge to the choice of suitable convenience foods in Refsum's disease. *J Hum Nutr Diet*, 1993, **4** 295–305.

18 Coppack SW *et al.* Can patients with Refsum's disease safely eat green vegetables? *Brit Med J*, 1988, **296** 828.

19 Poulos A, Sharp P Plasma and skin fibroblast C26 fatty acids in Infantile Refsum's disease. *Neurology*, 1984, **34** 1606–1609.

20 Wanders RJ, Heyman HS, Schutgens RB Poll-The BT, Saudebray JM, Tager JM *et al.* Peroxisomal functions in classical Refsum's disease: comparison with the infantile form of Refsum's disease. *J Neurological Sciences*, 1988, **84** 147–155.

CHAPTER 20

X-linked Adrenoleukodystrophy

X-linked adrenoleukodystrophy (ALD) is a serious progressive disorder where the adrenal cortex and myelin of the nervous system are affected leading to adrenocortical insufficiency and progressive central nervous system demyelination [1]. The biochemical defect in ALD is an impaired ability to oxidise very long chain fatty acids (VLCFA) thought to be due to a deficiency of peroxisomal lignoceroyl – CoA ligase necessary for VLCFA activation [2]. This results in an accumulation of saturated VLCFA, particularly $C24:0$ and $C26:0$, in the brain, adrenal tissue, testes, plasma, liver, erythrocytes and leukocytes [3].

ALD affects only males, although a small number of female carriers may develop a milder form of the disease. The first case report of a child with ALD was published in 1923. At the age of six and a half years a boy became disturbed in his speech and his gait deteriorated. He then became spastic, was unable to walk or swallow and died at the age of seven years [4]. In 1963 Fanconi and colleagues [5] established that it was an inherited disease, probably with a sex-linked transmission. The name of ALD was first suggested in 1970 by Blaw. The disorder has been reported in all races; the incidence is unknown, but it is estimated to be a minimum of 1.1 per 100 000. The phenotype of X-linked ALD is more varied than had been originally thought and at least seven clinical subtypes have been identified in males, the commonest being the childhood form affecting boys [6]. Even members of the same family may present with different subtypes of the disease.

SUBTYPES OF ALD

Childhood ALD

Approximately half the patients have this phenotype and this cerebral form is associated with a poor prognosis. The age of onset of symptoms is usually 3–10 years. Initial symptoms may include behavioural changes, ranging from withdrawn behaviour to bizarre aggressive outbursts; failing memory and poor school performance; dysarthria and dysphagia [7]. Visual impairment is an early sign in one third of patients and in the later stages of the disease vision may be totally lost [6]. Some 35–40% of childhood ALD patients have adrenal insufficiency. The progression of symptoms is usually rapid, leading to a vegetative state within one year [8], although the child may continue to survive in this state for over five years.

Adolescent ALD

Adolescent onset ALD has been identified as a separate phenotype [6]. Although the symptoms occur between 11 and 21 years, the symptoms resemble those seen in the childhood form.

Adrenomyeloneuropathy (AMN)

This form of the disease affects 25% or more of the patients with ALD. It usually affects men in their twenties or thirties and it affects the adrenal cortex, the spinal cord, and the peripheral nerves rather than the cerebral white matter [9]. The vast majority of patients with AMN will also have Addison's disease and AMN may be present as Addison's disease in childhood [6]. Some 40–50% of AMN patients develop evidence of cerebral involvement in magnetic resonance (MRI) and cortical function tests [10]. The rate of progression in AMN cerebral patients appears to be more rapid than in those with pure AMN.

Symptom free patients with the biochemical defect

A number of boys have been found to have the biochemical defect of ALD, but are free of symptoms. They are detected as a result of being tested following the diagnosis of a symptomatic relative. It is not known whether these individuals will later develop symptoms.

Symptomatic female carriers

Although female carriers are usually asymptomatic, at least 15–20% of women carriers develop symptoms [6] that resemble AMN, but which is milder and of later onset. Progressive spastic paraparesis, moderate vibratory sense loss and peripheral neuropathy may develop in the third or fourth decade of life.

Diagnosis of X-linked ALD

The diagnosis can be made by demonstrating high concentrations of the saturated VLCFAs hexacosanoic

(C26:0) and/or tetracosanoic (C24:0) fatty acids in cultured skin fibroblasts, plasma or red blood cells. In contrast, the levels of dodecosanoic acid (C22:0) or those with shorter chain lengths are not increased. This results in abnormally high ratios of C26:0/C22:0 and of C24:0/C22:0 fatty acids. Abnormal computed tomography (CT) and MRI scans, adrenal function tests, electroencephalogram (EEG) and nerve conduction studies may help lead towards the diagnosis of ALD. Carriers for ALD can also be detected by VLCFA measurements, but the accuracy of this varies from 80% to 93% according to whether levels in plasma or cultured fibroblast are measured. If the results are equivocal, DNA probes can be used to confirm carrier status [9].

TREATMENT

When neurological symptoms of ALD have already started there is little that can be done to halt the rapid progression of the disease. Although a number of possible treatments are being evaluated they are a long way from guaranteeing a successful outcome.

Replacement therapy for adrenal insufficiency

Adrenal steroid hormone replacement therapy for adrenal insufficiency is effective in relieving the adrenal dysfunction, but does not alter the progression of the neurological disability.

Bone marrow transplantation (BMT)

Although it is not clear how BMT works in ALD, it is hypothesized that functional bone marrow cells from the donor cross the blood/brain barrier and exert a favourable effect on slowing down or inhibiting the mechanisms leading to demyelination [11]. As there is a 20–30% mortality rate associated with BMT, Moser recommends that BMT is reserved for patients with mild and early symptoms, rather than for patients with advanced symptoms [10]. It would appear to have no role to play for patients with severe neurological impairment.

Table 20.1 Nutritional composition of glycerol trioleate oil

Nutritional analysis	Per 100 ml
Energy kJ (kcal)	3330 (810)
Fat g	90
Fatty acid profile	**g/100 g of fatty acids**
C14:0	0.02
C16:0	0.66
C16:1	0.07
C17:0	0.18
C17:1	0.13
C18:0	3.03
C18:1	88.7
C18:2	4.87
C18:3/C20:1	2.24
C20:0	0.10
C21:0	undetectable
C24:0	"
C26:0	"

Immunosuppression and plasmaphoresis

Immunosuppression and plasmaphoresis have been tried as possible treatments, but neither on their own has proved to be effective [12].

DIET THERAPY AND ITS EVOLUTION

Plasma levels of saturated VLCFA are elevated by as much as five times normal in ALD and AMN patients and by up to three times normal in female carriers. Several types of diet therapy have been tried through the years.

1984 Low C26:0 diet
1986 Low C26:0 diet and glycerol trioleate oil
1989 Low fat diet and Lorenzo's oil
1990 Low C26:0 diet and Lorenzo's oil.

Low C26:0 diet

Interest was generated in the possibility of using diet therapy in ALD in the early 1980s when it was reported that there was clinical benefit in Refsum's disease when a low phytanic acid diet was given and Kishimoto and colleagues reported that between 4% and 90% of the C26:0 in postmortem ALD brain was derived from C26:0 administered during the preceding 100 days [13]. A diet restricting VLCFA, specifically low in C26:0, was developed at the Kennedy Institute in Baltimore [14]. It limited C26:0 to less than 3 mg per day. The normal intake in an American diet is 12–40 mg daily. The diet was given to eight patients, six symptomatic with ALD, one adult with AMN and one presymptomatic. The period on diet varied from four months to two years. Unfortunately, the diet neither lowered plasma VLCFA nor did it appear to alter the clinical course of the disease, except in the one adult patient with AMN who reported improved ability to stand and walk. The asymptomatic patient developed symptoms nine months after the initiation of the diet [15].

The explanation for the failure of this diet was that it was not completely free of C26:0. Also there is evidence to suggest that saturated VLCFA in ALD appears to be derived both from exogenous and endogenous synthesis [16,17]. A fall in plasma C26:0 levels was seen in two patients when it was totally excluded from the diet [17]. However, neither patient

was able to tolerate the diet for more than three months.

Low C26:0 diet and glycerol trioleate oil

Methods to try and reduce endogenous synthesis of VLCFA were actively investigated in the mid 1980s. It was demonstrated that the C26:0 content of cultured skin fibroblasts from ALD patients was lowered *in vitro* by their incubation in the presence of monounsaturated fatty acids, especially oleic acid (C18:1) [18]. It was hypothesized that the administration of monounsaturated fatty acid might reduce endogenous synthesis of saturated VLCFA by competing for the same enzyme elongation system. From this work, a new diet therapy was devised aiming to reduce both the endogenous synthesis and exogenous sources of saturated VLCFA.

In 1987, Rizzo and co-workers reported treating five adult patients with AMN and two female carriers with a diet moderately low in C26:0 (10 mg daily) and supplemented with oleic acid in the form of 60 ml glycerol trioleate oil. Glycerol trioleate oil consists of 89% oleic acid (Table 20.1). Total plasma C26:0 levels decreased by 50% [19]. Moser's group also tried a similar therapy on 36 patients with various subtypes of ALD and AMN. They gave a low C26:0 diet (less than 3 mg daily) and gave 25% of the energy intake from glycerol trioleate oil. Reductions in plasma VLCFA were reported in 25 out of the 36 patients. However, the combination of the glycerol trioleate oil and low C26:0 diet had three limitations:

(1) It failed to stem the rapid progression of the disease in symptomatic boys.
(2) It took 30–90 days before there was a significant reduction in VLCFA.
(3) It failed to return VLCFA concentration to normal [14].

Lorenzo's oil and a low fat diet

As glycerol trioleate oil was ineffective at lowering plasma VLCFA to normal, it was hypothesized that diet therapy could be improved by combining oleic acid with longer chain monounsaturated fatty acids [1]. This would divert enzymatic activity from saturated to monounsaturated fatty acids, not only at the level of the C18:1 – elongase, but also that of elongases active at higher levels of the chain and, therefore, be a more potent inhibitor of saturated VLCFA elongation. C22:1 (erucic acid) was chosen because it had already been established that this fatty acid would inhibit C26:0 synthesis *in vitro* and lower the C26:0 content of ALD fibroblasts to normal [3].

Rizzo gave a product called Lorenzo's oil in combination with a low fat diet to a group of 12 newly diagnosed patients with ALD. Lorenzo's oil is a mixture of 70% oleic acid (C18:1) and 20% erucic acid (C22:1). It is named after a boy with ALD whose parents have been instrumental in researching this diet therapy. Twenty per cent of the patients' total energy intake was given from Lorenzo's oil and 20% from a low fat diet. C26:0 from fruit and vegetables was not restricted [20]. It was demonstrated that plasma C26:0 levels decreased to normal within four weeks of starting the diet therapy and by four months the C26:0 composition of erythrocyte lipids, plasma sphingomyelin and plasma phosphatidylcholine became normal. However, it is still not known whether Lorenzo's oil in this dosage is sufficient to lower saturated VLCFA accumulation in the brain or adrenal tissue. Unfortunately, six of the twelve patients with moderate or advanced disease continued to deteriorate neurologically although two mildly affected patients remained clinically stable for several months [20]. Similar results were reported by Uziel and co-workers using the same diet therapy [21]. They have also recently reported that six asymptomatic patients are still free of symptoms almost two years after the start of therapy [15].

Lorenzo's oil and a low VLCFA diet

The Kennedy Institute in Baltimore now recommend a combination of Lorenzo's oil and a low VLCFA diet for patients with ALD [22]. By the end of 1991, they had had over 200 patients on Lorenzo's oil and a low VLCFA diet. The majority of these patients are older and have AMN, although they have had a number of presymptomatic children on diet. Twenty per cent of the energy intake is given in the form of Lorenzo's oil and 15% as fat. C26:0 from fruit and vegetable sources is restricted, although the allowance of C26:0 has been increased from 3 mg to 5–8 mg daily. The rationale for choosing such a strict diet therapy is the suggestion that some of the abnormal fatty acids accumulated in the brain are of dietary origin [10]. Moser has demonstrated that plasma C26:0 levels

decrease to normal levels within one month of diet therapy in more than 80% of the patients. He has also reported increased plasma erucic acid levels and lower plasma cholesterol levels. He has shown an improvement in peripheral nerve function in AMN patients and 30 patients who had no neurological abnormalities at the beginning of therapy have not developed symptoms after 18 months on the diet. However, in 60% of childhood ALD patients with neurological symptoms the diet has done little to halt the rapid deterioration [10,22].

CURRENT RECOMMENDED DIETARY MANAGEMENT

The type of patients who may benefit from a trial of diet therapy are given in Table 20.2. The current diet consists of:

- Lorenzo's oil
- glycerol trioleate oil for cooking
- low fat/low C26:0 diet
- vitamin and mineral supplementation
- essential fatty acids
- energy supplementation.

Lorenzo's oil

Lorenzo's oil is a blend of 4 parts glycerol trioleate oil (GTO) and one part glycerol trierucate (GTE) (Table 20.3). The GTE component is a solid fat at room temperature. It is about 93% erucic acid which is purified from rape seed oil. When GTO and GTE are combined together, a clear yellow liquid is produced, although the GTE can solidify and form a white sediment if it is kept in a warm environment. Lorenzo's

Table 20.2 ALD patients who may benefit from diet therapy

Groups of patients which may benefit from diet therapy	Groups of patients which have had no proven benefit from diet therapy or diet therapy has not been tried
• Patients with biochemical defect	• Patients with symptomatic childhood ALD
• AMN Patients	
• Symptomatic female carriers	• Female carriers without symptoms

Table 20.3 Nutritional composition of Lorenzo's oil

Nutritional analysis	Per 100 ml
Energy kJ (kcal)	3312 (806)
Fat g	89.5
Fatty acid profile	**g/100 g of fatty acids**
C12:0	<0.1
C14:0	0.03
C16:0	0.5
C16:1	0.1
C17:0	0.1
C18:0	2.4
C18:1	72.2
C18:2	5.1
C20:0	0.5
C20:1	0.8
C22:1	18.4

Table 20.4 Daily dose of Lorenzo's oil for different age groups of boys over the age of 3 years

Age of boys	Estimated average requirements (EARs) for energy [23]		Estimated daily dose of Lorenzo's oil
	kcals/d	MJ/d	ml
3 years	1230	5.15	30
4–6 years	1715	7.16	45
8–10 years	1970	8.24	50
11–14 years	2220	9.27	55
15–18 years	2755	11.51	70
19–50 years	2550	10.66	65

oil is 90% fat providing 8 kcals (34 kJ) per ml. It is recommended that 20% of the total energy intake is given from Lorenzo's oil. Although this dose normalizes plasma C26:0 levels, the figure of 20% appears to be quite arbitrary. Suggested daily quantities of Lorenzo's oil for boys and males of different ages based on estimated average energy requirements is given in Table 20.4. It is recommended that Lorenzo's oil is not given to boys below the age of three years due to uncertainty about potential long term effects.

It is recommended that the quantity of Lorenzo's oil is divided into 2–3 daily doses throughout the day. Moser's group suggest that Lorenzo's oil should be taken with meals, although there is no evidence to say that it is less effective if taken at different times to meals or in a single dose, although patients may develop diarrhoea if all the oil is taken in one dose. It is difficult to disguise the oily taste or consistency of Lorenzo's oil. Many patients take their measured dose of Lorenzo's oil as a medicine, without any additional flavouring. Some patients prefer to take it mixed with skimmed milk and milkshake flavouring or fruit juice. Unfortunately, the oil does not mix particularly well in either medium and it increases the volume of fluid that needs to be taken. It may be easier to take the mixture in a covered cup or beaker to help mask the smell and the poorly dispersed fat. Other patients mix the oil with yoghurt or other low fat desserts with similar consistency.

It is not recommended that Lorenzo's oil is used for cooking. It may not be stable at very high temperatures. Also there is no guarantee that a patient will have taken his full daily dose if it is used for frying foods as some will probably be left in the cooking pan.

Adverse effects of Lorenzo's oil

There have been some concerns about the routine use of Lorenzo's oil and any toxic effects it may have in humans. Rats have a limited ability to metabolize monounsaturated fatty acids with 22 carbon atoms. Excess amounts in the diet have been found to cause a transient accumulation (lipidosis) of triacylglycerol in the heart and other tissues, but not in the liver, of pigs [13]. In humans, cardiac complications have been reported. Lorenzo's oil appears to be associated with a moderate reduction in platelet count [8,19]. The reduction does not appear severe enough to warrant discontinuation of the diet, but careful monitoring of the platelet count is recommended. It is important that any adverse effects that appear to be associated with the administration of Lorenzo's oil are carefully monitored and documented.

Glycerol trioleate oil

Glycerol trioleate oil is often used in addition to Lorenzo's oil specifically as a cooking oil. It is a pale yellow oil free of hexacosanoic acid (C26:0) and rich in oleic acid. Like Lorenzo's oil it is 90% fat providing 8 kcals (34 kJ) per ml. It is useful in the preparation of margarine substitutes, salad dressings, GTO oil cakes and biscuits and for frying potatoes, crisps, fish and meats. It should be stored at 4°C under dry conditions. It is not currently available on prescription in the UK and is quite expensive to buy. It may be cheaper for parents/patients to buy this by special arrangement directly from the supplier, Scientific Hospital Supplies Group UK Limited, than order it through a retail chemist. Recipes for this condition may be obtained from the author, Anita MacDonald, at her place of work (see Contributors list at the front of this volume).

Although Lorenzo's oil is effective in returning plasma C26:0 levels to normal, some degree of dietary restriction is thought to be necessary, although this is not as yet proven.

Management by low C26:0 diet

The Kennedy Institute in Baltimore designed the original low VLCFA diet. One of their goals of diet therapy was to reduce the dietary intake of C26:0, the primary VLCFA, to less than 3 mg daily. The C26:0 content of a large range of foods was analysed and C26:0 was found to be in two main food sources: foods high in fat; and fruits, vegetables, nuts and some starches. They found VLCFA in the cutin or outer covering of plants. This source of VLCFA has been referred to as 'cutilar' lipids [24]. Examples of the

Table 20.5 Examples of C26:0 content of foods

Food	C26:0 mg/100 g
Cereals/breads	
Rice Krispies	1.067
Shredded Wheat	2.014
White bread	1.486
Rice	0.273
Vegetables/fruit	
Tomato (no skin or seeds)	0.071
Tomato (with skin and seeds)	0.289
Peas	0.181
Boiled potato (peeled)	0.096
Chips cooked in lard or oil	7.465
Grapes (unpeeled)	0.643
Strawberries	0.163
Apple (unpeeled)	0.500
Apple (peeled)	0.045
Cabbage (fresh raw)	2.185
Meat/fish/dairy products	
Beef (lean)	0.083
Chicken breast	0.060
Tuna	0.090
Egg white	0.067
Cottage cheese	0.117

C26:0 content of foods are given in Table 20.5. Fruits and vegetables which are particularly high include tomatoes with skin and seeds, grapes, spinach, apple with peel, banana, broccoli and dried apricots. Wholemeal cereals, bread and pasta are higher in C26:0 than refined varieties.

The Kennedy Institute advise patients to consume:

(1) A very low fat diet including skimmed milk, lean meats, cottage cheeses and low fat yoghurts. Glycerol trioleate margarine is used instead of ordinary margarine. Butter and egg yolks are avoided completely. Glycerol trioleate oil is used as a cooking oil. Obviously fatty foods such as chocolate, crisps, cream, toffees, ice cream and mayonnaise are omitted.

(2) An intake of C26:0 less than 3 mg daily from fatty, vegetable, fruit, nut and starchy sources. Patients are given a series of C26:0 exchanges for protein, starch, vegetables, fruit, dairy and snack foods.

Patients are expected to calculate their own daily allowance of C26:0 using measured quantities of foods from the exchange lists. The diet is quite complex and patients/carers have to be very motivated and intelligent to adhere to this exchange system. Some dietitians in Britain who have used the Kennedy Institute diet have modified it to make it easier for the patient/carer to follow. In addition to avoiding high dietary fat sources, simple lists of high C26:0 sources (fruits, vegetables and starchy foods) which should be avoided are given. An example of British dietary guidelines is given in Table 20.6.

The Kennedy Institute has now relaxed the diet since Lorenzo's oil has been found to be so effective at reducing plasma C26:0 levels. Patients are now permitted to consume 5–8 mg of C26:0 daily and 15% of the total energy intake comes from dietary fat sources. Although this allows a wider variety of fruits and vegetables to be taken, the same intricate exchange system is still used; 15% energy from fat also involves the same rigid fat restriction as described above.

Low fat diet

Since the introduction of Lorenzo's oil there have been reports of at least two other centres advising patients on a low fat diet only in order to reduce their exogenous intake [20,21]. Rizzo recommends that

Table 20.6 Adapted low C26:0 diet

Foods allowed	Foods not allowed
Meat and poultry	
Extra lean beef, lamb, turkey, chicken, liver, kidney, lean ham, extra lean pork, lean bacon	Fatty meat, sausages, hamburgers, black pudding, chopped ham and pork, corned beef
Fish	
White fish not fried, tuna fish in brine, smoked haddock and cod, shellfish	Fish canned in oil, herring, mackerel, kippers
Eggs	
Egg white only	Egg yolks
Milk and dairy products	
Skimmed milk, cottage cheese	Whole milk, semi-skimmed milk, evaporated milk, cream, all other cheese
Fats	
Glycerol trioleate margarine	All fats, oils, butters and margarines
Flour and cereals	
All white flour, plain and self raising flour, cornflour, rice, semolina, tapioca, sago, rice flour, arrowroot, custard powder	Wholemeal flour, bran, barley, oats, lentils, dried savoury rice, brown rice
Breakfast cereals	
Cornflakes, Rice Krispies, Ricicles, Frosties	Bran cereals, e.g. All Bran, Bran Flakes, muesli type cereals, Porridge, Weetabix, Weetaflakes, Sugar Puffs, Shredded Wheat, cereals with dried fruit and nuts Wholegrain/wholewheat cereals
Bread, cakes, biscuits, pastry	
White bread, white rolls Rich Tea biscuits	Wholemeal bread and rolls. Pitta bread, rye bread. All other proprietary cakes and biscuits, all pastry
Pasta	
All white pasta. Tinned spaghetti in tomato sauce	Wholemeal, egg and spinach (verde) pasta. Tinned, frozen and dried pasta dishes
Puddings and desserts	
Jelly, sorbet. Tinned peaches, pears Milk pudding made with skimmed milk Natural low fat yoghurt	All tinned fruit except peaches and pears. Full cream yoghurt. All low fat yoghurts except peach, pear and apple. All proprietary desserts – tinned, dried and

Table 20.6 *Continued*

Foods allowed	Foods not allowed
Apple, peach, pear low fat yoghurt	frozen, e.g. gateaux. Instant Whip type puddings, trifle. Dumplings, suet pudding, pastries, tarts
Sugar, preserves and spreads	
Sugar – all kinds Jelly jam and marmalade, syrup, honey, lemon curd	Jams and marmalades with skins, seeds, peel. Chocolate spread, peanut butter
Fruit and fruit drinks	
Peeled apples, pears, peaches, grapes, plums, cherries, watermelon, tinned fruit cocktail, strawberries, pineapple Fruit juices, squashes, fizzy drinks Lemon juice, tomato juice	Skins on fruits. All tinned fruit except those mentioned on allowed list All dried fruit. Oranges
Vegetables	
Potatoes (peeled), chips cooked in GTO Carrots, broccoli stalk, mushrooms, tomatoes (peeled – no seeds), turnip, peppers, cucumber, lettuce	No jacket potatoes or other vegetables No chips cooked in lard or ordinary oil
Drinks	
Tea, coffee, milk shake flavouring syrup. Oxo, Bovil, Marmite	Malted drinks, cocoa, drinking chocolate
Confectionery/Snacks	
Plain boiled sweets, peppermints, ice lollies, barley sugar, fruit gums, pastilles, jelly beans, gum drops, marshmallows	Chocolate, toffee, fudge. Any sweet containing nuts and/or dried fruit, crisps, nuts

20% of the energy intake should come from low fat foods in addition to 20% of the energy intake from Lorenzo's oil. This degree of dietary restriction is still effective in achieving normal plasma C26:0 levels and at the same time has helped to increase variety in the diet, which ultimately will aid dietary compliance. Although it is not exactly clear how restrictive the VLCFA dietary intake should be, it would appear that it is possible to achieve normal plasma C26:0 levels by using a low fat diet providing 15–20% of dietary energy from food sources (including any glycerol trioleate oil used in food preparation) and 20% of the energy intake from Lorenzo's oil. Furthermore, some initial results from a small trial on presymptomatic children in Birmingham would indicate that the introduction of C26:0 dietary sources from fruit, vegetables and starch has not adversely affected C26:0 levels.

Energy intake

Although a fifth of the total energy intake is given from Lorenzo's oil, and glycerol trioleate oil can be incorporated into many recipes and dishes, energy intake may be low due to both a low fat and a low C26:0 diet as the foods allowed on these diets are quite limited. This may adversely affect energy intake and, therefore, growth. It is essential that the nutritional intakes of patients are assessed at regular intervals, and energy supplements are given if needed. Useful energy supplements include glucose polymers, glucose drinks such as Polycal Liquid and Hycal and milkshakes made from skimmed milk, glucose polymer, Build Up or low fat milkshake flavouring. Children soon become bored with such a limited diet and imaginative use should be made of all freely allowed foods to try to prevent anorexia or cheating.

Vitamin and mineral intake

Due to the limited nature of the diet, particularly if the diet is restricted in all the sources of VLCFA, the intake of several trace elements may be reduced. Principle nutrients affected include the fat-soluble vitamins A, D and E, and vitamin C and folic acid. Some parents are so anxious about the diet therapy that they try and limit any source of dietary fat and restrict the quantity of lean meats allowed, thereby reducing the dietary source of iron and zinc. If a child has a poor appetite, a comprehensive vitamin and trace mineral supplement such as Paediatric Seravit, Seravit or Forceval Junior capsules may be advisable. If a patient is on a low fat diet only, and eating lean meat and white fish, fruit, vegetables and cereals, a vitamin supplement containing a source of fat soluble vitamins may be all that is needed. The dose and type of vitamin and mineral supplement should be specific to meet the nutritional needs of the individual patient.

Essential fatty acid supplement

If a very low fat diet is advocated, an essential fatty acid supplement is now recommended for ALD patients providing a source of linoleic acid (C18:2ω6) and alpha-linolenic acid (C18:3ω3) in the ratio of between 4:1 and 10:1. Although glycerol trioleate oil

contains some linoleic and alpha-linolenic acids and Lorenzo's oil contains some linoleic acid, the overall quantity of essential fatty acids a child will obtain from a low fat diet and Lorenzo's oil is estimated to be approximately only 2% of total energy intake. Moser has suggested that the reduction of platelet count seen in some patients on diet is linked with essential fatty acid deficiency [10]. It is likely that a new formulation of Lorenzo's oil containing essential fatty acids will be available in the future. This will alter the ratio of GTO to GTE in the Lorenzo's oil and will probably be 2.5:1 instead of 4:1. It is not known how this change in the proportion of GTO to GTE will affect plasma C26:0 levels.

Tube feeding

Once a patient with childhood ALD has developed symptoms, a diet will do little to halt their rapid progression. There is probably no point in trying Lorenzo's oil and a low C26:0 diet at this stage. However, many parents are understandably desperate to do anything they can to help their children, and if they ask that their child be tried on Lorenzo's oil and the diet in these circumstances, most physicians will

Table 20.7 Summary of dietary protocol for adrenoleukodystrophy

Pre-diet
- Assess normal energy and nutrient intake using a three day recorded diet diary
- Assess growth, i.e. height, weight and mid arm circumference

Diet
- Give 20% of the total energy intake in the form of Lorenzo's oil as a drink in two doses with meals
- Give a low C26:0 diet by reducing dietary fat to 15–20% of energy intake (+ restriction of C26:0 to 5–8 mg daily)
- Use glycerol trioleate oil for cooking
- Supplement the diet with a vitamin/mineral supplement as necessary to achieve dietary reference values for nutrients
- Supplement the energy intake with a glucose polymer, or glucose drink, if energy intake is low
- Give essential fatty acid supplements.

Review
- Assess dietary intake and growth every three months
- Repeat plasma monitoring of VLCFA every three months

consider it acceptable to respect and support their request. Unfortunately once symptoms have started, it is usually only a matter of months before the child can eat very little orally and is reliant on tube feeding to supply his total nutritional requirements. There is no proprietary nasogastric feed which contains erucic acid. However, Scientific Hospital Supplies Group UK Limited produce a nutritionally complete enteral feed, Code 660, in which 80% of the fat is oleic acid (C18:1). It is recommended that the feed is made up at a 23% concentration, which will provide 1 kcal/ml (4.2 kJ/ml) and an osmolality of 355 mOsm/kg water. Initially the feed should be given at quarter strength, and gradually increased to full strength over 3–4 days. It is very difficult to give erucic acid with a tube feed. Erucic acid is solid; however, if it is melted it will pass down a tube. It is recommended that 5% of the total energy intake is given in the form of erucic acid, approximately 7–12 ml per day along with Code 660. The quantity of erucic acid needed is, therefore, small.

A summary of the dietary protocol for use in children with ALD is shown in Table 20.7.

REFERENCES

1 Odone A, Odone M Lorenzo's oil: a new treatment for adrenoleukodystrophy. *J Pediatr Neurosciences*, 1989, **5** 55–61.

2 Lazo O *et al.* Peroxisomal lignoceroyl-CoA ligase deficiency in childhood adrenoleuko-dystrophy and adrenomycloneuropathy. *Proceedings Nat Acad Sci USA*, 1988, **85** 7647–7651.

3 Rizzo WB *et al.* X-linked adrenoleukodystrophy: biochemical and clinical efficacy of dietary erucic acid therapy. In: Uziel G, Wanders RJA, Cappa M (eds.) *Adrenoleukodystrophy and other peroxisomal disorders: Clinical, Biochemical Genetic and Therapeutic Aspects.* Amsterdam; Elsevier Science Publishers, 1990.

4 Simerling E, Creutzfeldt HG Bronzenkrankeriheit and Sklersierende Encephanlomyelitia. *Arch Psychiatr Nervenkr*, 1923, **68** 217–244.

5 Fanconi A *et al.* Morbus Addison mit Hirnsklerose im Kindesatter Ein Hereditares Syndrom mit X-Chromosomaler Vererbung. *Helve Paediatr Acta*, 1963, **18** 430.

6 Moser HW, Moser AB Adrenoleukodystrophy (X-Linked). In: Scriver CR *et al.* (eds.) *The Metabolic Basis of Inherited Disease II.* New York: McGraw-Hill, 1989.

7 Schaumburg HH *et al.* Adrenoleukodystrophy. A clinical and pathological study of 17 cases. *Neurol*, 1975, **32** 577–591.

8 Green S Adrenoleukodystrophy. *Arch Dis Childh*, 1991, **66** 830–832.

9 Del Mastro RG, Bundey S, Kilpatrick MW Adrenoleukodystrophy: a molecular genetic study in five families. *J Med Genetics*, 1990, **27** 670–675.

10 Moser HW *et al.* Adrenoleukodystrophy: phenotypic variability. Implications for therapy. *J Inher Met Dis*, 1992, **15** 645–664.

11 Auborg P *et al.* Reversal of early neurologic and neuroradiologic manifestations of X-linked adrenoleukodystrophy by bone marrow transplantation. *New Eng J Med*, 1990, June, 1860–1866.

12 Murphy JV *et al.* Treatment of adrenoleukodystrophy by diet and plasmaphoresis. *Ann Neurol*, 1982, **12** 220.

13 Kishimoto Y *et al.* Adrenoleukodystrophy: evidence that abnormal very long chain fatty acids of brain cholesterol esters are of exogenous origin. *Biochem Biophys Res Commun*, 1980, **96** 69–76.

14 Moser AB *et al.* A new diet therapy for adrenoleukodystrophy: Biochemical and preliminary clinical results in 36 patients. *Ann Neurol*, 1986, **21** 240–249.

15 Uziel G *et al.* Adrenoleukodystrophy: a three years experience of dietary treatment with erucic acid. *SSIEM Abstracts.* London, 1991: 155.

16 Van Duyn MA The design of a diet restricted in saturated very long chain fatty acids: therapeutic application in adrenoleukodystrophy. *Am J Clin Nutr*, 1984, **40** 277–284.

17 Brown FR *et al.* Adrenoleukodystrophy: effects of dietary restriction of very long chain fatty acids and of administration of carnitine and clofibrate on clinical status and plasma fatty acids. *John Hopkins Med J*, 1982, **151** 164–172.

18 Rizzo WB, Watkins PA, Philips MW Adrenoleukodystrophy: very long chain fatty acid metabolism in fibroblasts. *Neurology*, 1986, **34** 163–169.

19 Rizzo WB *et al.* Adrenoleukodystrophy: dietary oleic acid lowers hexacosanoate levels. *Ann Neurol*, 1987, **21** 232–239.

20 Rizzo WB *et al.* Dietary erucic acid therapy for X-linked adrenoleukodystrophy. *Neurology*, 1989, **39** 1415–1422.

21 Uziel G *et al.* Dietary treatment with erucic acid for patients with X-linked adrenoleukodystrophy. *5th International Congress on Inborn Errors of Metabolism*, June 1–5th, 1990.

22 Moser H *et al.* Dietary treatment of adrenoleukodystrophy. *5th International Congress on Inborn Errors of Metabolism*, June 1–5th, 1990.

23 Department of Health Report on Health and Social Subjects no 14. *Dietary Reference Values for Food Energy and Nutrients for the United Kingdom.* London: HMSO, 1991.

24 Kolattukudy PE, Croteau R, Brown L Structure and biosynthesis of cuticular lipids. *Plant Physiol*, 1974, **54** 670–677.

Childhood Cancers

CHAPTER 21

Nutritional Support: Leukaemias, Lymphomas and Solid Tumours

Childhood cancers differ from those seen in adults in both type and outcome [1]. In comparison with therapies used to treat adults, multimodal therapy and combination chemotherapy have been effective in vastly improving the outlook for children with cancer. Children have tumours that are chemotherapy responsive and they tolerate chemotherapy better than do adults [2]. Children differ metabolically as well and continued growth and development is desired throughout therapy that often spans several years. Therefore, with more curable children being treated for what is much of the time a chronic disease, the more children there are that are subject to the nutritional problems caused by their disease and treatment.

TYPES OF CANCERS SEEN IN CHILDHOOD

The types of cancers seen in children can be divided into three main groups:

- leukaemias
- lymphomas
- solid tumours.

Leukaemias

Leukaemia is the commonest neoplastic disease of infancy and childhood accounting for 30–45% of all childhood cancers [3,4]. Acute lymphoblastic leukaemia (ALL) is the commonest form of the disease in childhood, followed by acute myeloid leukaemia (AML) and then chronic myeloid leukaemia (CML). The cure rate (i.e. five year survival without relapse) is 58% with ALL and 20% with AML [3,4].

The leukaemias are fatal unless treated. At presen-

tation pallor, fever, fatigue and aches and pains are the commonest features. Haemorrhage, apart from easy bruising, is not common unless infection is also present. Enlargement of the spleen and lymph nodes may be present [3].

Lymphomas

Lymphomas account for 9–15% of all childhood cancers [3,4]. In children the types of lymphomas seen are virtually limited to three types [5]:

- Hodgkin's disease which affects the lymph glands causing them to enlarge
- non-Hodgkin's lymphoma (NHL) which is a monoclonal neoplastic proliferation of lymphoid cells, usually B or T cells. It is more malignant than Hodgkin's
- Burkitt's lymphoma which is a maligant lymphoma of poorly differentiated lymphoblastic type masses of immature lymphoid cells.

Solid tumours

Solid tumours account for 40% of childhood cancers [4]. The most common solid tumours seen in children are listed below [5]:

- brain tumours, of which *medulloblastoma* is the most common. It is a tumour arising in the posterior fossa
- Wilm's tumour, also known as *nephroblastoma*, is a congenital highly malignant kidney tumour and can be bilateral
- *neuroblastoma* is another highly malignant tumour arising from the adrenal medulla from tissue of

Table 21.1 UKCCSG registrations for children aged under 15, by diagnostic group, 1977–91

Diagnosis	Diag year															Total
	77	78	79	80	81	82	83	84	85	86	87	88	89	90	91	
ALL	99	230	232	254	250	285	283	279	296	289	305	318	308	42	126	3595
ANLL	20	56	56	28	55	55	41	59	59	64	64	61	68	3	21	710
Hodgkin's disease	18	43	30	47	39	51	41	42	50	56	33	41	31	5	17	544
NHL	25	54	55	57	46	49	44	59	62	60	60	75	66	4	22	738
Burkitt's lymphoma	2	4	0	4	6	6	4	5	2	6	4	8	5	0	2	58
Medulloblastoma/PNET	9	32	26	32	39	27	48	27	40	32	47	46	42	2	18	467
Neuroblastoma	27	44	44	59	82	79	72	79	70	75	98	110	90	5	30	964
Retinoblastoma	2	4	6	6	6	9	21	21	30	35	45	29	42	3	17	276
Wilm's tumour	22	55	43	59	50	70	75	67	68	73	87	81	72	5	28	855
Osteosarcoma	2	10	22	13	23	20	20	13	16	22	19	21	15	0	1	217
Ewing's sarcoma	7	10	24	23	26	19	24	24	23	20	22	19	21	0	8	270
Rhabdomyosarcoma	18	29	41	50	52	50	48	66	65	54	69	56	56	3	34	691

ANLL – acute non-lymphoblastic anaemia
United Kingdom Children's Cancer Study Group Scientific Report, 1992

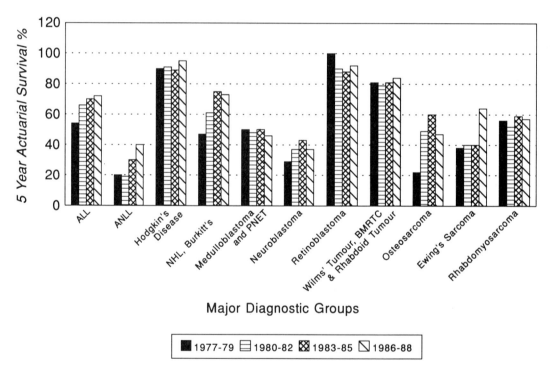

Fig. 21.1

sympathetic origin. It can also arise from some parts of the abdominal, thoracic, pelvic or cervical chains of sympathetic ganglia

- *rhabdomyosarcoma* is a malignant tumour of striated muscle most commonly found in the orbital region, nose, mouth or pharynx
- *osteosarcoma* is a malignant tumour arising from the bone. Any bone can be affected, but it usually occurs in the legs
- *Ewing's sarcoma* is a very malignant tumour which can develop anywhere in the body, but usually starts in the bones, most commonly the pelvis, upper arm or thigh. It can also develop in the soft tissue near bones
- *primitive neuroectodermal tumour (PNET)* is a highly malignant tumour of neuroepithial origin and can be thought of as being very similar to a Ewing's sarcoma [6].

Incidence rates and survival rates for these tumours are given in Table 21.1 and Fig. 21.1.

THE AETIOLOGY OF MALNUTRITION IN CHILDREN WITH CANCER

To a certain extent the problems of malnutrition seen in children with cancer are no different from the problems of any child who has an inadequate intake for demand. The majority of the malnutrition is iatrogenic; the consequence of the treatment and its complications, however, metabolic factors and psychological factors also play a role [7,8,9].

Malnutrition at diagnosis may be more common than previously thought due to nutritional assessment being based upon measurement of height and weight, which may not be appropriate for assessing children with cancer. Many children with cancer have large tumour masses which inevitably add to their body weight, therefore weight to height ratios are distorted and, consequently, are unlikely to be a sensitive indicator of malnutrition. Height for age is also a poor indicator, as the history of ill health in children with cancer is usually brief, therefore height for age, an index of chronic malnutrition, is unlikely to be depressed. The use of arm anthropometry gives a more reliable indication of the presence of malnutrition at diagnosis and indicates that malnutrition is more common at diagnosis than previously realized [10].

Metabolic factors

There are two main abnormalities of carbohydrate metabolism: increase in glucose turnover and impairment of peripheral glucose disposal [11]. Carbohydrates provide a major source of the energy requirements of tumour metabolism and glucose is metabolized in tumour tissue mainly by anaerobic glycolysis. One of the consequences of anaerobic metabolism is the release of lactate by tumour cells into the circulation which is then transported to the liver and kidney cortex to produce glucose in an energy requiring process [12,13]. This cycle from glucose to lactate and back to glucose, known as the Cori cycle, has been estimated to account for a 10% increase in energy expenditure in the tumour bearing host [14].

There is also found to be an abnormality of glucose tolerance and a decrease in insulin sensitivity in more than 60% of cancer patients [11]. A combination of increased glycogenolysis and gluconeogenesis suggests that glucose is utilized at increased rates in cancer patients [15]. This helps to explain the frequently elevated basal metabolic rate seen in cancer patients despite a reduced food intake.

Abnormalities in protein metabolism are also present with total protein turnover being accelerated due to an increase in both protein synthesis and degradation. There appears to be an alteration in the flow of amino acids and the synthesis of muscle protein is generally reduced. Increased catabolic enzyme activity and increased protein turnover have also been reported [13]. This results in a reduction in skeletal muscle mass and hypoalbuminaemia, both of which are common in cancer patients.

A significant increase in plasma free fatty acids (FFA) has also been reported in patients with cancer. This increased availability of FFA and ketones as metabolic fuel also inhibits glucose oxidation and impairs tissue responsiveness to insulin.

Malignant cachexia, therefore, appears to be a state of insulin resistance with glucose intolerance, increased gluconeogenesis, activated lipolysis and a possible increase in amino acid degradation. If the active process persists then the patient utilises adipose tissue and muscle mass as a source of energy, resulting in loss of lean body mass and general weight loss. This inefficient energy metabolism can result in a rapid nutritional deterioration in the growing child.

Table 21.2 Side effects relating to treatment seen in paediatric oncology patients

Side effect		Causative chemotherapeutic agent
Infection	Both chemotherapy and radiotherapy are known immune depressants; malnutrition also has an effect on immunity. The malnourished child with cancer and an uncontrolled infection can further deteriorate nutritionally from the side effects of cancer and infection leading to a vicious cycle [16]	
Diarrhoea	This is the commonest side effect and can be due to mucositis and consequent malabsorption; tumour infiltration of the bowel; infection and prolonged use of antibiotics. Children are especially sensitive to the effects of drugs and radiotherapy to the intestinal tract	Actinomycin 5-Fluorouracil Methotrexate (high dose)
Nausea and vomiting	This is another common side effect and some of the chemotherapy drugs are powerful inducers of vomiting [17]	Adriamycin Cyclophosphamide Procarbazine
Stomatitis mucositis	Stomatitis or mucosal damage is a common side effect of chemotherapy and can be severe enough to prevent an adequate oral intake	Actinomycicn Adriamycin 5-Fluorouracil Methotrexate Vinblastine
Renal damage and nutrient loss	A large number of chemotherapy drugs cause renal damage and hence significant protein and mineral losses	Ifosamide Cisplatin Carboplatin
Dysgeusia	This is often seen in advanced cancers, but is more often seen in adults	
Xerostomia	Xerostomia and poor oral hygiene can both be serious deterrents to an adequate oral intake	
Constipation	Occasionally this can be a problem in children with cancer	Vincristine

Complications of disease and treatment

Most of the malnutrition seen is a direct consequence of the disease progression and treatment. Table 21.2 shows the side effects which result in an increased risk of malnutrition.

Psychological factors

Learned food aversions associated with treatment have been demonstrated in children with cancer and part of this behaviour is the phenomenon of anticipatory vomiting [18,19]. Parents can often become preoccupied with getting their children to eat. However, this preoccupation may reduce the child's appetite further and cause him to rebel against the parent and purposely not eat.

IDENTIFICATION OF NUTRITIONAL RISK

Determination of the nutritional risk of a child with cancer can be associated with the diagnosis of certain tumours and stages of disease [20], by the treatment used and by nutritional assessment (Table 21.3) [21].

A nutritional assessment on diagnosis looking at the child's weight for age, height for age and weight/height ratio should be done routinely. However, it is important to remember, as previously mentioned, that a large tumour mass at diagnosis may mask a low body weight in relation to height and that treatment aimed to reduce tumour mass will also exaggerate deterioration in perceived nutritional status. Any fluid retention present at diagnosis will also give a false impression. In view of this arm anthropometry, e.g. skinfold thickness and mid arm circumference, es-

Table 21.3 Types of childhood cancers associated with high or low nutritional risk

High nutritional risk	Low nutritional risk
Advanced diseases during initial intense treatment	Good prognosis acute lymphoblastic leukaemia
Stages III and IV Wilm's tumour and unfavourable histology Wilm's tumour	Non-metastatic solid tumours
Stages III and IV neuroblastoma	Advanced diseases in remission during maintenance treatment
Ewing's sarcoma	
Pelvic rhabdomyosarcoma	
Some non-Hodgkin's lymphoma	
Multiple relapse leukaemia	
Acute non-lymphoblastic leukaemia	
Some poor prognosis acute lymphoblastic leukaemia	
Medulloblastoma	

pecially in solid tumour patients is a more reliable indicator [10].

Serum protein levels, in particular C-reactive protein, serum prealbumin and retinol binding protein which have short half-lives, are more sensitive indicators of malnutrition and will help to determine whether or not malnutrition is already present [22]. Transferrin is another protein with a relatively short half-life. However its synthesis is induced by iron deficiency and it also acts as an acute phase reactant so there may be too many variables present to allow it to be a consistent indicator of nutritional status [13].

A dietary history at diagnosis of the disease should be taken to determine the child's current intake, but a retrospective dietary history prior to diagnosis is also useful to compare whether the disease is affecting the child's current appetite and intake.

The consequences of malnutrition are multiple and include a poorer outcome compared with children who are well nourished at diagnosis [23]; a reduced tolerance to therapy and more complications [24]; and an increased susceptibility to infection.

NUTRITIONAL SUPPORT

The main aims of nutritional support are to reverse the malnutrition seen at diagnosis, prevent the malnutrition associated with treatment and to promote weight gain and growth rather than weight maintenance [25].

One of the questions that is often addressed in feeding cancer patients is the possibility that the nutrients given to replete the host may stimulate further growth of the tumour mass [11]. Numerous studies using different experimental cancers suggest a stimulatory effect of nutrients on tumour growth. This stimulatory effect of specific nutrients on cancer cell replication has been reported to enhance tumour response to chemotherapy or radiotherapy.

In clinical studies the efficacy of nutritional intervention with improved nutritional status in children has shown no evidence of enhanced tumour growth or decreased long term survival in the child [7]. Children have increased nutrient requirements for growth and development which must be met despite extended periods of cancer treatment [25]. Therefore, nutritional support should be considered a major part of therapy in order to prevent or reverse the effects of protein energy malnutrition and to increase the well-being of the child. If this is achieved then the aim of nutritional support has been reached even if the overall prognosis remains the same.

Oral feeding

In patients with a low nutritional risk, unless complicated by factors such as relapse, sepsis or major abdominal procedures, oral feeding is the best method if they are able to consume sufficient nutrients. However, the majority will need high energy supplements and specific advice on eating problems related to the side effects of their treatment (Table 21.4). Ideally there should be flexibility with regard to menu choice, meal times and parental involvement. Unfortunately, in the hospital environment this is not always possible. Fluids and foods consumed should be recorded accurately in order to assess nutrient intake.

Advice with regard to the use of high energy foods and small frequent meals should be given routinely to parents for when the child is at home. Advice on the use of supplements should be given and how to modify them in order to improve their palatability is useful as it is often found in this group of patients that

Table 21.4 Advice on nutritional problems associated with cancer and its treatment [26,27]

Problem	Suggested dietary advice
Loss of appetite	Offer small frequent meals/snacks 5–6 per day Avoid rich fatty foods A soft diet may be better tolerated Avoid drinking just before and during mealtimes
Nausea	Offer small amounts of food at a time Cold food may be better tolerated Avoid fatty or greasy foods Offer dry foods e.g. crackers, plain biscuits or toast Avoid very sweet foods Avoid hot and spicy foods Serve meals attractively Avoid favourite foods as the child may then develop a permanent dislike for them Sips of a cool, fizzy drink may help, e.g. soda water or ginger ale
Vomiting	Give mouth washes to help to remove the taste Avoid fluids or food until vomiting is controlled and then introduce clear fluids Avoid favourite foods Dry foods may be better tolerated
Sore mouth/throat	Offer soft, moist foods e.g. mashed potato, scrambled egg, custard, yoghurt, ice cream If severe blended/puréed foods may be more appropriate Use straws for drinking Keep foods moist by using butter, sauces, cream or yoghurt Avoid citrus fruits and fruit juices, spicy or salty foods Avoid rough or very dry foods
Dry mouth	Offer frequent drinks Crushed ice or cubes to suck may be useful Sucking fruit drops or boiled mints may stimulate saliva production Keep foods moist by using butter, sauces, cream, yoghurt, gravy
Taste changes and loss of taste	If the child complains of a 'metallic' taste when eating meat, then try poultry, fish, eggs or cheese instead Experiment using herbs and spices to flavour food Try cold sharp foods Offer foods familiar to and liked by the child Flavour gravy with Bovril, Marmite, soy and sweet and sour sauces Vary the colour and texture of the foods Emphasize the aroma of food

Table 21.4 (continued)

Problem	Suggested dietary advice
Diarrhoea	Avoid foods high in fibre Ensure the child continues to drink plenty, but avoid chilled drinks straight from the fridge Avoid any specific foods known to aggravate the diarrhoea
Intermittent constipation	Encourage foods high in fibre and plenty of fluids
Malabsorption	A low fat, low residue or lactose free diet as appropriate for the type of malabsorptive problem In some cases the enteral route will need to be avoided and the child will require total parenteral nutrition
Food aversion	Avoid favourite foods prior to chemotherapy Give carbohydrate based meals prior to chemotherapy rather then protein based meals Avoid making a big issue of the child's nutritional intake

their appetites for certain tastes change very frequently. Useful supplements include those shown in Table 25.2.

Enteral nutrition

Whenever nutritional intervention is indicated it is highly preferable to use the enteral route. Enteral nutrition has numerous practical and psychological advantages over parenteral nutrition including a low risk of infection and other catheter related complications; more normal play activities; and a lifestyle that provides a positive way for both parent and child to be involved in the child's care. In addition enteral feeding is more economical [7].

Previously it was thought that enteral feeding regimens were not effective in reversing or preventing protein energy malnutrition in high nutritional risk patients (e.g. those with Stage IV Wilm's tumour, or Stage IV neuroblastoma), and indeed several studies have shown this. There is now some degree of conflict as to which is the best feeding route in high nutritional risk patients. However, earlier studies compared parenteral feeding with oral feeding programmes in children with advanced Wilm's tumours and neuroblastomas and concluded that oral feeding failed to promote a good intake and reversal or prevention of protein energy malnutrition. The oral feeding programmes included the use of supplements, but not nasogastric feeding which was dismissed as being psychologically too traumatic for use in children [24, 25,28]. Other more recent studies report that nasogastric supplementary nutrition benefits children with malignancy and indeed a recent pilot study showed that nasogastric feeding is practical, acceptable and tolerated in children with newly diagnosed advanced malignancy who are commencing intensive treatment protocols. It improved their energy intake, wellbeing, and there was significant improvement in their nutritional status as measured by mid upper arm circumference. Therefore, even in advanced malignancies, whereever possible the enteral route should be used [28].

Generally a whole protein feed will be tolerated. However following chemotherapy a hydrolysate or elemental feed may be more appropriate if malabsorption occurs. If the child has had total parenteral nutrition he may not tolerate a whole protein feed initially when transferring to enteral feeding, so again a hydrolysate feed may be useful (Table 6.13).

The majority of children on enteral feeding will require it throughout their intense treatment, but once they go onto maintenance treatment their appetites generally improve and a conscious effort should be made to try and wean them off their feeds.

If enteral feeding at home is required it is desirable to feed the child overnight only in order not to disturb everyday life further. However, in some cases this may not be possible due to a very poor oral intake during the day and the child not being able to tolerate the high feed volumes required to provide adequate nutrition over this shorter period of time.

When deciding to feed the child with cancer enterally it is also important to establish whether he has minimal gastrointestinal complaints and that the passing of the tube will not cause bleeding due to a low platelet count. Continuing support is essential.

Parenteral nutrition

Parenteral nutrition should be reserved for those whose enteral feeding regimens cannot provide adequate nutrients, or for those patients with abnormal gastrointestinal function related either to their tumour or following chemotherapy or radiotherapy treatments.

Parenteral feeding is both safe and effective in children with advanced cancer; in those who are already malnourished, or likely to become so, it may be the most effective feeding method [24]. Curtailment of parenteral nutrition support before reversal of protein energy malnutrition and completion of intensive treatment will reduce the benefits of previous nutritional support. Parenteral nutrition should ideally be continued for several days beyond the cessation of chemotherapy or radiotherapy, which often induce both nausea and vomiting. In most cases this will not be possible as if the child is well enough to go home for a few days after therapy, then parenteral nutrition will need to be discontinued. Discharge from hospital is often cut short by the development of febrile neutropenia. Children receiving intensive chemotherapy experience a prolonged neutropenia (neutrophil count $< 1.0 \times 10^9$/l), often associated with fever. This febrile neutropenia renders the child especially vulnerable to developing infections. If the child has a fever of 38°C or above, or has a strong history of fever or rigors, urgent hospitalization is necessary for investigation and treatment as the child can deteriorate rapidly in this state [29].

The nutritional benefits from effective parenteral nutrition are maintained after completion of intense treatment unless complicating factors, such as relapse, sepsis or major abdominal procedures occur in the patient's clinical course. Although parenteral nutrition is an appropriate method for renourishing children with advanced cancer, some patients may not benefit from parenteral nutrition support because of overwhelming medical problems which may limit fluid and nutrient intake, interruptions of nutrient delivery or rapidly progressive disease.

The possibility that parenteral nutrition in excess of host repletion stimulates tumour growth again needs to be considered, but clinically has not been observed when aggressive cancer treatment is given simultaneously. In fact, parenteral nutrition may beneficially stimulate cell replication and increase the effectiveness of cell cycle drugs.

Metabolic complications of parenteral nutrition are well documented and are not significantly different between children with malignancies and other children requiring parenteral support. Monitoring of the patient's weight, fluid balance and biochemical parameters is essential. It is extremely important to check electrolyte levels daily, especially if the child has had or is receiving a course of chemotherapy containing drugs which impair renal function. In this case, certain electrolytes will be required above normal maintenance levels (Table 21.5) [30].

Table 21.5 Effect of chemotherapy drugs on electrolytes

Electrolyte affected	Side effect	Chemotherapy drug
Potassium	Muscular weakness Confusion Cardiac arrhythmias	Ifosamide Cisplatin Carboplatin
Phosphate	Anorexia, weakness, bone pain, joint stiffness Further symptoms include muscle weakness, tremor, paraesthesia, confusion and coma	Ifosamide Cisplatin Carboplatin
Calcium	Tetany Fitting Lethargy Osteomalacia	Ifosamide
Magnesium	Muscle weakness Fasciculation Tetany Vertigo Depression	Cisplatin Carboplatin

BENEFITS OF NUTRITIONALLY SUPPORTING THE CHILD WITH CANCER

The benefits from nutritional support are inherently important, independent of potential benefit related to improved survival. Proper nutritional support in children with cancer has value in improving growth and wellbeing. Current data suggests that chemotherapy-induced bone marrow suppression may be attenuated and chemotherapy tolerance improved with the use of adequate nutritional support in children with advanced cancers [7].

The organ systems most affected by protein energy malnutrition are those most sensitive to anticancer treatment, including the immune system. Data suggests that impaired immune competence and a decreased ability to fight infections are associated not only with the intensity and kind of anticancer treatment, but also the efficacy of nutritional support.

NUTRITION AND THE CHILD WITH CANCER UNDERGOING BONE MARROW TRANSPLANTATION

For children with AML, Stage IV neuroblastoma or relapse, or ALL undergoing bone marrow transplant

or autograft, there are further nutritional problems. The priming chemotherapy used causes severe nausea, vomiting and oral ulceration. The total body irradiation used immediately following priming chemotherapy also causes severe nausea and vomiting along with malabsorption and a very dry mouth. In addition to this, the patient is severely neutropenic and needs to keep to a clean diet in order to prevent gastrointestinal infection from food-borne pathogens. The provision of a clean diet is described elsewhere (Chapter 2).

ALTERNATIVE DIETS

There are various alternative or 'fad' diets advised by religious or philosophical groups which claim to treat or cure cancer and are used either in conjunction with or instead of conventional cancer treatments. Examples include the Bristol diet, the Kelly anticancer diet and the Macrobiotic diet.

Most of these diets claim to rid the body of unnatural chemicals, to restore the efficiency of and strengthen the body's immune system by maximizing the mineral, vitamin and enzyme systems. They are usually strictly vegetarian or vegan and, ideally, organic. The diets exclude all animal products, salt and refined carbohydrate and allow only very small quantities of fat. They often involve taking large amounts of vitamin and mineral supplements. They are therefore very bulky, low in energy, low in protein and totally inappropriate for most children, let alone the child with cancer. Children with a loss of appetite, nausea and vomiting will find it extremely difficult to eat a high fibre, raw food diet.

These diets are also very time consuming and costly to prepare and the high doses of vitamins and minerals may be harmful. Any parent contemplating putting a child on such a diet should be advised strongly against it.

The benefits of nutritional support for the child with cancer are extremely important. Proper nutritional support can improve growth, organ function and appears to improve treatment tolerance and quality of life.

REFERENCES

1 Van Eys J Nutritional therapy in children with cancer. *Cancer Res*, 1977, 87 2457–2461.
2 Van Eys J Malnutrition in pediatric oncology. In: Newell

GR (ed.) *Nutrition and Cancer: Etiology and Treatment.* New York: Raven Press, 1981.

3 Eden OB Paediatric oncology. *Hospital Update*, 1983, March 779–788.

4 United Kingdom Children's Cancer Study Group *Scientific Report*. London: UK CC SG, 1992.

5 Bury CL *Paediatric Pathology*, 2e. Berlin: Springer-Verlag, 1989.

6 Holland J *Cancer Medicine*. Boston: Lea & Febiger, 1982.

7 Mauer AM *et al.* Special nutritional needs of children with malignancies – a review. *J Parent Ent Nutr*, 1990, **14**(3) 315–323.

8 Carter P Energy and nutrient intake of children with cancer. *J Am Diet Assoc*, 1983, **82** 610–615.

9 Van Eys J A clinical trial of hyperalimentation in children with metastic malignancies. *Med Pediatr Oncology*, 1980, **8** 63–73.

10 Smith DE *et al.* Malnutrition in children with malignant solid tumours. *J Hum Nutr Diet*, 1990, **3** 303–309.

11 Rossi-Fanelli F *et al.* Abnormal substrate metabolism and nutritional strategies in cancer management. *J Parent Ent Nutr*, 1991, **15**(5) 680–683.

12 Dewys D Pathophysiology of cancer cachexia: current understanding and areas for future research. *Cancer Res*, 1982, **42** 7215–7265.

13 Jaffe N Nutrition in cancer patients. In: Grand, Stephen, Dietz (eds.) *Paediatric Nutrition – Theory and Practice.* London: Butterworth, 1987.

14 Danisheesky I *Biochemistry for Medical Sciences*. Boston: Little, Brown, 1980.

15 Brennan MF Metabolic consequences of nutritional support of the cancer patient. *Cancer*, 1984, **54** 2627–2634.

16 Holcomb C Nutrition and cancer in children. *Surg-Annu*, 1990, **22** 129–142.

17 Donaldson SS Effects of therapy on nutritional status of paediatric cancer patient. *Cancer Res*, 1982, **42** 729s–736s.

18 Bernstein IL Learned taste aversions in children receiving chemotherapy. *Science*, 1978, **200** 1302–1303.

19 Bernstein IL Physiological and psychological mechanisms of cancer anorexia. *Cancer Res*, 1982, **42** 715s–720s.

20 Rickard KA The value of nutritional support in children with cancer. *Cancer*, 1986, **58** 1904–1910.

21 Rickard KA Advances in nutrition care of children with neoplastic disease – a review of treatment, research and application. *J Am Diet Assoc*, 1986, **86** 1666–1675.

22 Carter P Nutritional parameters in children with cancer. *J Am Diet Assoc*, 1983, **82** 616–622.

23 Donaldson SS A study of the nutritional status of pediatric cancer patients. *Am J Dis Child*, 1981, **135** 1107–1112.

24 Rickard KA Short and long term effectiveness of enteral and parenteral nutrition in reversing or preventing protein–energy malnutrition in advanced neuroblastoma. *Cancer*, 1985, **56** 2881–2887.

25 Rickard KA Effectiveness of enteral and parenteral nutrition in the nutritional management of children with Wilm's tumours. *Am J Clin Nutr*, 1980, **33** 2622–2629.

26 *Postman Pat Says 'Eating Well Will Keep You Well'.* South Glamorgan HA/Bristol Myers Oncology, 1989. Available from Bristol Myers-Squibb Pharmaceuticals Ltd, 141–149 Staines Road, Hounslow TW3 3JA.

27 *Postman Pat's 'Eating Well Will Keep You Well' – follow on book.* Dietetic Department, St James's University Hospital NHS Trust, 1991. Available from Bristol Myers-Squibb Pharmaceuticals Ltd, as above.

28 Smith DE An investigation of supplementary naso-gastric feeding in malnourished children undergoing treatment for malignancy: results of a pilot study. *J Hum Nutr Diet*, 1992, **5** 85–91.

29 Sweetenham JW *et al. Clinical Oncology*. Oxford: Blackwell Scientific Publications, 1989.

30 Grant A, Todd E *Enteral – Parenteral Nutrition*. Oxford: Blackwell Scientific Publications, 1987.

Eating Disorders and Obesity

CHAPTER 22

Anorexia Nervosa and Bulimia Nervosa

Eating disorders generally occur most commonly in females aged 15–25. The most common of these are bulimia nervosa, anorexia nervosa, overeating and obesity. In children eating disorders are less common but manifest in a wider range, including anorexia nervosa, food avoidance emotional disorder, food fads, selective eating and food refusal, pervasive refusal syndrome, poor appetite secondary to illness, failure to thrive, and the over eating conditions such as obesity and Prader-Willi syndrome. The latter two disorders and failure to thrive are dealt with in other chapters and in this chapter we will focus on the remainder.

ANOREXIA NERVOSA

The term anorexia nervosa is a misnomer in that frequently there is no loss of appetite, but rather an avoidance of weight gain. In children the characteristic features of anorexia nervosa differ from those of the older age group [1]. For example disturbances of menstruation or loss of secondary sexual characteristics, which always occur in adults, are not likely to be relevant in many children. We have found the most common features to be:

(1) Determined food avoidance.
(2) Significant degrees of weight loss.
(3) Any combination of the following:
   - preoccupation with body weight
   - preoccupation with dietary energy
   - distorted body image
   - fear of fatness
   - self-induced vomiting
   - excessive exercising
   - laxative abuse
   - secretive eating.

In about one third of cases there is a past history of feeding problems, about a quarter have obsessional symptoms, and about a half are at some time during the illness depressed. However, it should be emphasized that there is no absolutely typical presentation of anorexia nervosa in children, and very commonly many of the features described are concealed and denied. This is all the more surprising to the parents since prior to the illness such children have usually been considered to be absolutely perfect, conscientious, hard working, popular and successful.

The cause of anorexia nervosa is unknown but is very likely to be multifactorial [2]. Genetic and personality factors appear to predispose to the illness, as does living in a relatively prosperous society where food is plentiful but slimness is considered desirable. The most obvious precipitating factor is the impending or recent onset of puberty. However, not uncommonly the illness commences after a chance remark is made about being overweight or after contact with someone who is already dieting. Sexual abuse or other major traumas may well be relevant in a number of instances. Family problems such as marital conflict, over involvement between a parent and child, or a prohibition on the expression of anger may also predispose towards or precipitate the illness. Once the illness has started other factors can perpetuate it, including a failure to recognize that the child is ill or a failure to treat the problem seriously, as well as the persistence of individual and family difficulties.

In summary it is essential to realize that there is an interaction between multiple factors, the end point of which is anorexia nervosa. For this reason treatment, discussed below, is complex and involves far more than simply giving dietary advice.

The incidence of anorexia nervosa is unknown but is probably in the order of 1–2 per 1000 of adolescent females. The incidence is lower in children, but of interest is the sex ratio. In the older age group, females outnumber males by 9:1, whereas girls outnumber boys by only 4:1. The disorder is more common in the upper income groups but this discrepancy is diminishing with time. Similarly there is a gradual increase in the incidence in the immigrant population. The prognosis is poor with only about one third making a full recovery and one third remaining ill for several years.

BULIMIA NERVOSA

Bulimia nervosa is a variant of anorexia nervosa that is very rare in children, although affecting as many as 1% of late-adolescent and young adult women. It is characterized by the same preoccupation with energy intake and body weight but, as well as a tendency to restrict food intake, there are times when food is consumed in excess, sometimes known as 'binge eating'. Binges are usually followed by self-induced vomiting. Because of its rarity in children we will not discuss it further in this chapter but the same cautionary comments as those made about the aetiology and treatment of anorexia nervosa also apply to bulimia.

FOOD AVOIDANCE EMOTIONAL DISORDER (FAED)

This condition was first described by Higgs *et al.* [3] and has some similarities to anorexia nervosa in that food avoidance is a prominent symptom. However, the diagnostic criteria for anorexia nervosa are not all present and, in particular, the most characteristic features of distorted body image and fear of fatness are absent. Other symptoms such as depression, obsessions, phobias and anxiety are more prominent than in anorexia nervosa. Occasionally a phobia of swallowing may be recognized, or a complaint made that there is a lump in the throat that makes swallowing difficult. There is usually a past history of feeding difficulty and there is no evidence of other disease. It may be that FAED is a less severe variant of anorexia nervosa with a better prognosis.

FOOD FADS, SELECTIVE EATING, AND FOOD REFUSAL

These problems take a variety of forms and are fairly common in children, especially in the younger age group [4]. Most young children pass through a phase of food faddishness in which they eat only a very small range of foods. For example the diet may consist of only fruit drinks, sweets, crisps and baked beans. Such faddishness is rarely long lasting and does not seem to have any adverse effect on the child. It is usually the mother who suffers most, with her understandable anxiety that the diet is inadequate.

Occasionally this problem persists into later childhood and, albeit rarely, into adult life. Surprisingly this selective eating, which is commonly carbohydrate-based, does not seem to be associated with any delay in growth and usually the children (or adults) are of normal weight. They are not preoccupied with their appearance and seem to function well in most other respects. The only associated problem is that of social functioning, as concern is often expressed that the child may find it difficult to negotiate situations which might necessitate eating foods outside the restricted range. However, that concern is usually not felt by the child prior to adolescence, and if parental concern can be contained the problem often slowly resolves before the teenage years.

Food refusal is also a common feature of early childhood. Such children may display relatively normal eating behaviour in one situation, for example at school or at a friend's house, whilst not eating in another, such as at home, or vice-versa. Alternatively they may eat normally on one day and totally refuse to eat on another. Such behaviour is usually temporary, often an attempt on the child's part to develop some autonomy and, providing it is managed sensibly, usually resolves with time.

PERVASIVE REFUSAL SYNDROME

This condition has been described by Lask *et al.* [5] and is characterized by the child's refusal not only to eat but also to talk, walk or care for herself in any way. She shuns all contact and appears both terrified and furious. It is believed that pervasive refusal may be a form of post-traumatic stress disorder. It is a life threatening condition that always requires hospitalization and artificial feeding. The prognosis is poor.

POOR APPETITE SECONDARY TO ILLNESS

A natural consequence of any form of ill health, be it localized or systemic, is diminished appetite. Generally normal appetite returns coincident with restoration of good health. Chronic illness may lead to persisting poor appetite and exacerbation or perpetuation of the disease, with a complex vicious cycle. Depression, either secondary to ill-health or as a primary disorder, is an important cause of diminished appetite and must always be considered. It is usually accompanied by disturbed sleep, impaired concentration, tearfulness, and lethargy. Less commonly, childhood depression is accompanied by behaviour problems.

TREATMENT OF EATING DISORDERS

There are no simple or certain paths to recovery from serious eating disorders. The successful treatment of children needs to be multifaceted, reflecting the complex aetiology. Flexibility is also essential, as different approaches are appropriate for different individuals, at different stages of the illness. Despite many years of research, there is still little certain information on what constitutes effective therapy, although a number of basic principles are widely applied.

Serious food refusal and obsession with weight is usually a late step in the development of emotional problems, and may be seen as a frantic effort to camouflage or defend against those problems. This means that simply trying to deal with the mechanics of the illness (persuading the child to eat more or to stop vomiting) is unlikely to lead to a 'cure'. At some point, the focus of intervention must shift away from food intake onto the issues that may have lead initially to the development of symptoms and, more importantly, onto those issues which are keeping the symptoms going.

Somewhat simplistically, we can divide treatment into two main areas: treatment tackling physical issues and treatment tackling psychological issues [6].

Physical issues in treatment

As outlined above, eating disorders in children can lead to serious physical problems and a few children even die from anorexia nervosa and its complications.

For such potentially serious disorders, treatment must be rapidly initiated, intensive and comprehensive. Where the patient's physical state is a serious concern, treatment must focus directly on the physical issues (e.g. dehydration, low serum potassium levels, oesophageal tears). Where the child's physical state has not yet deteriorated to a worrying degree, treatment can focus more immediately on the underlying emotions.

Whether or not a child should be hospitalized is an early and important decision. Hospital admission should be considered if the following signs are present:

- extreme weight loss (weight less than 80% weight for height for age)
- dehydration
- signs of circulation failure
- persistent vomiting or vomiting of blood
- marked depression or other major psychiatric disturbance.

If a child is admitted to a paediatric ward as a medical emergency, an individualized but clear and firm medical regimen is essential, preferably carried out by staff who have some experience of children with eating disorders. At very low body weights a patient may be prescribed certain definite amounts of high energy liquid nourishment, with the possibility of nasogastric tube feeding as an alternative. Children who persistently vomit need warnings of the extreme danger of this practice and should be helped to tolerate the anxiety of eating while being prevented from vomiting. It is important that skilled psychological help is begun or continued during the medical admission so that emotional issues are not neglected, although if a child is at very low body weight it may be impossible to do much therapeutic work.

Strict behavioural regimens are far less popular nowadays on medical or psychiatric wards for eating-disordered patients, since it is widely recognized that fast weight gain achieved by staff coercion is not a substitute for genuine recovery.

For longer term and more comprehensive treatment an admission to a child or adolescent psychiatric unit may be advised. Such units take children whose physical state is poor, but also children for whom parental and professional efforts to resolve the destructive struggle around food has failed on an outpatient basis.

When children remain as outpatients, the most important element in treatment is a clear message to parents about the importance of their taking charge of the child's health, including what he or she eats. If the diagnosis is anorexia nervosa or bulimia nervosa, the potential seriousness of the illness must be spelt out and the need for relieving the child of the burden of controlling so destructively his or her own food intake. Since eating disorders often occur precisely because children feel that they have little or no control over their lives, and strive for one area of successful self-control – eating – children will invariably object vigorously to parents taking charge. The child should therefore retain some control of some areas of his or her life, like clothing, and the issue of appropriate kinds of control must be addressed directly in therapy.

Parents generally find it hard to intervene firmly, even forcibly, without a great deal of encouragement and support. They often fear that being firm will upset the child and worsen the situation. By failing to challenge the child, parents may inadvertently be maintaining the problem. Professionals need to help them to see this while not giving them the unhelpful impression that they are to blame.

Parents are frequently at odds over the management of their eating-disordered child, believing that the other parent is too lax or too strict. Frequently the child is sided with by one parent against the other. Issues over which parents may well disagree, and therefore need help to resolve, include expectations over what their child should eat, what should be done in the event of persistent refusal, whether or not they wish to accept treatment at all. The professional's role here is not to take sides but rather to offer advice and help the parents to reach agreement, preferably without being adversely influenced by their child's protests. As well as trying to reach joint decisions, parents should be helped to think about the sharing of responsibility for cajoling their child into eating, and the need for both parents to be involved in this often painful and frustrating process.

Adults should generally try not to get into interminable discussion around weight and calories with children who have eating disorders. However, it is often helpful to discuss briefly and clearly with the child what is a safe weight and, for girls, at what weight menstruation is likely to occur (roughly 94% weight for height for age). It is hard to be exact about a healthy weight, so a weight range is more meaningful. It is wise to set a target of 95–100% weight for height. This may need to adjusted upwards if menstruation fails to occur. The child and parents should also be reminded that, as the child gets older and – hopefully – grows, the actual weight that represents

95–100% will increase. For some children a weight chart is helpful, with a variety of target weights clearly marked. These target weights could indicate when various physical activities that have been suspended during illness can be resumed.

Treatment of psychological issues

As we have stressed, preoccupation with weight is usually the surface presentation of underlying difficulties. For each child the particular constellation of psychological issues at stake will be unique, but common themes often emerge: chronically low self-esteem, lack of assertiveness, high expectations, poor differentiation of feelings and needs, fear of separating from parents. The family as a whole may have difficulty in facing up to and trying to resolve conflicts, and it is often noted that the families of anorectic children have problems in coming to terms with change. A child's entry into adolescence (often the trigger for the onset of an eating disorder) is just such a change that needs negotiating. The initial causes of the difficulties are probably impossible to track by the time the symptoms have developed, but there is plenty of scope for tackling current patterns of thinking and communicating which are contributing to the maintenance of the symptoms.

There exist a number of therapeutic approaches tackling these issues for individuals under 18 years. The treatment of choice is currently family therapy [7]. Therapeutic work with the child's family can begin at the time when issues of control and conflict are addressed in discussing food intake. For a family where open disagreement is frowned on, it may be hard for the child to voice a contrary point of view or express any 'negative' emotions like anger or jealousy – except, indirectly, by refusal of food.

Family therapy can lead to the child making first steps in emotional separation and independence. This may be hard for the parents unless they are offered support and help through a time of change. They may complain about the child's lack of maturity and self-reliance but still need help in permitting her to change, and in finding new satisfactions for themselves once they begin to 'let go'. The child may have to be helped out of a 'triangulated' position between parents who experience mutual difficulties in intimacy and trust.

Individual therapy can be an important adjunct to family meetings, especially for older children who are keen to preserve some areas of private concern. In individual sessions, the focus is often on helping the child to recognize needs, to express feelings and to interact more assertively. Individuals with eating disorders have often been eager and obedient children who, when faced with increasing demands for self-reliance in adolescence, reveal a deep but hidden sense of incompetence, isolation and dissatisfaction.

In individual sessions it is also very important to do some gentle exploration of any possible traumatic experiences, including sexual abuse. Schooling issues may also need confronting in both family and individual work, perhaps involving consultation with teachers. Eating-disordered children often impose on themselves unrealistic and perfectionist standards in their school work, while deriving little pleasure from the work except in so far as it pleases others. They may also experience difficulties in being assertive in peer relationships and may feel pushed around and imposed on by others.

For children with specific food-related fears (e.g. fear of vomiting, fear of trying new foods, fear of eating in public) the discussion of general emotional issues remains important but can be coupled with therapy directly targetted at coping with the feared situations. This usually involves gentle graded exposure to the feared object or situation in the presence of a trusted therapist who helps the child to try and tolerate the anxiety until it subsides naturally.

It can be seen that to provide effective treatment it is often essential to work within a multidisciplinary team. Different professionals will be needed to think about the physical issues, the child's mental state, family interactions, peer relationships and school issues. It is often important for a social worker to provide expertise and statutory powers when abuse is suspected, or on the rare occasions when parents decline treatment for the sick child.

In treating children with eating disorders, parents and professionals often experience strong feelings of frustration and anger as the child seems to reject all help and a prolonged battle of wills is joined. Parents need to be warned, however, that as the child begins to recover, eating will be less the area of conflict, and oppositional behaviour will become more evident in other areas of life. In particular, the child is likely to go through a phase of expressing a great deal of hostility towards her parents. Parents can be helped to view this positively as a sign of the child's growing awareness of her own impulses, wishes and needs. In time this negative behaviour is replaced by a more age-appropriate expression of feelings and the child learns to discuss these with others.

THE ROLE OF THE DIETITIAN

When a serious eating disorder of non-organic origin is suspected the dietitian is ill-advised to work alone: recovery will be hampered or delayed if no psychological help is sought. The dieitian should be part of a multidisciplinary team and involved in discussions on care, not just called in to advise on the energy content of the diet. Some children and young people find it easier to accept advice over food intake from a dietitian, who may be seen as neutral and objective, rather than from a member of the psychiatric team with whom they discuss emotional issues. The dietitian thus needs to build a working relationship with the patient, the care staff and the parents.

The main dangers for the dietitian when dealing with eating-disordered patients are a feeling of frustration, anger and irritation at the patient's apparent inability to help herself; the misrepresentation to other carers by the patient of information given by the dietitian in order to avoid eating; and the danger of over involvement. The young female dietitian may share some of the patient's beliefs and aspirations regarding thinness, come from a similar background and have experienced similar pressures at the same age.

Communicating with the patient

A core experience of eating disordered people is low self-esteem. It is helpful therefore to act in a way that promotes self-esteem: give time to letting the patient express her opinions; give the message that you understand, even if you have to disagree. It must also be acknowledged that panic about increased eating and weight gain often leads the child to tell untruths about how much food has been consumed. This should be anticipated and the dietitian should let the young person know that she understands how hard it is to speak honestly about food. It is particularly important that the dietitian is honest also; it is not acceptable to try to introduce 'hidden' energy into the diet in the form of glucose polymers or protein supplements unless the patient is aware that this is happening.

It can be helpful for the dietitian to take the 'medical' approach and discuss food as if it were medicine, an essential requirement of the body.

Practical management

Intravenous feeding is usually not indicated unless as a short term measure to correct dehydration. Children may be so resistant to eating that they require naso-gastric feeding; others may accept oral nutrition with the knowledge that tube feeding will be introduced if weight gain does not proceed satisfactorily. An agreed rate of weight gain, with intermediate and final target weights, needs to be agreed. It is sometimes believed that a rapid build up to an intake of 3000–4000 kcal a day is essential to ensure that the child is swiftly helped into an adequate physical and intellectual condition to undertake psychotherapy. In fact after such a harsh experience of refeeding the young person may be very reluctant to use psychotherapy and may even resort to more physically dangerous ways of losing weight – vomiting or laxative abuse. Weight gain and psychotherapy should occur in parallel, so that at each stage of weight gain the patient will have time and psychological space to come to terms with what is happening to her body.

Energy intake should initially be the Estimated Average Requirement (EAR) for age, but this is likely to require upward or downward adjustment depending on weight gain. The day's eating should be planned round a structure of three meals and three snacks. Weight gain through regular meals is preferable to chaotic eating, which feels dangerous and wrong. The suggested menu should contain foods which are familiar and foods which the child is already eating or likes. Although dislikes can be taken into consideration where reasonable (e.g. dislike of offal, fish or a specific item) foods generally considered to be staple, such as bread, potato, pasta or rice must be included in the diet. Too many choices should not be offered to a young person who already has difficulty making decisions. Do not expect the child to welcome much variety: what may seem boring and repetitive to others may be the only safe and acceptable one to the patient.

Fortified drinks such as sip feeds may be useful if there is difficulty in managing adequate amounts of ordinary food. These contain added vitamins and minerals, and supplements may not be necessary if these are included; a multivitamin supplement such as Ketovite tablets and liquid (Paines and Byrne) or

Forceval capsules (Unigreg Ltd) are indicated if the patient is already malnourished or is eating an inadequate diet.

It is important to ensure an adequate fluid and fibre intake if laxatives are not prescribed, as constipation is a common problem in eating disorders. The patient may be unwilling to drink even water if she feels it will increase weight, and will need reassurance about this.

It may be helpful, especially in the early stages, to use foods which come in standard portions or which are easily measurable, and whose energy value is easily calculated. If ward staff are inexperienced in estimating the energy content of meals, a chart indicating standard portions (e.g. tablespoons, cups) of common foods and their energy content should be made available where food is served and eaten. Alternatively food may need to be pre-weighed in the diet kitchen or bay before being sent to the ward. Clear guidelines should be agreed between the dietitian, care staff and patient about which items need not be consumed and which foods must be replaced by an equivalent amount of energy if rejected. This prevents confusion and arguments at meal times. Once the general framework has been agreed with the dietitian, the young person will probably need considerable help and guidance over the details, usually from members of staff involved in her day-to-day care. She may find it reassuring to discuss a whole day's intake to see which were the points of real difficulty. The child should be encouraged to write out her own menu within the agreed framework, as this may engender a greater sense of being in control and will emphasize the need for her to take responsibility. At all times, however small the achievements may be, the child will need plenty of praise for her courage.

Maintaining a safe weight

Once a safe weight has been achieved the struggle to maintain it begins and may go on for many years, if not a whole lifetime. While it is important that medical follow-up and psychotherapy continue for some time after satisfactory weight gain, some young people also find it helpful to have continued advice from a dietitian as they return to a more normal and flexible eating pattern. Many eating-disordered people go on counting calories for years and, whilst this is not encouraged, it may be realistic to accept that it helps them to feel more in control. Others shift the focus of the need to exercise control over their eating by changing to an alternative dietary practice such as veganism, and they and their parents may need help to plan a balanced diet within the constraints of such regimens.

REFERENCES

1 Fosson A *et al*. Early onset anorexia nervosa. *Arch Dis Childh*, 1987, **62** 114–118.
2 Wren B, Lask B Aetiology. In: Lask B, Bryant-Waugh (eds.) *Children with Anorexia Nervosa and Related Eating Disorders*. London: Laurence Erlbaum Associates, 1993.
3 Higgs J, Goodyer I, Birch J Anorexia nervosa and food avoidance emotional disorder. *Arch Dis Childh*, 1989, **64** 346–351.
4 Bryant-Waugh R, Kaminski Z Clinical presentations of early onset eating disorders. In: Lask B, Bryant-Waugh R (eds.) *Children with Anorexia Nervosa and Related Eating Disorders*. London: Laurence Erlbaum Associates, 1993.
5 Lask B *et al*. Children with pervasive refusal. *Arch Dis Childh*, 1991, **66** 866–869.
6 Lask B Overview of treatment. In: Lask B, Bryant-Waugh R (eds.) *Children with Anorexia Nervosa and Related Eating Disorders*. London: Laurence Erlbaum Associates, 1993.
7 Russell G *et al*. An evaluation of family therapy in anorexia nervosa and bulimia nervosa. *Arch Gen Psych*, 1987, **44** 1047–1056.

CHAPTER 23

Obesity

SIMPLE OBESITY

Obesity is a relatively common problem in childhood and adolescence, which presents a difficult task and challenge for the clinician and dietitian to manage.

Obesity may be defined as 'an excess of adipose tissue, considered to be undesirable, or reach levels above those set arbitrarily, and based on a suitable anthropometric measurement' [1]. British figures for the prevalence of childhood obesity range from 2–11% depending on age and sex [2]. It is more common in adolescence with 2.9% of girls and 1.7% of boys aged six years being overweight, compared with 9.6% and 6.5% respectively for 14 year olds [3].

Aetiology

The aetiology of obesity is complex and multifactorial. Organic causes of obesity such as Cushing's syndrome and hypothyroidism are rare; Prader-Willi syndrome is associated with obesity and this condition is dealt with separately.

Both genetic and environmental factors contribute to the development of obesity. Many studies support the theory that obesity tends to run in families [4,5]; children of non-obese parents have a less than 10% chance of being obese, whereas this probability increases to 40% and 80% respectively when one or both parents are obese. In a more recent study heredity and the degree of obesity in childhood and adolescence were found to have major influences on prognosis. Excessive overweight during puberty was associated with higher than expected morbidity and mortality in later life [7].

Lifestyle in the past few decades has changed considerably and this is reflected in eating habits, which tend to include more high energy 'fast foods' [8,9].

The advent of television viewing, computer games and other sedentary activities and the decrease in priority of physical education in schools means that many children are less physically active than in previous years. Obese children are less active than their leaner peers [10]; they are less fit and may feel embarrassed and uncomfortable when taking part in sporting activities.

Assessment

At the first clinic visit baseline anthropometry should be obtained: weight and height measurements should be plotted on centile charts (e.g. Tanner and Whitehouse, 1975). Skinfold measurements, preferably taken by the same individual, using calipers will give a more accurate estimate of fatness and can be compared with centile charts [11]. Generally a weight of more than two centiles higher than the height, or a weight for height index greater than 120% is considered to constitute obesity. Measurement of body mass index (weight/height^2) is little used in children as the values are dependent on height centile and age, and it is difficult to monitor progress using this equation, although it has been suggested that weight/height$^{2.8}$ may be a useful measure of obesity in school-age children [12].

It is most important to get a detailed dietary history from both the child and his parents. Other details such as age of onset of obesity, eating pattern and family dynamics are also helpful. A recall diet history is most frequently used to determine current intake. It is advisable to ask specifically about snack foods and drinks consumed between meals since these are often overlooked. In addition friends may share their food outside the home.

Management

To be successful the child over school age must want to lose weight, but this requires support and co-operation from the parents, grandparents, siblings and all who come into contact with the child. It is necessary to educate the child and his family so that they understand the aims of management, which is that overweight children eat more than they require and must reduce their intake in order to lose weight. A suitable diet should be constructed, taking into account the child's current intake, age, social circumstances and family income.

A target weight should be agreed, and a timescale planned for achieving this. In mild to moderate childhood obesity the aim should be for the weight to remain static so that the child will 'grow into' his weight. In the severely obese child the aim is to restrict the dietary intake so that weight loss is achieved without causing impairment of normal growth.

Frequent reinforcement is necessary in order to maintain interest and motivation. This should be carried out weekly or fortnightly, and may be done by the school nurse, practice nurse or dietitian. Attempts have been made to run group sessions for overweight children, but on the whole these have not been successful, with a high drop-out rate.

Dietary treatment

Infants

It is difficult to overfeed a breast fed infant, but bottle fed infants can be persuaded to consume a greater volume than they require; in addition feeds can be made more concentrated than recommended or items such as cereal can be added to the bottle [13]. An infant is meant to be plump and naturally has more body fat than at other times in the lifespan; body fat content begins to decline after the first year of life. There is usually no need to restrict an infant's diet, but advice may be needed if feeding practices are inappropriate or a slowing of weight gain is thought to be necessary.

The following advice may be helpful:

(1) Make sure that parents react appropriately to the infant's crying: often crying is perceived as indicating hunger, when the baby is bored, tired or uncomfortable.

(2) Avoid any additions to the infant's bottle (e.g. sugar or cereal).

(3) Make certain that the feed dilution is correct and that the volume is appropriate for age.

(4) Solids should not be introduced before the age of four months.

(5) Weaning solids should have a low energy density (e.g. vegetables and unsweetened fruit).

(6) Skimmed milk can be used in the weaning diet (e.g. low fat yoghurts) in place of whole milk products.

(7) When a greater variety of foods are being consumed (e.g. lean meat, white fish and wholegrain cereals), the quantity of milk should be decreased.

(8) Infants should be introduced to a cup or teacher beaker from about 7–8 months and bottles omitted by one year, since more milk is generally consumed when feeding from a bottle.

(9) Whole cows' milk can be introduced at one year; whilst skimmed and semi-skimmed milk should not normally be used before the ages of five and two years respectively, these lower fat milks are a useful way of decreasing energy intake in the overweight toddler, and can be used from the age of one year. It is important that a supplement of vitamins A and D are given with these milks.

(10) Drinks of water should be offered with and in between meals, Pure unsweetened fruit juice, well diluted, can be given once daily, although if the vitamin C content of the diet is adequate there is no nutritional need for this.

The pre-school child

In the under-fives a strict 'calorie counted' regimen is not usually appropriate. Written advice should be given to the parents on the avoidance of high energy foods (Table 23.1) or on a balanced 'healthy' diet (Table 23.2). It is important that the whole family changes its eating habits and hopefully prevents the pattern of obesity from continuing into later life.

Too much emphasis on diet in front of the child can lead to a feeling of victimization and resentment and he may become very self-conscious about his size. It may be wise to send the child to play during part of the dietetic consultation.

Physical activity should be increased among the less active families: on occasions parents may be seen who still use a pushchair for an overweight child of 3–4 years because he walks too slowly!

Table 23.1 General guidelines for reducing energy intake

1 Avoid fried foods (including chips and crisps), and added fat during cooking
2 Remove visible fat from meat and choose low fat product (e.g. low fat mince, sausages)
3 Use butter and margarine sparingly on bread and crispbread. A low fat spread is preferable. Do not add butter or alternatives to foods (e.g. cooked vegetables)
4 Avoid adding sugar to foods and drinks. An energy-free artificial sweetener (e.g. aspartame) may be used if required
5 Exclude as far as practical chocolate, sweets, cakes and biscuits
6 Give vegetables or salad at each meal
7 Use fruit (fresh, frozen, tinned in natural juice), low-calorie yoghurt and sugar-free jelly in place of desserts
8 Use low energy drinks and squash
9 Use semi-skimmed or skimmed milk (with care in children under five years). Do not exceed 600 ml daily
10 Use low fat cheese in place of full fat; use low fat fromage frais in place of cream
11 Avoid using diabetic foods except fruit squash

Table 23.2 Healthy intake for young children (1–5 years)

Milk – aim to give 300 ml daily, with a maximum of 600 ml. Semi-skimmed or skimmed can be used, provided that a supplement of vitamins A and D are given. Low fat yoghurts, milk puddings, white sauces, low fat hard cheese will all provide calcium if milk is disliked as a drink

Meat, fish, poultry, egg, cheese, beans and lentils – 1 to 2 portions should be given from this group daily. Low fat meats should be used, and meat should be grilled or baked, not fried

Cereal foods: breakfast cereal, wholemeal bread, brown rice, wholegrain pasta and crackers – at least one portion should be included at each meal. Avoid adding extra fat and sugar

Vegetables and fruit – at least four portions daily, raw or cooked

Sample menu

Breakfast	Wholegrain unsweetened cereal, porridge or muesli with milk (no sugar)
	Bread or toast with small amount of spread
	Milk or unsweetened fruit juice
Snack	Plain cracker or piece of fruit
	Water or low calorie squash
Lunch	Roll or bread, filled with tuna, meat, egg, low fat cheese or peanut butter/baked beans on toast
	Chopped salad or cooked vegetables
	Low calorie yoghurt or fruit
Snack	Fruit, raisins or small sandwich
	Water or low calorie squash
Evening meal	Meat, fish, cheese or pulse dish
	Vegetables or salad
	Potatoes, rice or pasta
	Fruit or low energy dessert
Bedtime	Milky drink (unsweetened)

Other advice which may be offered includes the following:

- crisps, sweets, chocolate and sugar should be avoided
- do not give food or sweets to a child as a reward or to console him.

Children over five years

The main aim of the diet must be to re-educate the eating habits of the child. The diet prescribed is based on the current intake, and for a child whose consumption of chocolate, sweets, biscuits, crisps and chips is high, then general guidelines (Table 23.1) are often initially all that is required. The establishment of a sensible eating pattern and regular physical activity should be the goal.

In moderate to severe obesity, a more formal approach is necessary. The reducing diet advised varies and those most frequently used are 800–1500 kcals (3.3–6.3 MJ) daily. Diets of less than 800 kcal are not usually advised. Most school-age children will lose weight on 1000 kcals (4.2 MJ) [14].

The diet constructed needs to be flexible, and provide variety and sufficient food to stop the child pilfering or cheating. If the regimen is too strict the treatment will fail. Parents should be advised that weight loss is greatest in the first few weeks on the diet, but thereafter the rate of weight loss declines. A realistic and achievable target weight should be set at each visit, usually 1–2 kg per month.

High energy foods outlined in Table 23.1 should be avoided. Foods such as fruit, vegetables and whole grain cereals and bread should be encouraged. Many children unfortunately refuse to eat vegetables and fruit and parents may need advice on different forms of presentation. Home-made vegetable soup or vegetables incorporated into pasta sauce or casserole dishes may be more acceptable than plain vegetables; often one or two vegetables such as peas, sweetcorn kernels or tinned tomatoes will be eaten, and maximum use should be made of these.

There are also a wide range of sugar-free and low energy products such as low calorie yoghurts, sugar-free jellies and low calorie soups which provide variety in the diet.

It is important to ensure normal growth occurs when dietary intake is restricted. Adequate quantities of protein, vitamins and minerals should be taken; some children who dislike certain foods and do not consume a nutritionally adequate diet may need a supplement of vitamins or minerals (particularly iron and calcium). A reducing diet should provide at least 60% of the theoretical EAR for the child's age [15].

Written information in the form of a diet sheet, a list of unrestricted foods and a list of foods allowed should be given to the parents and child (Tables 23.3 and 23.4).

The question of school dinners should be addressed. Many overweight children regularly consume chips and pastry items for lunch at school. Fruit and low calorie yoghurt can replace desserts and the child should be advised to avoid second helpings. However the use of a 'treat' on a weekly or daily basis if necessary can help the child psychologically and pro-

vide motivation. It is easier to provide suitable food in the form of a packed lunch, although a certain amount of 'swapping' of items often takes place.

The suggestion that money previously spent on sweets, chocolate etc. can be used for other items of the child's choice (e.g. games, books, clothing) is sometimes useful, particularly for indulgent grandparents.

Social eating

Eating out is usually a pleasurable activity and with a little planning and forethought this should still be possible on a reducing diet. An invitation to tea with friends should not be turned down because of the diet, since a suitable choice of foods can usually be arranged.

For birthday parties pastries, crisps and chocolate can be replaced with sandwiches, vegetable and fruit cocktail sticks, sugar-free jellies and unsweetened fruit. Low calorie drinks can be used for all. Prizes for games can be toys, notebooks, pencils, crayons, novelties in place of sweets.

Table 23.4 Low energy foods allowed freely

Vegetables

All green varieties and salads	Courgettes	Peas
Brussel sprouts	Celery	Peppers
French beans	Fennel	Swede
Runner beans	Leeks	Turnip
Cauliflower	Mushrooms	Tomato
	Onions	

Fruit

Bilberries	Gooseberries	Raspberries
Blackberries	Grapefruit	Redcurrants
Blackcurrants	Lemon	Rhubarb
Cranberries	Loganberries	Strawberries

Miscellaneous

Artificial sweeteners e.g. saccharin, Nutrasweet	Mineral and soda water
Coffee	Sugar-free drinks
Tea	Sugar-free jelly and chewing gum
Herbs	Stock cubes
Spices	
Seasonings	
Vinegar	

Table 23.3 Reducing diets

Meals should be chosen from the following foods

Lean meat	Vegetables	Fruit
Poultry	All varieties of	All varieties, fresh, frozen,
Fish	vegetables and salads	stewed without sugar,
Eggs		tinned in natural juice
Cheese		
Pulses		

Drinks
Low calorie squash and carbonated drinks
Mineral and soda water
Coffee, tea without sugar

Daily allowances
300–600 ml milk
30 g Margarine or butter
... slices of bread or equivalent exchanges depending on energy content of diet

Exchanges for 1 slice of bread: 70 kcal (290 kJ) approximately

1 potato – baked, boiled or mashed
or 1 tablespoon boiled rice/spaghetti
or 3 tablespoons unsweetened breakfast cereal
or 1 Weetabix
or 2 Crispbreads
or 2 Crackers/large water biscuits
or 1 Digestive biscuit/2 Rich tea

Adolescents

This group presents the dietitian with the greatest challenge. The dietary prescription will depend on age and sex, with teenage boys requiring more energy generally than girls. Peer group pressure for consumption of snack foods is high and suggestions for alternative lower energy items is necessary. Adolescent girls may be at risk of developing anorexia nervosa or bulimia, and an awareness of this is vital.

In general slimming foods and drinks as a replacement for a meal are not appropriate, as they generally contain insufficient protein, minerals and micronutrients to meet the high requirements for this age group. Very low calorie diets (around 400–600 kcal) are specifically contraindicated.

Increasing energy expenditure

Increased physical activity on a regular basis should be encouraged in conjunction with the diet. Studies have shown that subjects treated with diet and exercise programmes continued to lose weight for longer than children treated by diet alone in the follow-up period [16,17].

Physical exercise usually promotes a feeling of well-being and, in addition, will keep the child/teenager occupied and avoid boredom. Walking, swimming and jogging are useful activities for those who dislike team games or who are embarrassed by their appearance.

Whatever the cause of obesity, successful treatment demands a sustained commitment and effort from the whole family and the dietitian must endeavour to maintain a positive attitude and motivation towards weight control.

PRADER-WILLI SYNDROME

Prader-Willi syndrome (PWS) is a rare congenital disorder, the main characteristics of which are hypotonia, short stature, hypogonadism, a degree of mental retardation and an insatiable appetite leading to gross obesity if not controlled. Behavioural problems are encountered most often during adolescence [18] which add to the difficulties of treatment. The prevalence has been estimated at 1 in 25 000 births [19] making PWS the most common syndromal cause of obesity.

At birth infants present with hypotonia and feeding

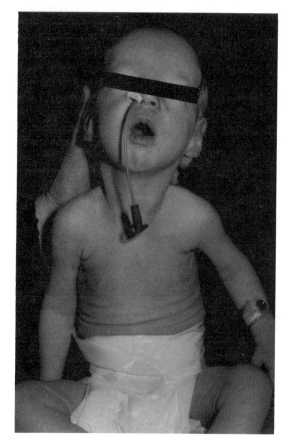

Fig. 23.1 Infant with Prader-Willi syndrome

difficulties and subsequently fail to thrive (Fig. 23.1). Tube feeding may be required during this period. Parents should be made aware of the two phases which are characteristic of the syndrome, namely from birth to approximately two years of age when weight gain is poor and from two to three years onwards when weight is likely to escalate. It is important that dietary intervention and advice is given at the onset of weight gain in order that excessive weight gain is curtailed. Consistent dietary advice from all professionals must be given to parents and carers and the need to adhere to this explained. This can prove very difficult because of the hyperphagia. Gross obesity often occurs during adolescence (Fig. 23.2) but can be controlled with comprehensive management. Crnic *et al.* believe that maintenance of a lower body weight will improve intellectual performance [20].

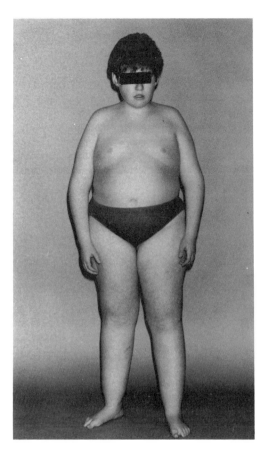

Fig. 23.2 Adolescent with Prader-Willi syndrome (same boy as in Fig. 23.1). With kind permission of Dr JK Brown

Dietary treatment

The child with PWS requires a considerably lower energy intake than his normal peers. In order to achieve weight loss, energy intake must be 50% or less than expected for age (Table 1.2). Attempts should be made to check any potential sources of food (e.g. from neighbours or friends).

Much encouragement is required, but weight loss can be achieved with great vigilance. Weight should be monitored at monthly or three-monthly intervals.

The diet presents great difficulty for the child, family, carers and school, due to the insatiable appetite; food is uppermost in the thoughts of most people with PWS. Bray *et al.* found that, when food was unrestricted, six of their adolescent patients consumed a daily average of 5167 ± 503 kcal (21.7 ±

2.1 MJ). Foraging for food is common and parents should be advised to lock the kitchen, cupboards and refrigerator. Many children get up during the night to eat and inappropriate foods such as bread for the birds or dog and cat foods are commonly eaten. Interestingly, however unsuitable the foods are that may be eaten, stomach upsets are rare.

Dietitians must be aware that medical and other health workers may not have encountered PWS previously and may lack the understanding necessary to give proper support to the family. Communication with other health professionals is essential to avoid misunderstanding.

Some activities are physically difficult for the PWS child due to poor muscle strength; however walking and swimming can be accomplished by most and should be encouraged to increase energy expenditure. Contrary to some views it has been shown that during exercise individuals with PWS require as much energy as others with simple obesity for the same level of work [21].

Multidisciplinary management, which includes dietary advice, behaviour modification and family support is advocated as an effective form of treatment [22]. A parents' self-help group exists, which parents may find helpful and supportive.

REFERENCES

1 Taitz LS *Textbook of Paediatric Nutrition*, 3e. Edinburgh: Churchill Livingstone, 1991: 485.
2 Wilkinson PW *et al.* Obesity in childhood: a community study in Newcastle upon Tyne. *Lancet*, 1977, **i** 350–352.
3 Stark O *et al.* Longitudinal study of obesity in the National Survey of Health and Development. *Brit Med J*, 1981, **283** 13–17.
4 Borjeson M The aetiology of obesity in children: A study of 101 twin pairs. *Acta Paediatr Scand*, 1976, **65** 279–287.
5 Stunkard AJ *et al.* An adoption study of human obesity. *New Eng J Med*, 1986, **314** 193–198.
6 Garn SM, Clark DC Trends in fatness and the origins of obesity. *Paediatrics*, 1976, **57**(4) 443–456.
7 Mossberg HO 40-year follow-up of overweight children. *Lancet*, 1989, **ii** 491–493.
8 Olsen L *Food Fight; A Report on Teenage Eating Habits and Nutritional Status*. San Francisco: Citizens Policy Centre, 1982: 124.
9 Young EA *et al.* Fast foods update: nutrient analysis. *Ross Laboratories Dietetic Currents*, 1986, **13**(6).
10 Durnin JV Physical activity by adolescents. *Acta Paediatr Scand*, 1971, **217**(Suppl) 133–135.

11 Tanner JM, Whitehouse RH Revised standards for triceps and subscapular skinfolds in British children. *Arch Dis Childh*, 1975, **50** 142–145.

12 Keiller SM, Colley JRT, Carpenter RG Obesity in school children and their parents. *Annal Hum Biol*, 1979, **6** 443–455.

13 Taitz LS *The Obese Child*. Oxford: Blackwell Scientific Publications, 1983.

14 Brooke OG, Abernethy E Obesity in children. *Hum Nutr: Appl Nutr*, 1985, **39a**(4) 304–314.

15 Bentley D, Lawson M *Clinical Nutrition in Paediatric Disorders*. London: Bailliere Tindall, 1988: 191.

16 Epstein LH *et al.* Effect of diet and controlled exercise on weight loss in obese children. *J Paediatr*, 1985, **107** 358–361.

17 Reybrouck T *et al.* Exercise therapy and hypocaloric diet in the treatment of obese children and adolescents. *Acta Paediatr Scand*, 1990, **79** 84–89.

18 Whitman BY, Accardo P Emotional symptoms in Prader-Willi syndrome adolescents. *Am J Med Genetics*, 1987, **28** 897–905.

19 Bray GA *et al.* The Prader-Willi syndrome: a study of 40 patients and a review of the literature. *Medicine*, 1983, **62** 59–80.

20 Crnic KA *et al.* Preventing mental retardation associated with gross obesity in the Prader-Willi syndrome. *Paediatrics*, 1980, **66** 787–789.

21 Holm VA, Pipes PL Food and children with Prader-Willi syndrome. *Am J Dis Childh*, 1976, **130** 1063–1067.

22 Wodarski LA, Bundschuh E, Forbus WR Interdisciplinary case management: a model for intervention. *J Am Diet Assoc*, 1988, **88**(3) 332–335.

USEFUL ADDRESS

Prader-Willi Syndrome Association (UK)
30 Follett Drive, Abbots Langley, Herts WD5 0LP.

Other Conditions Requiring Nutritional Support and Advice

CHAPTER 24

Epidermolysis Bullosa

INTRODUCTION

Epidermolysis bullosa (EB), comprises a rare group of inherited skin blistering disorders which are characterized by extreme fragility of the skin and mucous membranes and recurrent blister formation.

Broadly speaking, EB falls into 3 main types: junctional (lethal and non-lethal), dystrophic and simplex – depending on the site of cleavage of the epidermal layers within the skin. At least 16 subtypes of EB have also been identified. Diagnosis is made by electron microscopy of a skin biopsy or antigen mapping by immunofluorescence [1]. Nutritional problems occur mainly, but not exclusively, in lethal and non-lethal junctional EB (JEB), recessive dystrophic EB (RDEB) and the Dowling-Meara subtype of simplex EB.

The different forms of EB are caused by a variety of structural defects in the skin which allow separation of the layers, resulting in blistering and ulceration. Blisters (bullae) may be present at birth or occur soon after, spontaneously and as a result of mechanical trauma. The structure of the skin is such that blister margins spread indefinitely if they are not burst as soon as they are detected. To minimize the area of the resultant raw lesion, carers are taught to burst blisters, usually with a sterile needle. Dressings are applied to damaged areas of skin and to areas vulnerable to knocks and self-inflicted damage. In RDEB especially, prolonged and recurrent blisters with subsequent scarring lead to tautness of the healed skin known as a contracture. This is most disabling when it occurs at joints causing walking difficulties, and when fingers become fused making self-feeding difficult. Specialized surgery is available to separate the fingers. Contractures in the mouth can severely limit mouth opening and immobilize the tongue. Scarring in the oesophagus leads to strictures, and in the anus to fissuring and extremely painful defecation. The de-velopment of skin or mucous membrane malignancy is a complication of severe adulthood RDEB: the tumours metastasize readily and the prognosis is poor.

In simplex EB other than the Dowling-Meara subtype, affected skin is generally confined to hands and feet, with no oral, oesophageal or anal involvement. Some of these patients become overweight because their physical activity is limited, especially in hot weather when the feet can become extremely sore leading the sufferer to depend on a wheelchair for mobility.

Lethal JEB is usually, but not always, fatal within the first year of life, sufferers frequently succumbing to overwhelming infection and acute laryngeal obstruction [2]. Non-lethal JEB patients experience similar skin problems to those of RDEB sufferers, but tend not to experience the oral, laryngeal and oesophageal complications to the same degree.

The exact incidence of EB is unknown and difficult to assess. This is due to the rarity of the condition and the fact that mild cases may go undiagnosed, whilst the severely affected may die before a skin biopsy can confirm the diagnosis. There are an estimated 2500 sufferers of all types in the United Kingdom. EB affects the sexes equally and occurs in all races. Mental development is normal. Prenatal diagnosis, by means of a fetal skin biopsy, is available to mothers who have previously given birth to a DEB or JEB baby. The earliest stage at which this can currently be undertaken is 15 weeks gestation.

The main factors leading to malnutrition and growth failure in severe EB are:

The hypercatabolic state induced by open skin lesions with blood and plasma loss, increased protein turnover, heat loss and frequent infections. As in the burns patient, energy needs reflect the severity of skin lesions [3] and this also seems likely to be the case for protein.

Reduced nutrient intake through oral, oesophageal and gastrointestinal complications, dental disease and hand deformities. Oral problems include fixed tongue and small mouth opening (due to contracted scar tissue tethering the tongue and preventing effective chewing) leading to painful, tiring and tedious eating. Oesophageal strictures and anal fissures demonstrate gastrointestinal involvement. Some RDEB sufferers experience periods when they are unable to swallow even their own saliva, and require hospitalization for rehydration. Chronic constipation and painful defecation are extremely common and (see later section) frequently cause apathy and secondary anorexia. Recent studies have demonstrated inadequate dietary intakes and abnormal haematological and biochemical findings [3,4]. There is no consensus amongst experts as to whether the intestinal mucosa is affected in some types of EB. Some consider the abnormality to be confined to stratified epithelium, i.e. skin, mucous membranes, oesophagus, bronchus and anus [5]. Others suggest that gastrointestinal tract lined by columnar epithelium may also be affected [6]. Dental disease is likely in EB children because of their high sucrose intake (see later section) and the difficulties experienced in carrying out dental hygiene routines.

These interactions between causes and effects of nutritional problems in EB are illustrated in Fig. 24.1.

The tendency to develop skin lesions may decrease in teenage and adulthood. Although some DEB patients report an improvement in dysphagia during adult life, many children and adults can tolerate only puréed food and liquids.

Until relatively recently, malnutrition and growth retardation were regarded as inevitable consequences of the severe forms of EB. However, research suggests that optimizing nutrition from birth along with regular nutritional assessment and appropriate intervention can significantly improve growth. Accelerated wound healing, decreased susceptibility to infection and an enhanced feeling of wellbeing are further likely consequences of improved nutrition. The value of early nutritional intervention, better skin care (prevention of infection, dressings, topical treatments), physiotherapy and dental care has yet to be appraised, but it is hoped that a multidisciplinary approach will lead to reduced impact of complications. However, the aetiology of the condition is such that these are inevitable to some extent, and some forms of EB are amongst the most physically disabling and disfiguring of all diseases. Despite a claim that EB can be cured by a complicated exclusion diet combined with topical and systemic treatments, this was not borne out in an open study to evaluate the regime [7]. Nevertheless,

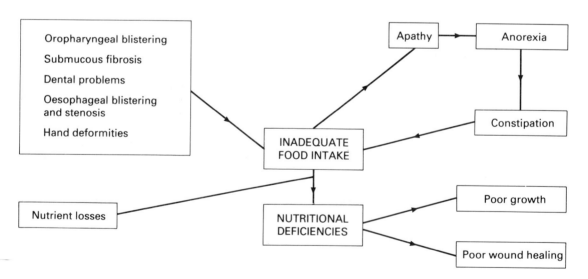

Fig. 24.1 Interactions between causes and effects of epidermolysis bullosa (EB). After Allman 1990

the holistic nature of this approach warrants consideration [8].

Nutritional requirements

Sufferers with widespread areas denuded of skin appear to require up to 150% of the estimated average requirement (EAR) for energy and as much as 200% of the reference nutrient intake (RNI) for protein in order to grow normally, and to permit the healing of skin lesions. Supplementary vitamins, iron and zinc are generally also indicated to a similar degree.

Assessment of growth

Measurement of weight and height velocity is the most practical means of assessing growth. Babies' weights (ideally nude) should be recorded on alternate days whilst a feeding routine is established in hospital. This can be reduced to once weekly and then less frequently once the baby is discharged. Values should be plotted on a growth chart so that any 'fall-off' can be detected early and appropriate measures taken to modify the feeds accordingly.

Older children should be weighed and measured 3–6 monthly, preferably on the same scales each time, and ideally by the same dietitian so that a rapport can be established between them.

Since within a given type of EB, severity of the disease and associated complications can vary widely, the information which follows in this chapter is mainly arranged under headings of age and requirements for specific nutrients, rather than EB type.

BABIES

Energy requirements appear to range between 130 and 180 kcal/kg actual body weight/24 hours (115–150% EAR), protein requirements between 2.5 g and 4 g/kg, (115–200% RNI), and fluid requirements from 150–200 ml/kg. Babies with extensive blistering lose significant amounts of fluid from these open areas and may require correspondingly larger volumes of feeds.

Breast feeding an EB baby is possible and, if it permits normal weight gain, should be encouraged for the many benefits it confers [9]. Blistering of the baby's tongue and mouth should not be the main deciding factor in whether or not to breast feed. Oral blisters usually burst during suckling (those which do not should be burst with a sterile needle) and upset babies far less than than their mothers. Babies should be allowed to suckle on demand.

For all but mild cases of EB, however, breast feeds alone frequently fail to satisfy increased requirements, demonstrated by failure to gain weight. As soon as possible, measures should be taken to provide a fortified feed, (see also section on babies with lethal junctional EB). There are several ways in which this can be done (see Tables 1.9 and 1.10).

If facilities permit, the mother's own expressed breast milk (EBM) can be fortified with a proprietary whey-based powdered infant formula e.g. Premium at a rate of 5 g per 100 ml. A glucose polymer such as Caloreen can also be added at a rate of 2–5 g per 100 ml to increase further the energy content. Because of the small quantities of additions involved, fortifying EBM in this way may be practical only if a reasonable volume of milk can be treated each time.

Formula feeding

A 'low birthweight formula' babymilk, e.g. SMA Low Birthweight Formula can be used in hospital to 'top-up' or replace breast milk. This can be fortified with glucose polymer to a total carbohydrate content of 10–12 g per 100 ml. It should be noted that low birthweight formulas available in the community have a lower energy content than those supplied to hospitals.

A powdered whey-based infant formula can be made up in a 15% or even 17% dilution. Extra energy can be added as a glucose polymer as above, and as a fat emulsion (e.g. Calogen).

Supplementing or concentrating the feed as suggested above is done as a therapeutic measure. This must be explained to parents and community medical and nursing personnel to avoid misunderstandings and conflicting advice. The baby's growth and the adequacy of the feed should be reviewed regularly.

Bottle fed babies with a sore mouth or tongue may benefit from having the hole in the teat enlarged with a sterile needle. Sucking may be easier from a specialized teat such as an orthodontic teat by Milupa [Hillingdon, UK] or one of the several fast-flow teats on the market. Silicon teats tend to be favoured for their softness. Babies who cannot suck from a teat may need to be fed from a spoon or dropper.

Nasogastric feeding is best avoided because of trauma to the nasopharynx whilst passing the tube and whilst the tube is *in situ*. If a tube is used, it should be as soft and of as narrow a gauge as possible, e.g. Silk enteral feeding tube, 6 French gauge (2.1 mm), [E. Merck, Alton, UK] and it should not be resited at every feed but left in place. Tubes must never be fixed to the baby's skin with sticky tape, because skin will be removed with the tape. It is possible to keep tubing in place with non-adhesive dressings such as Tubifast [Seton, Oldham, UK]. The tube can be secured by winding it around a length of Tubifast where the tube enters the nostril. The ends of the dressing are then tied together behind the head. Alternatively, Tubifast can be fashioned over the face 'Balaclava-style', with the feeding tube secured to the inside of this, out of the baby's reach. If a long term feeding problem seems likely, insertion of a gastrostomy should be considered (see later). Dummies are discouraged because of their tendency to cause blistering of the lips, tongue and soft palate.

Constipation

Chronic constipation with painful defecation can occur in all types of EB and is especially common in RDEB. The passing of even a moderately bulky stool can tear the delicate skin around the anus causing fissuring and extreme pain with subsequent bowel movements. It should be treated without delay if a vicious cycle (Fig. 24.1) of pain, conscious witholding of the stool and anorexia is to be avoided [9].

Constipation seems more common after weaning than before, when it may be a consequence of a reduced fluid intake (see later section on older children). Extra fluid should be offered in the form of water, or if this is refused, one teaspoon of fresh fruit juice diluted in 100 ml water or ready-to-feed baby juice diluted with an equal volume of water. If these measures fail to provide relief, one teaspoon of sugar should be added to feeds for several days. A prophylactic dose of lactulose may be required as a preventive measure, even after a wholegrain breakfast cereal, fruit and vegetables have been introduced.

Vitamins and minerals

Vitamins

Babies who thrive on breast milk or normally reconstituted formula feeds tend to be those with minimal skin lesions, and their requirements for vitamins are unlikely to be greater than those of normal babies. As a safeguard though, they should receive five drops daily of Mother's and Children's Vitamin Drops A, D and C (Hough, Manchester, UK) [10]. More severely affected infants are very likely to require increased amounts of all vitamins [4,11] especially vitamin C, whose roles in enhancing iron absorption [12,13] and in collagen synthesis [14] are recognized.

Research has yet to establish the extent to which vitamins should be supplemented, so approximately 150–200% of the RNI is recommended. Babies taking feeds containing an increased concentration of babymilk powder will be receiving correspondingly increased amounts of all nutrients, possibly nearing 150% RNI if large volumes are consumed. If a satisfactory intake is in doubt, a comprehensive preparation such as Ketovite Liquid and Tablets (Paines & Byrne, Greenford, UK) should be prescribed. Ketovite tablets can be crushed, mixed with a small amount of feed or water and given from a syringe or spoon. If this is not tolerated, a liquid preparation such as Abidec drops (Warner Lambert, Eastleigh, UK) can be used, although this will not provide a complete range of vitamins. These preparations should be given at the normal recommended dose for age unless intake from other sources is substantial. When considering vitamin D intake, even fortified feeds may barely meet the normal RNI and it should be remembered that the skin of these babies may be largely covered with dressings and therefore rarely exposed to sunlight.

Iron

Despite blood loss from open skin lesions and the upper gastrointestinal tract, iron deficiency anaemia may not occur under six months in babies who were full term, presumably because of good iron stores at birth and an adequate intake of iron and associated nutrients from fortified babymilk and weaning foods. Unless it is indicated biochemically, i.e. by reduced haemoglobin, mean corpuscular volume (MCV) and ferritin, and elevated total iron binding capacity (TIBC), it is our practice not to give routine supplementary iron under six months because of its apparent tendency to cause or aggravate constipation (see later section) and the possibility that it may interfere with zinc absorption [15,16]. If extra iron is indicated, a liquid form is preferable, for example Sytron [Parke-Davis Medical, Eastleigh, UK] 1–5 ml daily, in two divided doses (5.5–27.5 mg iron). There is evidence from animal studies [17] that iron absorption is enhanced when administered on alternate days (see below). There may also be a reduced incidence of undesirable side effects, including constipation or gastric irritation.

Zinc

Zinc has important roles in wound healing, growth and immunocompetence [18]. Zinc supplementation is usually considered necessary in babies with severe blistering, on the basis of inadequate oral intake or reduced serum zinc concentration. It is best given as 5–10 ml zinc sulphate solution (30 mg zinc in 5 ml).

Where both zinc and iron supplementation is indicated, it may be beneficial to give one supplement on one day and the other on the next. This may aid absorption [17], reduce the constipating effect of iron and reduce competition for absorption between zinc and copper [19].

Babies with lethal junctional EB

The prognosis for this type of EB is extremely poor, death usually occurring within the first year of life, and often within weeks of birth. Weight gain may initially take place on breast or normally reconstituted infant feeds, but almost invariably gives way to failure to thrive, as new areas of skin become denuded, infection sets in and respiration becomes more difficult. Nutritional intervention (as outlined above), should be offered as a means of enhancing the quality, rather than the quantity, of life. Mothers who have established breast feeding and wish to continue should be encouraged to do so even if weight gain is poor, as this is one of the few positive things they can do for a terminally ill baby. From the point of view of nutritional management parents, medical and nursing staff should be discouraged from weighing the baby, as the disappointing result only adds to an already very distressing situation. However, since pain relief is an important aspect of terminal care, the baby may need to be weighed before the best regimen can be agreed.

Weaning

Severely affected EB sufferers should receive a fortified, modified infant formula until at least one year of age. A 'follow-on' formula or a paediatric enteral feed may be appropriate after one year. Solids should be introduced at the same time as for normal babies, i.e. 4–6 months. Weaning foods of a suitable texture for normal babies are usually suitable for EB babies. However, extra care should be taken to ensure that sharp items such as hard rusks or crisp crusts are not given as these may damage the mouth and gums. Parents should be advised regarding ways of increasing the protein and energy values of the diet, without increasing its bulk. For example if the baby is receiving a supplemented milk, this should be used to mix with dried baby food and rusks instead of cows' milk. (see *Nutrition for Babies with Dystrophic Epidermolysis Bullosa*, DEBRA publication). There is, as yet, no evidence to suggest that long term adherence to a liquid or puréed diet necessarily influences the course of dysphagia and oesophageal stricture, and failure to encourage chewing may impair speech development. However, babies who demonstrate swallowing problems from early on may be best to remain indefinitely on foods of a very soft consistency.

THE OVER ONES

Assessment and advice

A dietary assessment usually reveals that a child with oral and oesophageal complications seldom achieves even the EAR for most nutrients using normal foods. Some RDEB sufferers experience periods of severe dysphagia. Liquidised foods, unless large volumes are consumed, tend to be low in all nutrients.

Advice, in the first instance, should aim to improve the nutritional value of the child's normal food intake, where this is practical (see *Diet for Epidermolysis Bullosa – for Children over 1 Year*, DEBRA publication). Skin care and dressing changes can take up to four hours each day, so dietary modifications must be realistic and not overly time consuming. The emphasis should be on increased protein and energy intakes, with improvements in vitamin and mineral intakes as indicated by dietary assessment and haematological and biochemical indices. In practice, milk often figures prominently in the diets of EB children, and protein and calcium intakes are generally satisfactory. On the other hand, the intakes of those who dislike milk and who have difficulties chewing and swallowing meat invariably fall below the normal RNI.

Many EB children are unable to consume adequate quantities of normal foods and must rely heavily on multinutrient supplements such as Build-Up, Fresubin and Fortisip to make up the deficit. In the UK, the Advisory Committee on Borderline Substances (ACBS) authorizes the prescription of many of these products in cases of dysphagia. Glucose polymers and fat emulsions are not routinely used, but are useful for the child who requires an increase in energy intake only. These are not prescribable in EB, but most general practitioners are willing to do so. Children consuming multinutrient supplements on a regular basis will generally receive extra vitamins from these. This should be taken into consideration before a further vitamin supplement is prescribed. Those with EB of anything more than the mildest degree should receive extra vitamins [4] e.g. 150–200% of the RNI for age (see section on vitamins).

Older EB children whose nutritional status has been compromised by the condition can be sceptical of the potential value of nutritional intervention (as can their medical/surgical advisors!) and need considerable support and frequent reinforcement if they are to persevere with recommended dietary modifications and supplements.

Anaemia

Low plasma iron levels have been demonstrated in RDEB patients [11] and JEB patients [20]. Iron deficiency anaemia is common and ideally iron status should be checked six monthly or at least annually. The results of Allman *et al.* [4] showed that the usual pattern is a combination of low haemoglobin, low serum iron and a normal to raised TIBC. They suggest that this implies an iron deficiency anaemia combined with 'the anemia of chronic disorders' [21], which is unlikely to respond to iron supplementation alone. Other aspects of management such as optimal skin care, improved general nutrition and treatment of infection must also be addressed. Supplementary iron can be prescribed as a liquid preparation, e.g. Sytron 5 ml twice daily (27.5–55 mg). A modified-release preparation, e.g. Feospan [Smith Kline & French, Welwyn Garden City, UK], may be prescribed (one capsule contains 47 mg iron) although the therapeutic advantage of such preparations is controversial [22].

As previously mentioned, administration of iron on alternate days may be beneficial.

Biochemical and haematological estimations

In the absence of hard data regarding the requirements of EB patients, laboratory monitoring should be undertaken in addition to measurement of height and weight velocities. Ideally, the investigations detailed in Table 24.1 should be carried out six monthly or annually, depending on the age and condition of the patient.

Dental caries and sugar consumption

The oral complications of JEB and RDEB such as small mouth opening and tongue fixation due to the accumulation of scar tissue, often make it impossible to clean the teeth either by tongue or toothbrush. Enamel dysplasia seems to occur more frequently in these two groups of patients than in the dominant dystrophic and simplex forms [23]. The oral mucosa of many patients is too delicate to allow the use of a normal brush. Plaque collects around the teeth, leading to chronic marginal gingivitis. The removal of badly decayed teeth from a mouth with very poor opening may be extremely difficult even under general anaesthesia and may result in increased oral ulceration and scarring [24].

A diet sufficiently high in energy to permit normal growth in EB generally necessitates the ingestion of considerable quantities of fermentable carbohydrate, especially sucrose, at regular intervals throughout the day. The frequent consumption of such foods, especially in the presence of the complications noted

Table 24.1 Nutritional monitoring in epidermolysis bullosa (EB)

Plasma calcium and phosphate	Haemoglobin
Plasma amino acid profile	Serum iron and ferritin
Serum albumin and total protein	Total iron binding capacity (TIBC)
Plasma alkaline phosphatase	Serum folate
Plasma urea	Red cell folate
Serum immunoglobulins	Erythrocyte sedimentation rate (ESR)
Serum zinc, copper and	Reticulocytes
selenium	Mean corpuscular volume (MCV)
Free erythrocyte protoporphyrin (FEP)	

above, is conducive to the development of dental caries.

This apparent conflict of interests between dietitian and dentist can lead to contradictory advice to the child and his carers. However, compromise is possible, and families must be taught from early on of the importance of oral hygiene, initially using moistened cotton buds, and later a soft-bristled toothbrush or sponge-tipped stick, in conjunction with a recommended plaque-inhibiting mouthwash. Appropriate mouth and tongue exercises should be encouraged to reduce immobility (see *A Guideline to Physiotherapy for Parents of Children with Dystrophic Epidermolysis Bullosa*, DEBRA publication). Sticky sweets and chocolate biscuits should ideally be restricted to the end of mealtimes and continuous sipping of sugary drinks outside mealtimes discouraged.

Constipation

Chronic constipation is one of the most frequent yet underestimated complications of EB, especially RDEB [25]. The situation appears to arise as a result of painful anal fissuring provoked by the disease, leading to fear of defecation and the gradual accumulation of faeces. The use of stool softeners and laxatives is largely unsuccessful [26]. At best they result in overflow and faecal soiling, leaving the problem of faecal impaction unresolved. Many EB sufferers mistake overflow for diarrhoea and reduce their laxative therapy, thereby unwittingly worsening the problem.

A vicious cycle involving deliberate ignoring of the gastrocolonic reflex and anorexia is rapidly established [4,9], and can have a devastating effect on appetite and on general quality of life. It is unrealistic to expect severely affected patients to consume a diet sufficiently high in non-starch polysaccharides to alleviate their constipation because of their oral problems, dysphagia and requirement for a low bulk, nutrient-dense intake.

Substantial relief of the problem can be achieved using a liquid fibre-containing supplement such as Enrich. Children with faecal impaction or megarectum demonstrated by abdominal x-ray should have their bowel emptied by a bowel-prep solution such as Klean-Prep [Norgine, Oxford, UK], before the introduction of Enrich, in order that the feed has the best chance of taking effect quickly and so encouraging future compliance; 500–750 ml Enrich daily is usually required to maintain comfortable and regular defecation and patients should be warned that 2–6 weeks may elapse before a regular bowel habit is established [26].

ALTERNATIVE FEEDING TECHNIQUES

The numerous complications of severely affected EB sufferers may preclude their ever achieving a nutritional intake sufficient to avoid malnutrition and support normal growth. More invasive feeding techniques are indicated [4].

Nasogastric feeding

This is generally contraindicated for the reasons cited in the earlier section describing baby feeding. Equally importantly, in a condition which already attracts stares and questions from strangers, many older EB children are understandably unwilling to have a nasogastric tube *in situ*.

Gastrostomy feeding

A number of RDEB patients have received gastrostomies, through which they are fed nocturnally over 8–10 hours, using a pump. Although the 'button' gastrostomy is aesthetically superior to the conventional type, we have experienced problems such as slight leakage around the entry site. This has been reported in other centres and tends to be only a short term problem. The leakage may be due to our not providing these children with a conventional-style gastrostomy in the first instance, until a channel is established in the abdominal wall. Supplying nutrition by gastrostomy appears to be an extremely promising method of establishing increased growth velocities. Equally importantly, from the parents' point of view, it has lifted the seemingly impossible burden of nourishing the child adequately. Patients should be encouraged to sit at the table for meals with their families, eating what normal foods they can, and receive the bulk of their nutrition overnight.

Oesophageal dilatation

We strongly advise against routine oesophageal dilatation as a treatment for dysphagia. It is an extremely hazardous procedure to undertake in EB, and the often short term benefits do not justify the considerable mortality risks [27,28]. Colonic interposition is also contraindicated [27].

REFERENCES

1 Eady RAJ The classification of Epidermolysis Bullosa. In: Priestley GC *et al*. (eds.) *Epidermolysis Bullosa: A Comprehensive Review of Classification, Management and Laboratory Studies*. Berkshire: Dystrophic Epidermolysis Bullosa Research Association (DEBRA), 1990.
2 Davies H, Atherton DJ Acute laryngeal obstruction in junctional epidermolysis bullosa. *Pediatr Dermatol*, 1987, 4(2) 98–101.
3 Lechner-Gruskay D *et al*. Nutritional and metabolic profile of children with epidermolysis bullosa. *Pediatr Dermatol*, 1988, 5(1) 22–27.
4 Allman SM *et al*. Nutrition in dystrophic epidermolysis bullosa. *Pediatr Dermatol*, 1992, 9(3) 231–238.
5 Orlando RC *et al*. Epidermolysis bullosa: gastrointestinal manifestations. *Ann Int Med*, 1974, 81 203–206.
6 Sehgal VN *et al*. Dystrophic epidermolysis bullosa. Interesting gastrointestinal manifestations. *Brit J Dermatol*, 1977, 96 389–391.
7 Haber RM, Ramsay CA, Boxall LBH Epidermolysis bullosa. Assessment of a treatment regimen. *Int J Derm*, 1985, 24 324–328.
8 Atherton DJ The Pavel Kozak Institute – reflections of a visiting paediatric dermatologist. An article written for DEBRA members, 1987.
9 Clayden GS Dysphagia and constipation in epidermolysis bullosa. In: Priestley GC *et al*. (eds.) *Epidermolysis Bullosa: A Comprehensive Review of Classification, Management and Laboratory Studies*. Berkshire: DEBRA, 1990: 67–71.
10 Department of Health and Social Security Report on Health and Social Subjects No 32. *Present Day Practice in Infant Feeding*. London: HMSO, 1988.
11 Fine JD, Tamura T, Johnson L Blood vitamin and trace metal levels in epidermolysis bullosa. *Arch Dermatol*, 1989, 125 374–379.
12 Bothwell TH *et al*. *Iron Metabolism in Man*. Oxford: Blackwell Scientific Publications, 1979: 431.
13 Seshadri A, Shah A, Bhade S Haematological response of anaemic preschool children to ascorbic acid supplementation. *Hum Nutr: Appl Nutr*, 1985, 39A 151–154.
14 Levene CI, Bates CJ Ascorbic acid and collagen synthesis in cultured fibroblasts. *Ann NY Acad Sci*, 1975, 258 288–305.
15 Meadows NJ *et al*. Iron supplementation impairs oral bioavailability of zinc. *Gut*, 1982, 23 A438.
16 Solomons NW, Jacob RA Studies on the bioavailablity of zinc in humans: effects of heme and non-heme iron on the absorption of zinc. *Amer J Clin Nutr*, 1981, 34 475–482.
17 Wright AJA, Southon S The effectiveness of various iron-supplementation regimens in improving the Fe status of anaemic rats. *Brit J Nutr*, 1990, 63 579–585.
18 Halstead JA Zinc deficiency in man, the Shiraz experiment. *Amer J Med*, 1972, 53 277–284.
19 Prasad AS *et al*. Hypocupricaemia induced by zinc therapy in adults. *J Amer Med Ass*, 1978, 240 2166–2168.
20 Hruby MA, Esterley NB Anemia in epidermolysis bullosa letalis. *Amer J Dis Childh*, 1973, 125 696–699.
21 Cartwright GE The anemia of chronic disorders. *Seminars in Hematology*, 1966, 3 351–375.
22 Hann IM Personal communication, 1992.
23 Nowack AJ Oropharyngeal lesions and their management in epidermolysis bullosa. *Arch Dermatol*, 1988, 124 742–745.
24 Winter GB Dental problems in epidermolysis bullosa. In: Priestley GC *et al*. (eds.) *Epidermolysis Bullosa: A Comprehensive Review of Classification, Management and Laboratory Studies*. Berkshire: DEBRA, 1990.
25 Atherton DJ Management of dystrophic epidermolysis bullosa. In: Happle R, Grosshans E (eds.) *Pediatric Dermatology*. Berlin, Heidelberg: Springer-Verlag, 1986.
26 Haynes L, Atherton DJ, Clayden GS (in preparation) Constipation in dystrophic epidermolysis bullosa: successful treatment with liquid fibre.
27 Atherton DJ Personal communication, 1992.
28 Gryboski JD, Touloukian R, Campanella RA Gastrointestinal manifestations of epidermolysis bullosa in children. *Arch Dermatol*, 1988, 124 746–752.

FURTHER READING

Information booklets published by DEBRA

Allman S *Diet for Epidermolysis Bullosa, For Children Over 1 Year*, 1989.
Haynes L *Nutrition for Babies with Dystrophic Epidermolysis Bullosa*, 1993. (This information may be suitable for babies with other types of EB)
Mullett F *A Guideline to Physiotherapy for Parents of Children with Dystrophic Epidermolysis Bullosa*, 1990.
Gascoine H *Guidelines for Parents on the Play and Developmental Needs of Children with Dystrophic Epidermolysis Bullosa*, 1990.

USEFUL ADDRESS

Dystrophic Epidermolysis Bullosa Research Association (DEBRA)
DEBRA House, 13 Wellington Business Park, Duke's Ride, Crowthorne, Berkshire RG11 6LS. Tel 0344 771961.

ACKNOWLEDGEMENTS

The author is in receipt of a grant from the Dystrophic Epidermolysis Bullosa Research Association.

The author is grateful for permission from Mrs S Allman to reproduce Fig. 24.1 and to Dr DJ Atherton for helpful comments on the text.

CHAPTER 25

Burns

The incidence of burns in children in the UK is not known; in similar environments, such as the United States, approximately 2 million people are treated for burns each year. Of these 100 000 are hospitalized, and 30–40% are under 15 years of age. The average age of children when burnt is 32 months, and two thirds of victims are male [1,2].

ASSESSMENT OF INJURY

Burns are assessed from an accurate history of the incident. This should include the type of burn (flame, scald, electrical or chemical) and whether there has been any smoke inhalation. Burns are classified as:

- partial thickness (superficial or deep dermal)
- full thickness.

Total burn surface area (TBSA) is determined using modified Lund and Browder charts [3]. While the percentage of the body surface area occupied by the upper body and feet remains constant, the proportions for the head and neck, thigh and calf vary with age (Fig. 25.1). In children a major burn is defined as >10% of total body surface area burnt or if there is smoke inhalation. Children with major burns will require resuscitation with intravenous fluids; those with minor burns do not usually require such resuscitation.

METABOLIC RESPONSE TO BURN INJURY

The metabolic response to burn injury has three phases, the ebb phase, the flow phase and the anabolic phase [5].

Ebb phase This may last from a few hours to two days post-burn. During this period fluid moves from the circulation into the tissues and the patient becomes oedematous. Other features include pallor, hypotension, thirst and reduced urine flow. Energy expenditure is depressed. Plasma and other fluids must be given intravenously to preserve blood volume and urine output.

Flow phase This phase lasts for weeks or months depending on the severity of the burn. It is characterized by an increase in energy expenditure and protein requirement. This is a result of an increased production of catabolic hormones (catecholamines, glucocorticoids and glucagon) which lead to hypermetabolism, increased protein and fat breakdown, negative nitrogen balance and altered carbohydrate metabolism.

Anabolic phase This is the final phase when nutritional intake can gradually return to normal. The aim of therapy is to promote growth, restore muscle mass and strength and a return to normal function.

Calculating energy and protein requirements

There are many different formulas designed to calculate the nutritional requirements of burned children. None are used exclusively and they should be used as a guideline only. Some formulas are illustrated in Table 25.1.

Children have a higher resting metabolic rate (RMR) than adults and exhibit a smaller rise in RMR in response to burn injury. Some centres use dietary reference values (DRV) [9] to calculate energy requirements on the basis that a child confined to bed will have a reduced energy output for activity which

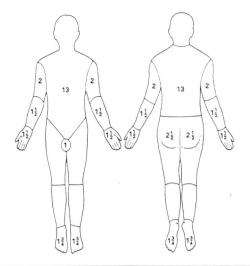

Area	Age (years)					
	0	1	5	10	15	Adult
Head and neck	21	19	15	13	11	9
Thigh	$5\frac{1}{2}$	$8\frac{1}{2}$	8	9	9	$9\frac{1}{2}$
Calf	5	5	$5\frac{1}{2}$	6	$6\frac{1}{2}$	7

Fig. 25.1 Percentage of different parts of the body at different ages

Table 25.1 Energy and protein requirements in the burned child

25.1(a) From Grotte *et al.* 1982 [6]

Age years	Energy kcal/kg/d (kJ/kg/d)		Nitrogen g/kg/d	
	<20% burns	>20% burns	<20% burns	>20% burns
0–1	125 (523)	150 (627)	0.45	0.5
1–8	100 (418)	125 (523)	0.3	0.45
8–15	75 (314)	100 (418)	0.25	0.3

25.1(b) From Solomon 1981 [7]

Age	Energy kcal/d (kJ/d)	Protein g/d
0–1 year Up to 9 kg	Normal requirement + 15 kcal (63 kJ) × percentage burn	Normal requirement + 0.75 g × percentage burn
1–3 years (10–13 kg)	Normal requirement + 20 kcal (84 kJ) × percentage burn	Normal requirement + 1.0 g × percentage burn
3 + years	Normal requirement + 30 kcal (125 kJ) × percentage burn	Normal requirement + 1.5 g × percentage burn

25.1(c) From Sutherland and Batchelor 1968 [8]

Age	Energy kcal/d (kJ/d)	Protein g/d
0–10 years	60 kcal (251 kJ)/kg + 35 kcal (146 kJ)/ % burns	3 g/kg + 1 g/ % burns

would offset the rise in RMR in response to burn injury. When total energy expenditure has been measured in burned children it is found to be much lower than predicted. Goran *et al.* [10] recommend measuring resting energy expenditure and multiplying by a factor of 1.2. They found that the formulas currently in use overestimate total energy expenditure by at least a factor of 1.6. Protein breakdown is elevated throughout the ebb, flow and convalescent phases of the response to burn injury. However, a significant net loss of nitrogen occurs only in the flow phase. During the convalescent phase there is net protein anabolism despite the continuing elevation in protein breakdown [11]. It is important, therefore, to ensure an adequate intake of protein.

A study in young children under three years concluded that efficient protein utilization for recovery will be achieved with energy provision of 120–200% RMR provided that there is a protein intake of at least 2.5 g/kg/day [12].

Vitamins and trace elements

Children with burns are likely to have an increased requirement above the DRV for vitamins because of their increased energy and protein requirements, their stressed state, and to allow for tissue healing. There are very few studies on which to base recommendations for supplementation. Most vitamins, particularly vitamins A, C, E and pyridoxine, affect immune function. Thiamin, pyridoxine, folic acid and vitamins C and B12 are essential for protein synthesis and wound repair [13].

Vitamin supplementation varies widely between units. The *UK National Feeding Guidelines for Burns Patients* recommends individual assessment of each patient. B vitamins should be supplied in proportion to energy and protein requirements. Other vitamins should meet the reference nutrient intake (RNI). Vitamin C should be supplemented in amounts up to 10 times the RNI [14]. Burns patients also have increased requirements for trace elements. This is to cover the increased losses in cases of large burns from urine, plasma and skin and to meet the increased requirements particularly during the anabolic phase. Again each child should be individually assessed and trace elements should meet the RNI. Care should be taken not to over supplement with one trace element as this may compete for absorption with others.

At risk patients, particularly those with large burns, should have serum levels monitored once a week [14]. Trace element depletion has been reported in burns patients. Hypomagnesaemia has been shown in patients following severe burns trauma despite achieving recommended intakes. Magnesium requirements increase during recovery from severe burns [15]. Selenium depletion has also been reported [16].

NUTRITIONAL SUPPORT

Minor burns

Children with minor burns (<10%) do not require fluid resuscitation and will usually start eating and drinking straight away. They will usually meet their requirements with a high protein high energy diet, use of between meal snacks and supplementary drinks. Choice of regimen will vary depending on the age of the child (Table 25.2).

Major burns

Children with major burns (>10%) are not usually fed during the active resuscitation period (36–48 hours post-burn). There have been several studies recently which suggest that early feeding (within six hours) is possible and indeed beneficial. Early feeding is said to prevent paralytic ileus and reduce the rise in catabolism [17,18].

Meeting nutritional requirements can be very dif-

Table 25.2 Choice of enteral feeds and supplements

Age (years)	Enteral feed	Supplements
0–1	Baby milk formula *or* Follow-on formula Concentrated + energy supplement if necessary	As for enteral feed
1–6	Paediasure Nutrison Paediatric	Paediasure Nutrison Paediatric Fresubin Ensure Plus* Fortisip* Build Up* Liquisorb*
7+	Standard adult enteral feed	Fortisip Fresubin Build Up Ensure Plus Liquisorb

* Not usually given below 3 years but depends on protein and energy requirements

ficult in burned children. There are many factors affecting food intake. These include pain, fear, sedation (e.g. for dressing changes), isolation, and the smell of burn injuries. There is also the length of time spent having physiotherapy and the time spent 'nil by mouth' for theatre procedures to consider. For these reasons many children will need to be enterally fed. Others will meet their requirements using a high protein high energy diet with supplements (Table 25.2).

The proportion of children who are fed nasogastrically varies widely. Some units routinely feed children with >15% burns nasogastrically. Others rarely use this type of nutritional support. Policy will be decided at a unit level taking into account local conditions such as flexibility of catering arrangements, staffing levels, choice of supplements and past experience. Continuous rather than bolus nasogastric feeding is usually undertaken using a feed appropriate to the child's age (Table 25.2). Volume of feed should be calculated to meet requirements, taking into account any oral intake.

Diarrhoea is perceived to be a major problem in burns patients. It has been shown to affect approximately 30% of patients and is associated with the use of antibiotics [19]. Current practice is variable.

Some centres introduce clear fluids before restarting feeds. Others use peptide-based feeds or feeds with low osmolarity. One study in adults has suggested that feed tolerance is improved by feeding early, using a low fat (<20% total energy) feed and having vitamin A supplementation [19].

Other studies in adults have also looked at changes in the composition of feeds to improve outcome for burns patients. One study has shown that branched chain amino acid supplementation reduced muscle protein breakdown [20]. Others have looked at varying the lipid content of feeds to improve outcome. Improved protein anabolism and attenuated protein catabolism has been achieved by the use of medium chain triglycerides and fish oils in burned rats [21]. Another study in burned guinea pigs compared the use of fish oil with lipid sources rich in linoleic acid and found lower resting metabolic rates, less weight loss and better cell mediated immune respones in the fish oil group [22]. New feeds may be developed in future to improve outcomes for burns.

Parenteral feeding may be necessary if a child's gut is inaccessible or not functioning or if enteral feeding cannot fully meet his requirements. Feeding can be either via central or peripheral lines. It may be as a sole source of nutrition or an adjunct to enteral feeding. It should aim to meet requirements. Fat-free feeding regimens are not encouraged as these rely on glucose as the major source of energy. Burns patients have a limited capacity to oxidize glucose. Excess glucose is then synthesized into fat which may lead to fatty infiltration of the liver. The use of fat as an energy source prevents this and also decreases the respiratory quotient to below 1.0, thereby reducing carbon dioxide production in patients who may have pulmonary insufficiency.

MONITORING

Monitoring is essential to ensure that feeding is adequate and that changes are made to the regimen to reflect changes in the child's requirements. *UK National Feeding Guidelines for Burns Patients* [14] recommend monitoring as follows.

- nutritional intake should be monitored daily from accurate records of food and fluid intake
- the child should be weighed weekly without dressings
- nitrogen balance should be measured at least once

a week as a measure of catabolism and imminent sepsis
- biochemical measurements:
  serum transferrin   – weekly
  serum albumin   – weekly
  C-reactive protein   – weekly
  urea and electrolytes   – weekly
- burned surface area should be reassessed at each dressing change and nutritional requirements recalculated
- changes in clinical condition (e.g. sepsis, pyrexia) should be monitored, and nutritional requirement adjusted.

REFERENCES

1 Herndon D *et al.* Treatment of burns in children. *Ped Clin North Am*, 1985, **32** 1311–1332.
2 Felle I, Keith JC National Burn Information Exchange. *Surg Clin North Am*, 1970, **50m** 1423–1436.
3 Lund CL, Browder ND The estimation of areas of burns. *Surg Gynecol Obstet*, 1944, **78** 352.
4 Harvey-Kemble JV, Lamb BE *Plastic Surgical and Burns Nursing*. Eastbourne: Baillière Tindall, 1984.
5 Cuthbertson DP Post shock metabolic response. *Lancet*, 1942, **i** 433–437.
6 Grotte G, Meurling S, Wretlind A Parenteral nutrition. In: McClaren DS, Burman D (eds.) *Textbook of Paediatric Nutrition*, 2e. Edinburgh: Churchill Livingstone, 1982.
7 Soloman JR Nutrition in the severely burnt child. *Progr Pediatr Surg*, 1981, **14** 653–679.
8 Sutherland AB, Batchelor ADC Nitrogen Balance in burned children. *Ann NY Acad Sciences*, 1968, **150** 700.
9 Department of Health Report on Health and Social Subjects no. 41. *Dietary Reference Values for Food Energy and Nutrients for the United Kingdom*. London: HMSO, 1991.
10 Goran MI *et al.* Total energy expenditure in burned children using the doubly labelled water technique. *Am J Physiol*, 1990, **259** 576–585.
11 Jahoor F *et al.* Dynamics of the protein metabolic response to burn injury. *Metabolism*, 1988, **37** 330–337.
12 Cunningham JJ, Lydon MK, Russell WE Calorie and protein provision for recovery from severe burns in infants and young children. *Am J Clin Nutr*, 1990, **51** 553–557.
13 Gottschlick MM, Warden GG Vitamin supplementation in the patient with burns. *J Burn Care Rehab*, 1990, **11** 275–279.
14 British Dietetic Association Burns Interest Group *UK National Feeding Guidelines for Burns Patients*. Birmingham: BDA, 1992.
15 Cunningham JJ, Anbar RD, Crawford JD Hypo-

magnesemia: a multifactorial complication of treatment of patients with severe burn trauma. *J Parent Ent Nutr*, 1989, **11** 364–367.

16 Hunt DR *et al*. Selenium depletion in burns patients. *J Parent Ent Nutr*, 1984, **8** 695–699.

17 McDonald WS, Sharp CW, Deitch EA Immediate enteral feeding in burn patients is safe and effective. *Ann Surg*, 1991, **213** 177–183.

18 McArdle AH *et al*. Early enteral feeding of patients with major burns: prevention of catabolism. *Ann Plast Surg*, 1984, **13** 396–401.

19 Gottschlich MM *et al*. Diarrhea in tube-fed burn patients: Incidence, etiology, nutritional impact and prevention. *J Parent Ent Nutr*, 1988, **12** 338–345.

20 King P, Power DM Branched chain amino/keto acid supplementation following severe burn injury: a preliminary report. *Clin Nutr*, 1990, **9** 226–230.

21 DeMichel SJ *et al*. Enteral nutrition with structured lipid: effect on protein metabolism in thermal injury. *Am J Clin Nutr*, 1989, **50** 1295–1302.

22 Alexander JW *et al*. The importance of lipid type in the diet after burn injury. *Ann Surg*, 1986, **204** 1–8.

CHAPTER 26

Nutrition for Children with Feeding Difficulties

Disability affects every aspect of a child's life, much of which can have a negative effect on nutrition. Children with a disability have been identified as a nutritionally vulnerable group. However dietetic practice has not focused on this particular problem, resulting in identification of nutritional problems at a later rather than an earlier stage of life. Webb [1] summarizes: 'Nutrition for handicapped children is not a subject which generates much discussion probably because it is a difficult problem on which to speak in generalities. Classifications of handicaps usually consider only the major handicap, and thus labelling a child as having a particular disability gives little information on the food and nutrition problems which may be present'.

Issues that dietitians should consider when working with children with feeding difficulties are discussed. The social and physical issues affecting the lives of these children, and the services they may receive, are highlighted. Together these provide a picture from which nutrition goals can be planned to help them achieve their potential.

In the text the term 'carers' describes parent, guardian, or staff in residential or educational locations.

Children with feeding difficulties require a multidisciplinary approach if the problems are to be assessed and managed successfully. The development of eating and drinking skills is important for several reasons, only one of which is nutrition:

- efficient eating is necessary if the child is to consume adequate nutrition orally
- oral control, the patterns of movement of lips, tongue, jaw and breathing are practised whilst eating; this strongly influences the development of precise movements necessary for speech and control of saliva
- mealtimes provide opportunities for the develop-

ment of posture, head control and eye/hand co-ordination
- mealtimes provide ideal settings for social interaction where rules and social behaviour are learned and rehearsed
- social integration into mealtimes and eating out is easier as a child's competence improves
- independence can be gained through providing choice and control at mealtimes, allowing the child to develop self-esteem and his own identity.

MAJOR NUTRITIONAL PROBLEMS

The major nutritional problems seen in these children are:

- failure to thrive
- low body weight for height
- constipation
- vitamin and mineral deficiencies
- dental caries.

Failure to thrive or low body weight has been well documented for children with developmental delay, neurological dysfunction and in particular for children with cerebral palsy [2,3,4,5]. However few studies have been published accurately describing food intake and consequently how this affects anthropometry [6,7,8]. Thus beliefs that it is 'normal' for children with severe disabilities, particularly those children with cerebral palsy, to have poor stature and low weights are accepted by many clinicians and carers. Bax, in an editorial addressing this issue [9], was 'shocked' by the number of young disabled people (40%) who had feeding problems. As a result a new clinical category of 'emaciated' was introduced to the study. In this study of 100 children, 11% were characterized as emaciated, 9% very thin. Other studies have shown that minimal oromotor dysfunction should be considered in non-organic failure to thrive [10]. Some of the issues that appear to be unresolved in this area are:

- can children with oromotor dysfunction who are failing to thrive or have low body weight for height achieve the accepted growth norms for children?
- should we therefore be using standard growth charts for children with these problems?

Special charts have been developed for children with Down's syndrome [11] but for no other groups. Therefore until studies show that children with specific problems (e.g. cerebral palsy) have innate growth problems it should be assumed that, given adequate nutrition, they can achieve heights and weights within the normal centiles.

Constipation is a common problem for children with feeding difficulties. It may be as a result of: inadequate fluid intake; excessive fluid loss via spillage or dribbling; immobility; poor gut motility; side effects of medication; or occasionally lack of dietary fibre. This problem appears to be accepted as 'normal' and medication, rather than assessment of the cause and appropriate management, might be the favoured treatment.

Studies on vitamin and mineral intakes and deficiencies for children with feeding problems are not well documented. However nutritional assessment based on good diet history will highlight inadequate intake due to poor variety, small quantities of food eaten and potential vitamin losses through liquidizing foods or long cooking methods.

Dental caries can be a problem for a number of reasons – poor dental hygiene due to hypersensitivity to teeth cleaning, medications, inability to clear the mouth of food after eating, reduced saliva production and frequent consumption of foods containing sugar. A dilemma exists in the management of children with feeding difficulties because small, energy-dense meals and drinks given regularly throughout the day are often contrary to the advice given to prevent dental caries. A compromise may be necessary and discussion with the child's dentist will not only help to prevent contradictory messages being given, but may offer alternative preventative dental treatment. Dental treatment can be dangerous, time consuming and very frightening for some children with disabilities and therefore prevention should always be considered. In addition a child with dental caries who cannot communicate his pain will more than likely exhibit negative behaviours around food and drink, thus increasing his feeding difficulties.

MEDICAL CONDITIONS CAUSING FEEDING PROBLEMS

Down's syndrome

A number of studies have been carried out to ascertain the frequency of feeding problems in children with Down's syndrome. Van Dyke *et al.* [12] review the American based studies and suggest that eating problems are common but are usually minor in nature. Surveys of parents [12] suggest that 60% are totally independent in feeding by early childhood and the most common problems are slight oral hypotonia, tongue thrust, difficulties in chewing, poor lip seal, and choking and gagging on food. However it is noted that this feeding success may be partly a direct result of feeding programmes and not simply a natural developmental step, thus reinforcing the need for assessment and management programmes. Other authors [13] suggest that normal motor development follows a systematic timetable.

The main reasons why children with Down's syndrome may experience feeding difficulties are due to multiple cranial skeletal differences. The palate is often short and narrow, and this underdevelopment of the maxilla may alter the position of the muscles used for chewing. The tongue may be large or appear large due to a small oral cavity secondary to midfacial hypoplasia. Many children with Down's syndrome are mouth breathers, due to a small oral cavity, enlargement of the tonsils, and/or decreased nasal passages. This will have an effect on the development of efficient oral skills. Generalized facial/oral hypotonia also contributes to poor lip closure, poor suck, poor tongue control, and difficulties with jaw stability. In addition, infants with Down's syndrome with congenital heart defects may have the combined problems experienced by infants with heart abnormalities (page 143) and poor oral skills stated above. Other medical problems that may be present that have a direct effect on nutrition assessment are compromised immune systems and hypothyroidism.

Anthropometric assessment of children with Down's syndrome is complicated because the disorder is associated with a number of abnormalities related to growth e.g. short stature, decreased head circumference, and altered growth patterns. Cronk [11,14] suggests that while heights in people with Down's syndrome are significantly lower that the norm, the period in which most significant growth failure occurs is during the first five years of life. Longitudinal studies [15] corroborate this but show that growth velocity of children aged 7–18 is not significantly different to the norm. Cronk [11] has produced growth charts for children with Down's syndrome based on these studies and Taylor Baer [16] has reviewed studies around these problems.

Cerebral palsy

Cerebral palsy is a disorder of movement, either athetosis, spasticity or ataxia, due to a lesion within the brain. The resultant type of cerebral palsy depends upon which part of the brain has been affected. A child may have one distinctive type, or more commonly a combination of two or three types. The main features of athetoid cerebral palsy are uncontrolled, continuous movements of the body. The movements can be slow and writhing or jerky and are accentuated by voluntary movement. At times the child may also be very floppy. A child with spastic type cerebral palsy usually has very little movement, resulting in tightness, limited range of movement and deformity. Children with ataxia appear clumsy, have poor balance, often have shaky hand movements and are poorly co-ordinated. The different parts of the body involved are described as: hemiplegia when one side of the body is affected; diplegia when the legs are affected more than the arms; and quadraplegia when all four limbs are affected. The nature of cerebral palsy is that it changes as the child develops and matures. The severity of the disorder can vary between muscle groups and different parts of the body and this will affect the severity of the feeding problems. Not all children with cerebral palsy will have a feeding problem.

Children with cerebral palsy often display both retained and abnormal patterns of movement, which are sometimes excessively strong or brisk. These reflexes prevent children developing more mature and controlled patterns of movement and will affect their feeding capabilities. Examples of these reflexes are extensor thrust, gag and bite reflex. A child with extensor thrust will throw his head back, spine arched, legs straight and arms tight. The result is that it is hard to position the child for feeding; assisted or self-feeding is more difficult in this stiff position; chin thrust prevents efficent swallowing and may cause choking; jaw thrust prevents mouth closure and interferes with normal sucking or chewing movements. The gag and cough reflex is a protective mechanism; however, an oversensitivity to food may cause frequent coughing and will override all other eating patterns. A brisk gag reflex at the front of the mouth reduces the tolerance to food. The bite reflex is typified by sudden jaw closure in response to front gums or teeth being touched. This results in an inability to open the mouth and co-ordinate jaw movement whilst introducing food into the mouth. An extended list of potential reflexes and reactions and their effect on feeding is described by Chailey Heritage [17]. Additionally children with cerebral palsy are often multiply disabled. They may have sensory difficulties (e.g. vision, hearing, touch); perceptual difficulties resulting in impaired interpretation of the senses; a degree of learning difficulty; difficulties in communication, breathing and oral skills; and epilepsy.

Cleft palate

Clefting is one of the most common birth defects and the most common affecting the face and oromotor mechanism. A cleft is a separation of parts of the mouth usually joined together during the early weeks of fetal development. A cleft lip is separation of one or both sides of the upper lip, and often the upper dental ridge. The cleft can be incomplete, affecting primarily the lip and not extending into the nasal cavity. A complete cleft includes separation of the dental ridge and the lip and extends through the nasal cavity. A bilateral cleft occurs on both sides of the nose.

Clefts of the palate may occur in the bony hard palate or in the soft palate at the back of the mouth. It may occur with or without a cleft lip. It can occur as a unilateral complete cleft through soft and hard palate on one side or bilaterally. A submucous cleft occurs when the tissue connecting the two sides of the hard or soft palate is incomplete even though the surface tissue is intact. The latter is invisible to the eye.

Clefts are repaired by surgery, and the timing is dependent upon the severity of the cleft, the child's condition and the surgeon's preference.

Feeding is the most immediate issue facing carers. Some infants have few feeding problems but others will experience great difficulty. The majority of infants will be fed orally; however the carer will require help to obtain adapted drinking utensils and the optimum feeding position to prevent choking. Bottle feeding is generally prefered to spoon feeding in the early months. Breast milk can be given as expressed milk and some mothers have managed to establish breast feeding [18].

The main problem experienced by the child is difficulty with sucking and maintaining an adequate suction. In addition, because the nose and mouth cavities are not fully separated by the palate, food may back up and run out of the child's nose causing coughing, choking, spitting or vomiting.

Weaning would normally occur in the same sequence as for other children; however as these transitions may occur before surgical closure of the cleft the infant will need to learn how to control lumps as they arrive at the palate opening. Infants with clefts will normally learn to eat proficiently with modifications for positioning, equipment and speed of presentation of food, as they will compensate for difficulties of the cleft. Children who do not may signal that other developmental problems may exist.

CAUSES OF FEEDING DIFFICULTIES

The main causes of feeding difficulties can be broadly divided into four groups:

- oral dysfunction resulting from either structural abnormalities such as cleft palate, high roof of the mouth, enlarged tongue or neurological disturbances such as cerebral palsy
- physical disabilities such as cerebral palsy where the child finds it difficult to co-ordinate the passage of food and fluids to and in the mouth
- sensory impairment where one or more of the senses are affected
- learning disabilities or developmental delay, where some children may take longer than their chronological peers to learn the skills necessary for eating and normal masticatory patterns.

As a guide the more severe the disability and the presence of multiple disabilities, i.e. two or more of the above, the greater the likelihood of feeding difficulties.

OTHER FACTORS RESULTING FROM DISABILITY WHICH HAVE AN EFFECT ON A CHILD'S NUTRITION

Subsidiary factors which often accompany disability and which have an effect on the child's nutrition are outlined below.

Medication

Some children may be on medication with side effects which directly or indirectly have a negative effect on their nutrition, e.g. some forms of anticonvulsant therapy affect appetite, induce nausea and gastrointestinal irritation, cause drowsiness and affect the utilization of vitamin D.

Ill health

Repeated periods of ill health (e.g. recurrent chest infections) may be common for some children. This affects not only the appetite, but it also decreases the opportunities for learning or practising eating skills and possibly increases nutritional requirements.

Social effects

The social effects which can affect a child's nutrition are obviously the same as for any other child, but disability heightens the effect. Financial commitments are greater in a family where a person has a disability. Eating socially, eating out in popular peer group venues, picnics, school meals, cookery classes are all limited for a child with feeding difficulties, thus reducing the opportunities to learn and eat the variety of foods and drinks available to other children.

Pressures on the carer

Pressures on the carer responsible for providing and delivering food and drink are enormous. Not only are they expected to provide an adequate, varied diet of the correct consistency and texture, but also to know how to help the child develop the necessary oral and motor skills. Time is a major consideration; it takes longer to feed a child with feeding difficulties. Some children may take up to an hour to eat a meal, leaving all concerned tired and bored with the event. As with all children, when learning skills initially it takes longer to complete the task. Consider a child who is developing according to normal milestones: for this child completing the goal – learning to eat and drink independently with a degree of dexterity – occurs within his first three years. For some children with developmental delay this period is extended and may be doubled or trebled; some may never achieve the goal. It is potentially a frustrating and messy business for both child and carer.

The time factor has to be weighed against all the other activities that carers are required to perform for their child. The more severe the disability, and particularly for those with multiple disabilities, the greater is the time and energy invested in the caring and educational role. Appointments with the multitude of professionals, specialists, researchers from all statutory and voluntary agencies can make the daily timetable very difficult to adhere to. Privacy can be a rare commodity in families where the child has input from a large number of people.

Communication

Requesting and signalling your needs and desires for food provide cues for the carer. An infant who is unable to cry for food, a child who is unable to demand food, is obviously placed at risk. In addition children with feeding difficulties may be incorrectly interpreted at meal times e.g. it is accepted that an infant of 4–6 months (without feeding difficulties) may initially reject lumpy food because he cannot yet manage the consistency; however an older infant, toddler or child (with undiagnosed feeding difficulties) doing the same may be misinterpreted as disliking the food, being fussy, stubborn, awkward or lazy. Generally carers do not report that the child has a feeding problem, but describe him as fussy or naughty at meal times. Thus it might appear that amongst the other problems that occur, carers just accept the feeding difficulties and do not ask for help. Without thorough investigation of exactly what the carer means by 'fussy' or 'naughty' the severity of the problem may be overlooked or even accepted as normal for that particular medical diagnosis.

A child with epilepsy and severe physical and learning disabilities could well be disadvantaged on most, if not all, of the above points.

NUTRITIONAL ASSESSMENT

Nutritional assessment is based upon the same principles as for other children. Dietary reference values for energy and nutrients can be used as broad guidelines, though they must be used with caution for the individual. Children whose growth and weight are severely stunted should have their nutritional requirements interpreted with care using current weight as the baseline. In conjunction with the nutritional assessment other observations and information will help in planning and implementing remedial and diet therapy.

Rarely can a dietitian extract this detail from an outpatient interview with a main carer. It requires communication with a number of people and observations at meal times. The broad areas that need to be identified in children with eating and drinking difficulties are food, utensils, positioning, sensitivity, techniques, behaviour/emotion and medical issues. All these form the basis for producing an individualized management programme.

Assessment observation/recall

The questions posed in the Assessment Checklist (see Table 26.1) are vital for formulating a feeding programme.

Food

Dietary assessment Recall on quantities of food is difficult if home food is liquidized. Food diaries provide more information but are time consuming to complete.

Appetite Does it fluctuate? Is it improving or deteriorating? Are there any medical or social trends that affect the child's appetite? How does he communicate his hunger/satiety?

Fluids How much does the child consume? How much does he lose? Does he have poor lip seal resulting in loss of fluids whilst drinking? How much is actually placed in his cup? How often is he offered a drink? How does he communicate his thirst?

Variety Does he have the opportunity to try a wide range of foods and drinks? Are meals repeated in the same day at home and at school? Does he have

Table 26.1 Assessment checklist

	Observation/recall
Food	Dietary recall
	Appetite
	Fluids
	Variety
	Taste
	Temperature
	Texture
Equipment	Utensils
	Plates
	Drinking cups
Positioning	Seating
	Position of feeder
Sensitivity	Sensory loss/impairment
	Sensitivity to foods/fluids
Techniques	Who feeds
	How
	Time
	Food loss
	Oral skills
	Motor skills
Behaviour and emotion	Venues for eating
	Eating with others
	Environment
Medical	Salivation
	Medication
	Dentition
	Medical history
Services	Professional/specialist input
	Expectation of service providers/carers

the same meal because he cannot say what he has had at school?

Taste Does the child like the food? Are his preferences known? How does he communicate them?

Temperature Does he have a preference for cold/ hot foods or drinks?

Texture Is the texture appropriate? Is it quick and easy to eat? Does it help or hinder development of oromotor skills? Is it a safe texture if the child has a poor or no swallow?

Equipment

Is he using the correct utensils, plates, plate guards to enable him to be successful at both oral and motor skills?

Positioning

Is the seating conductive to developing oromotor skills and safe swallowing? Is adapted seating required? What position has the helper adopted? Has the physiotherapist/occupational therapist assessed his positioning?

Sensitivity

Sensory loss Are any of his senses impaired? Do mealtimes consider his limitations and focus on using the other senses? Is he sensitive to particular tastes, temperatures or textures?

Techniques

Who feeds at meal times? Do they offer the same texture and quantity? Do they all use the same equipment, same prompts, same feeding techniques? Does he like everyone who feeds him?

Time How long does a meal take? Is the meal cold half way through? Is the preparation of food separate from other people's?

Food loss How much is lost during drinking/ eating? Is this as a result of poor oral or motor skills?

Oral skills Does he have a normal masticatory pattern? Does he have poor lip seal, tongue protrusion, bite reflex, immature tongue movements? Is he able to bite, chew or move food around the mouth? Does he swallow food or does it slip down his throat?

Motor skills Is he able to co-ordinate food to the mouth using hands, two fingers, spoon, fork? How much energy goes into this task? How successful is he?

Behaviour and emotion

Venues for eating These can include home, school, respite care, friends, eating out. What are the limitations for him and why?

Eating with others Does the child eat with the family or alone? In school who does he eat with?

Environment Does he find it noisy, cold, hot, distracting, friendly, embarrassing, boring, stimulating?

Medical

Salivation Does he lose fluids through excessive salivation, inability to swallow saliva or constant open lips? Does he suck his fingers/toys causing excessive saliva loss? Does he have a dry mouth?

Medication What type of medication is he on and what are the side effects? Does drowsiness occur as a result at mealtimes?

Dentition Is his dentition normal for chronological age? Has he dental caries? How does he communicate this? Has he recently lost teeth and does this affect his oral skills?

Medical history What is known about his medical history? What investigations have been carried out?

Services

What professionals/specialists and support does he receive? Are they communicating with each other? Is there an identified key person? Is there a consistent message? Does he have day care/respite/school? Is he with his main carer all the time?

Expectations What expectations do others have? Is he receiving treatment from other people who all expect certain outcomes? How many tasks/skills is he expected to master? Is it practical to add more? Can he learn the skill or is he being set up to fail? Does the skill need to be broken down into smaller components?

MANAGEMENT OF FEEDING

Multidisciplinary feeding assessment

This draws together the skills and expertise from carer, speech and language therapist, occupational therapist (OT), physiotherapist, dietitian and possibly psychologist. There are various models that can be used, all involving observing the child eat and drink: individual people assess independently and make recommendations; one or two key people observe the

child eating and drinking; the whole team observes the child eating/drinking; a video assessment is carried out. The latter seems to be the most beneficial and the least invasive to the child. It provides a visual record which can be analysed and discussed by the group and carer without the child being present or distracted by people watching him eat. It also provides an objective record for reviewing whether goals have been achieved. The carer can keep the video as a reminder of progress and to retain some confidentiality.

The venue, timing, health of the child and familiarity need to be considered carefully if a true picture of the child's capabilities is to be extracted. Sometimes videos of the child eating in two familiar places, such as home and school, can elicit useful information.

Identification of why the child is having difficulties with eating

Assessment will identify why the child is having difficulties with eating and will fall into one of three categories. Food or drink is difficult to:

- control in the mouth
- tolerate in the mouth as it causes sensitivity reactions such as gag reflex, grimacing or vomiting or gives little sensory stimulation to notify that food is present.
- load or keep on the spoon.

Thickness, texture, taste and temperature are the properties that will dictate the degree of ease of consumption of a particular food or drink. Each child will react individually. Table 26.2 provides a generalized picture to help choose the types of food to use in a management programme.

Challenging food/drinks

If a child is to develop oral skills, sensory tolerance or self feeding then foods that are liked but present a challenge to the child need to be incorporated into the meal. For some children the emphasis may be on ensuring a safe texture to reduce the risk of aspiration.

One approach identifies three methods of introducing challenging foods [17]:

- start with challenging food whilst appetite is strong and modify the food to easy

Table 26.2 Food textures

Challenging foods			Easier foods	
Thickness	Thin fluids	e.g. water, juice	Thick fluids	e.g. drinking yoghurt, milkshake, thin custard
	Thin and watery	e.g. thin yoghurt, thin gravy	Thick and creamy	e.g. creamed potatoes, semolina, ground rice, creamed pulses, thick sauces, thick gravy, thick custard, fromage frais, thick creamy yoghurt
	Swimming foods	e.g. sponge cake swimming in custard, carrots and meat in gravy. Overcooked lumpy scrambled egg		
	Thin and lumpy	Dilute Stage 2 baby food, thin rice pudding	Thick and lumpy	e.g. meat/fish and veg in thick sauces, macaroni cheese, sieved meals
Texture			Single texture	e.g. Stage 1 baby food, mashed vegetables, mashed bananas
	Crunch and crumble/splinter	e.g. crisp raw apple, raw carrot, crisps, cream crackers, nuts, digestive biscuits	Crunch and dissolve	e.g. cheese puffs, sugar puffs, wafers, sponge fingers
	Bite and stick	e.g. white bread	Bite and dissolve	e.g. sponge cake, chocolate buttons
	Hard chew	e.g. tough meat, dry fish, toffee, chewing gum	Soft chew	e.g. soft raw apple, boiled potato, boiled carrot, processed meat (e.g. corned beef) brown bread and spread
	Stringy and husky	e.g. spinach, runner beans, shredded meat, chicken, celery		
	Bite and slip	e.g. tinned peaches, oranges, jelly	Soft slip and swallow	e.g. tinned spaghetti, ice cream, mousse, Angel Delight
Temperature	Very hot/very cold		Warm	
Taste	Acid		Bland	
	Bitter		Mild	
	Savoury meat		Sweet	

- start with easy (to allay strong eating patterns and appetite) and then introduce challenging food
- alternate easy and challenging food throughout the meal.

It is important to remember when using this approach that the helper must persevere and keep offering the challenge even when unsuccessful in the initial periods. Whenever possible foods should be chosen which make challenges fun – for example, soft chocolate bars and jelly based sweets. A meal should never be offered that is all challenge; some easy food should always be included.

Texture

The food texture required by the child should be assessed by a speech and language therapist. One useful system for classifying food textures is shown in Table 26.2. The carer should be provided with numerous ideas on the foods within that group to help provide variety in the diet. Where the child requires thick, smooth, paste-type consistency, e.g. to ensure safe swallowing, the thickness required can be demonstrated by using easily available foods such as instant mashed potato or baby rice.

Presentation

The way food is presented to the child is important to success. Food should be given slowly and rhythmically allowing time for him to finish each mouthful and anticipate the next one. Small mouthfuls are more likely to be successful; however for some children the spoon needs to be heaped towards the tip of the spoon to provide sensory cues for his lips. The spoon should normally be presented horizontally from the front and, depending on the techniques being practised at the time, can be directed centrally or towards the side of the mouth when encouraging chewing. Scraping food off the spoon with the top teeth should be avoided. The speech and language therapist/OT can suggest other methods to help the child to learn to take food from the bowl of the spoon.

Fluids

Inadequate consumption or excessive loss of fluids is a feature common to many children with feeding difficulties. Advice should be based on careful assessment of why the child is not consuming adequate fluids. Sometimes the carer will offer the child the same number and quantity of drinks as other children, forgetting that a large percentage of the fluid offered is being lost. By simply reminding carers to offer a second cup, or more frequent drinks, this problem may be overcome. However this does add to the time taken to feed. The long term goal would be to help the child develop better oral skills, e.g. lip closure which reduces saliva loss and improves the movement of fluids to the back of the mouth.

Thickening drinks

For some children thickening drinks to the consistency of a 'thickshake' or thick sauce can enable them to be successful. Thin fluids are the most difficult consistency to manipulate in the mouth. The child with a poor or no swallow is more likely to aspirate thin fluids than thick ones. Numerous thickened milkshake type drinks are now commercially available; they are not only useful but are also acceptable to peers. Other fluids can be thickened using a range of familiar products such as thick yoghurts, ice cream, instant powdered desserts, instant sauce granules, smooth puréed fruit and jars of puréed baby food fruit

desserts. Cornflour, blancmanges and custard powder can be used, but are time consuming to prepare. A range of proprietary thickening agents are now available on prescription such as Instant Carobel, Nestargel, Thixo-D, Vitaquick and Thick and Easy, though these may not be prescribable or appropriate for use in infants or small children. The easy to mix type such as Thixo-D and Instant Carobel are the most likely to be acceptable and can be used in a range of drinks such as juices, tea, milk-based and proprietary drinks. Many carers have fears about offering thick drinks as they perceive these as 'not quenching his thirst'; their use should be fully discussed. For some children a compromise of thin and thick fluids will be more realistic and practical for the carer.

For children who manage food better than fluids, a method of increasing their fluid intake is to offer foods with a high water content between meals, e.g. fruit-based baby foods, puréed fruit, thick yoghurts, fromage frais, ice cream and ice lollies. Jelly can be useful, however it does dissolve immediately on entering the mouth, resulting in the same problems as thin fluids. Indicators that the fluid intake has increased will be incidentally reported by carers as: more wet nappies, fewer urinary tract infections, softer or more regular bowel movements. Assessment will identify the child's long term goals, e.g. working on oral skills to improve his lip seal, to enable him to drink with minimal fluid loss. This long term goal is broken into small steps which may include remedial work such as lip exercises designed by the speech and language therapist.

Increasing energy

This should be based upon the same dietetic principles as for other children who are failing to thrive or are underweight (page 7). However caution should be taken where failure to thrive occurs when epilepsy is evident or is associated with a particular syndrome as undocumented clinical experience suggests that some children with severe feeding difficulties and poor energy intakes may be ketotic. Thus suddenly increasing energy intake may increase the risk of epilepsy (page 173). Energy-dense foods of the correct consistency should be offered regularly throughout the day. Carers familiar with current healthy eating messages are often concerned about the use of high fat milks, the addition of margarine to foods or the frequent use of energy rich desserts e.g. chocolate mousses. Supplementation with a glucose polymer can often be the most practical method to increase energy intake. For some children the use of proprietary high energy drinks may be appropriate.

Enteral or gastrostomy feeding

This type of feeding may be indicated for some children, either as a partial or total source of fluid or nutrition. Differing opinions between professionals may make this difficult to initiate. In some cases the carers are against this option as it is perceived as yet another abnormal feature for their child. However many carers find that, once the decision to feed via this method is made, they are relieved [19] and pleased with the positive outcomes of weight gain, growth and lack of constipation. Multidisciplinary decisions and total participation of carers is crucial to success. Generally children who have feeding difficulties cannot initially tolerate the quantity required to provide adequate nutrition. Feeds should be commenced based upon current intake and gradually increased in volume and energy content. It may take many months to achieve optimum nutrition.

Increasing cereal fibre

The use of cereal fibre to help with constipation should only be considered if the child is consuming adequate fluids. High fibre breakfast cereals, e.g. Weetabix softened with hot milk or incorporated into desserts, or soft wholemeal breadcrumbs added to main courses, smooth savoury egg custards and sauces can be eaten by some children. The use of natural bran or high bran foods should be avoided and should only be considered in the most extreme cases with an older child who is known to be drinking more than adequate fluids and when all other sources of dietary fibre have been considered.

Equipment

The choice of equipment will have an enormous effect on whether or not the child is successful in feeding. Occupational therapists normally have the expertise to assess the child's needs and they have numerous catalogues from which to choose the appropriate pieces for each individual. For some children, standard equipment with slight adaptations will meet their needs, while for others a wide range of specialized equipment is available.

Spoons that are soft, strong and shatterproof, made of plastic or polycarbonate, are preferred. A flat or shallow bowled spoon facilitates removal of food with the lips and a small sized spoon helps direct the food to the side of the mouth. Hard metal, brittle or poorly shaped spoons can stimulate a bite reflex or cause discomfort. For some children it may be more appropriate to use a fork, spatula or fingers rather than a spoon as it is easier to direct food to the side of the mouth than with a broad or deep bowled spoon. Angled spoons help some children with limited hand or arm movement to achieve independent or assisted feeding. Children with a poor grasp can be assisted to develop independent self-feeding skills by using cutlery with built up or shaped handles to suit the child's hand; sometimes a strap may be used to maintain grasp. Training knives and forks with an indent for the index finger can be used to encourage correct holding of cutlery.

Plates to assist independent self-feeding include high sided plates or plate guards, sloping plates with a curved edge (e.g. the Mannoy plate). Divided and heated plates encourage better visual presentation and temperature of food. Divided plates also discourage the helper from mixing all flavours and textures together. Non-slip mats provide more stability for a child who finds the plate runs away from him when he eats.

The choice of drinking utensils is crucial to successful fluid intake. Experimentation with teats is necessary to find one that provides adequate stimulation. Bulbous cherry topped teats can stimulate swallowing but for some children they may produce a gag reflex. Extended use of bottles however can prevent the development of oral skills as it promotes an immature sucking action. Teats for children with cleft palates include long soft teats with enlarged holes allowing the milk to trickle into the mouth. The Rosti bottle, a soft plastic bottle with a teat shaped like a spoon or scoop, may be preferable for infants who have difficulty in sucking (Fig. 7.2).

A wide variety of commercially available training beakers are available. The correct balance has to be found between those that offer independent drinking e.g. a cup with a wide flat training nozzle with a lid, and those that develop immature drinking patterns e.g. beakers with drinking spouts. Soft plastic cups are more comfortable, particularly if the child has sensitive teeth. Slanted cups can facilitate good lower lip seal and control of unwanted tongue movements. Straws are sometimes the preferred choice and special straws are available for the child who has difficulty in maintaining lip seal.

Positioning

The child's position at meal times is vital to success. He needs to be secure and symmetrical to obtain optimum trunk, limb, head and oral control. The position should be assessed by the physiotherapist or OT and may be either on the carer's lap (infants and small children) or in adapted seating. For some children a personalized seating system is necessary. The helper needs to adopt a position that is comfortable, particularly if the meal takes a long time, and that facilitates the techniques necessary to help the child. Sometimes this will require the helper to experiment with different positions until they have the best arrangement for them both.

Eating with other people

This is important for children with feeding difficulties; however limitations may prevent this from happening, e.g. the special chair will not fit under the family table. The problems should be identified in the assessment and the physiotherapist/OT alerted to this problem. In some cases the carer finds it easier to give the child his meal before everyone else. Practical ways in which the child can join in on some family meals need to be identified, e.g. the time or stress involved with meal preparation can be reduced and this time spent with the child at the table; other members of the family can be asked to help feed the child. If it is the child's behaviour that is identified as the problem, then a psychologist's expertise would be indicated. Eating out may be a problem, however familiarization with popular commercial menus will provide ideas for the carer. For example, many venues serve thickshakes which, if transferred to the appropriate cup, can provide a perfect consistency for some children requiring thickened drinks.

Helpers

All people who could possibly be involved with feeding the child should be identified. Total reliance upon one main carer should be discouraged as this can be so frustrating. Other members of the family, grandparents, friends, respite care, social service family support, students, volunteers can all give support at mealtimes. The carer should be encouraged to let another person help with at least one meal a week. Liaison with the health visitor or social worker and statutory agencies, such as a meal at a family centre once a week, gives this needed respite. Training and support should be offered to the helpers and they can be involved in the assessment and review process.

Prompts

The use of prompts at mealtimes prepares a child for eating or drinking. It helps him to understand what is expected of him and he is therefore more likely to be successful. Prompts can be given visually e.g. an environment with other people eating, mirrors, seeing the food being prepared or arriving at the table. Physical prompts such as the smell of food, stroking the lower lip with the spoon or giving very small amounts allowing time for the child to experience the taste, texture and temperature of the food can all be used. Verbal prompts promote the awareness of the concepts of eating, telling the child what he is doing as it occurs. Repetitive phrases throughout the meal help the child know what he is doing e.g. 'bite', 'chew' and 'swallow.' Assessment will suggest which combination will be preferred by the child; however consistency by all helpers is important.

Documentation

A clear picture of the child's feeding capabilities should be documented. Assessment tools [20] based on normal development provide an excellent aid to identifying the movement and sensory patterns that create limitations. With this information precise short and long term goals can be set.

Small goals

Skills should be broken down into small short term goals as these are more likely to enable the child to succeed e.g. 'encourage him to chew by placing toys and hard foods such as sticks of carrot in the side of the mouth once a day' could be a goal to help him develop chewing skills. Regular review of the child's progress will provide the baseline for building upon these skills. Ideally more small goals will be added according to the child's needs, speed of learning, and opportunity to practise. When a child has been unable to achieve a goal it needs to be assessed whether he has been given long enough to practise, whether the task has been impractical for the carer to carry out and why, and whether the carer has understood the purpose of carrying out the task. If necessary the goal needs redesigning, checking that the carer feels able to carry it out. Possibly other carers, in school for example, can practise the skill with the child.

Demonstrating technique

A model of how the task is best carried out provides the carer with a clear picture of what is expected. Also this can increase the empathy of the demonstrator by giving a better understanding of difficulties experienced by the feeder at every meal.

Support literature

Pre-printed diet sheets rarely accommodate the needs of children with feeding difficulties. Individualized lists of foods of the correct consistency including suggestions and/or recipes for meals and snacks are the most useful to a carer. This is particularly important if a child cannot eat a commonly used food such as bread. Foods which can quickly be added to other staples like instant mashed potatoes, grated cheese, cream cheese, mashed tinned fish, corned beef, pâté, avocado pear, frozen chopped spinach all provide variety without too much preparation time. When lists of food/drinks are given, as many convenience foods as possible should be included. The main reason for this advice is to help reduce the time involved with the preparation of foods and also to help reduce the guilt that some carers may feel when relying heavily upon convenience foods. Carers should be helped to select value for money convenience foods that can be easily modified to the correct texture for the child.

Specific feeding techniques

These exist for a number of feeding problems. The management of these problems will normally be addressed by a speech therapist or OT. Detailed explanations of these techniques are provided in various publications [17]. They include passivity and slow oral response; spasm, grimace and gagging; chewing; swallowing and drinking.

Specialist approaches

These can aid in either assessment or in helping some children to develop awareness of certain oromotor skills.

Videofluoroscopy A video recording showing the passage of radiopaque substance from mouth to oesophagus.

Exeter lip sensor A visual or auditory feedback system to encourage partial or complete lip closure.

Orthodontic plate With roughened alveolar ridge or bead contact points, this can enhance awareness and tongue tip movement.

Palatal training device This device may help a child with sensory loss by stimulating swallowing, improve soft palate function and prevent tongue humping.

Electopalatography This individualized orthodontic plate with electrodes can provide a visual picture of tongue position and movements.

REFERENCES

1 Webb Y Feeding and nutrition problems of physically and mentally handicapped children in Britain: a report. *J Hum Nutr*, 1980, **34** 241–285.
2 Karle IP *et al.* Nutritional status of cerebral palsied children. *J Am Diet Ass*, 1961, **38** 22–26.
3 Krick J, Van Duyne M The relationship between oral-motor involvement and growth: a pilot study in paediatric population with cerebral palsy. *J Am Diet Ass*, 1984, **84**(5) 555–559.
4 Tobis J *et al.* A study of growth patterns in cerebral palsy. *Arch Phys Med*, 1961, **42** 475–481.
5 Thommessen M *et al.* Feeding problems, height and weight in different groups of disabled children. *Acta Paediatr Scand*, 1991, **80** 527–533.
6 Binns C Assessment of growth and nutritional status. *J Food Nutr*, 1985, **42** 119–125.
7 Patrick J *et al.* Rapid correction of wasting in children with cerebal palsy. *Dev Med Child Neurol*, 1986, **29** 734–739.

8 Shapiro BK *et al.* Growth of severely impaired children: neurological versus nutritional factors. *Dev Med Child Neurol*, 1986, **28** 729–733.

9 Bax M Editorial: Eating is important. *Dev Med Child Neurol*, 1989, **31** 285–286.

10 Matisen B *et al.* Oral-motor dysfunction and failure to thrive among inner-city infants. *Dev Med Child Neurol*, 1989, **31** 293–302.

11 Cronk CE *et al.* Growth charts for children with Down syndrome: 1 month to 18 years of age. *Pediatrics*, 1988, **81** 102.

12 Van Dyke D *et al.* Problems in feeding. In: Van Dyke DC *et al.* (eds.) *Clinical Perspectives in the Management of Down Syndrome.* New York: Springer-Verlag, 1990.

13 Alexander R *Early Feeding, Sound Production and Pre-linguistic Cognitive Development in their Relationship to Gross Motor Development.* Madison, WI: Curative Rehabilitation Center, 1980.

14 Cronk CE Growth of children with Down syndrome: Birth to age three years. *Pediatrics*, 1978, **61** 564.

15 Rarick GL, Seefedlt V Observations from longitudinal data on growth in stature and sitting height of children with Down's syndrome. *J Mental Deficiency Res*, 1974, **18** 63.

16 Taylor Baer M *et al.* Nutrition assessment of the child with Down syndrome. In: Van Dyke DC *et al.* (eds.) *Clinical Perspectives in the Management of Down Syndrome.* New York: Springer-Verlag, 1990.

17 Chailey Heritage *Eating and Drinking Skills for the Child with Cerebral Palsy.* North Chailey, East Sussex: Chailey Heritage, 1993.

18 La Leche League Establishing breastfeeding for a baby with a cleft lip. *Midwifery Digest*, 1991, **1**(1) 71. Also available from La Leche League.

19 Campbell A Tube feeding: parental perspective. *Exceptional Parent*, 1988, April, 36–40.

20 Evans Morris S *Pre-Feeding Skills. A Comprehensive Resource for Feeding Devleopment.* (Therapy Skill Builders). Buckinghamshire: Winslow Press, 1987.

USEFUL ADDRESSES

Chailey Heritage
North Chailey, East Sussex BN8 4EF.

Down's Syndrome Association
153 Mitcham Road, Tooting, London SW17 0PG.

La Leche League
BM 3424, London WC1N 3XX. Tel. 071-242 1278.

CHAPTER 27

Failure to Thrive

The term 'failure to thrive' (FTT) is applied to infants and young children who do not achieve a normal or expected rate of growth. FTT was described by Holt in 1897 [1]:

> The history in severe cases is strikingly uniform. The following is the story most frequently told 'At birth the baby was plump and well nourished and continued to thrive for a month or six weeks while the mother was nursing him; at the end of that period circumstances made weaning necessary. From that time on the child ceased to thrive. He began to lose weight and strength, at first slowly and then rapidly, in spite of the fact that every known infant food was tried. As a last resort the child, wasted to a skeleton, is brought to the hospital.'

Classically FTT has been subdivided into two areas, 'organic' and 'non-organic' failure to thrive. This dichotomy is no longer thought to be appropriate as undernutrition is the primary cause of failure to grow appropriately in all cases of non-organic failure to thrive and in the majority of organic causes [2]. In medical conditions such as gastrointestinal disease, neurological disorders and congenital heart disease growth failure is due to an inadequate nutritional intake compared with requirements. In cases of FTT associated with behavioural factors such as inadequate parenting (including neglect and abuse), growth failure is still due to a low energy intake, not emotional deprivation [3].

WHEN DOES GROWTH RETARDATION BECOME A CAUSE FOR CONCERN?

In general, FTT is defined as a downward deviation of weight gain trajectory; corrections for prematurity should be made when plotting trajectories. Recently it has been suggested by Edwards et al. that the child's maximum weight centile achieved between 4–8 weeks is a better predictor of the centile at 12 months than is the birth centile [4]. Birthweight centile is largely determined by maternal influences such as age, parity, nutrition, smoking and alcohol habits during pregnancy. The child's own genotype may exert a greater influence by 4–8 weeks of age. FTT may then be defined as a downward deviation in weight across two or more major centiles from the maximum centile achieved at 4–8 weeks for a period of a month or more.

Since length is not as rapidly affected by undernutrition as weight (page 3), a weight that deviates from the height centile, or is persistently more than two major centiles below height centile, may be considered as FTT. Weight, height and head circumference should be monitored longitudinally and plotted on centile charts in suspected cases of FTT.

Stunting of length and head circumference usually indicates more chronic and severe malnutrition which is more difficult to reverse, and is strongly associated with long standing psychosocial deprivation or chronic disease. Delay in nutritional intervention or inadequate treatment may mean lifelong deficit in head circumference, even if weight and height can be normalized [5]. In addition to the growth failure there may be slowing or disruption of emotional, behavioural and social development. The criterion that the child gains weight in hospital (particularly where there is no apparent organic cause of FTT) is generally no longer accepted. Some children may have such major feeding difficulties that they may even lose weight during their admission to hospital.

INCIDENCE OF FTT

It is suggested that between 1 and 5% of paediatric hospital admissions exhibit FTT. This figure is likely to be even higher in some large paediatric centres covering a wide range of paediatric specialities. A study in Birmingham showed that approximately 15% of admissions were wasted and a similar number severely wasted. When subgroups, such as patients with chronic respiratory, cardiac or gastrointestinal disease were examined the figures were considerably higher [6]. The incidence of FTT in the population is not known, though it is considered to be more common in deprived inner city areas.

DEVELOPMENT OF FTT

Failure to thrive can be multifactorial in origin and causes are summarized in Table 27.1. FTT which has its onset in children under one year of age is more likely to have a primary physiological cause which interferes with energy intake or energy utilization, or the infant may be being actively deprived of food. Gastrointestinal disorders may lead to failure to thrive, despite an often seemingly adequate intake, through malabsorption (e.g. coeliac disease), bowel obstruction or vomiting (e.g. reflux). Children with congenital cardiac or respiratory defects may show FTT due to decreased nutritional intake because of anorexia, breathing problems or increased energy requirements caused by their disease. Children with neurological dysfunction may have problems with oro-motor development which can affect the ability to suck and swallow. They may also suffer from oral hypersensitivity and therefore refuse to feed. Children with metabolic disorders can present with FTT as a result of poor feeding or inability to utilize energy correctly.

Young children with FTT as a result of organic disease or functional problems often respond quickly to adequate refeeding once the underlying organic disease or functional problem is diagnosed and appropriate nutritional treatment given, both in terms of nutrients required and route of administration, e.g. infants with oromotor dysfunction may require nasogastric or gastrostomy feeding.

Failure to thrive in older infants or toddlers may be more greatly influenced by behavioural feeding problems as a result of interactions between the child and primary caregiver. Children with FTT and emotional or physical deprivation may have such chronic feeding disorders leading to inadequate nutritional intake that they also show secondary stunting of linear growth and head circumference.

MANAGEMENT OF FAILURE TO THRIVE

Overall assessment

Because FTT is such a multifactorial disorder there is much to recommend a multidisciplinary team approach to its management [2,7,8]. This will allow for assessment of nutritional status, dietary intake, medical status, oral function, psychosocial and developmental components. Potential membership of a multidisciplinary feeding team is given in Table 27.2.

It is not necessarily practical or desirable to have all children with FTT assessed individually by all members of a feeding team. However the existence of such teams enables team discussions of individual cases and increases awareness of other areas of man-

Table 27.1 Multifactorial causes of failure to thrive

Organic causes	e.g.	Gastrointestinal Metabolic Neurological Congenital cardiac anomalies
Functional problems	e.g.	Suck/swallow incoordination Oral hypersensitivity
Behavioural		
Social		

Table 27.2 Multidisciplinary feeding team

Paediatrician	e.g.	Community paediatrician Gastroenterologist Neurologist
Dietitian		
Clinical psychologist		
Speech and language therapist		
Nurse		
Physiotherapist/Occupational therapist		
Social worker		
Health visitor		

Table 27.3 Failure to thrive – areas for assessment

Underlying organic disease

Nutritional status – anthropometry

Nutritional intake

Feeding history

Oromotor function

Feeding behaviour

Social assessment

Developmental assessment

agement. Areas for assessment in FTT are given in Table 27.3.

Treatment

The treatment of FTT has to be geared to the individual needs of the patient.

Underlying organic disease, when treated, may lead to improvement in nutritional status by either improvement in appetite by treatment of the underlying disorder (e.g. cardiac anomalies), correction of malabsorption (e.g. cystic fibrosis), or by treatment with correct diet (e.g. coeliac disease, certain metabolic disorders).

Many cases of FTT are not found to have any underlying organic cause. In addition, by the time of referral a proportion of children with underlying organic disease also have non-organic components to their problems, e.g. oral hypersensitivity, self-induced vomiting, food refusal. Treatment of such cases of FTT needs to recognize the varying components of the individual child's problem and be planned accordingly. The long term natural history of a particular disorder may need to be considered, e.g. handicapped children with severe oromotor dysfunction will continue to have this problem as efforts to improve oromotor function have not been shown to be successful [9] despite employing several techniques to improve feeding [10].

Nutritional management

Assessment of requirements

Following assessment of anthropometry and nutritional intake a strategy for catch-up growth has to be planned. Diets which only cover age-specific requirements (e.g. Department of Health Dietary Reference Values, 1991) for energy and protein will not normally provide for catch-up growth [7]. Diets based on normal requirements will usually allow for maintenance of growth along the centile to which the child has fallen. Additional protein and energy will be required for catch-up growth.

A formula for predicting energy requirements for catch-up growth in infants and young children has been suggested [10]:

$$\text{kcal/kg} = \frac{120 \times \text{ideal weight for height (kg)}}{\text{actual weight (kg)}}$$

This may mean an intake of 1.5–2 times the normal recommended energy requirements for age.

Additional protein above the reference nutrient intake (RNI) for age will be needed for periods of increased growth velocity. A minimum of 9% energy from protein has been shown to be necessary in order to achieve maximum nitrogen retention in malnourished children [11], although care must be taken when advising high protein intakes if there is any risk of renal insufficiency.

Vitamins, minerals and trace element requirements are increased during periods of rapid growth, and a suitable supplement should be included if the diet is thought to be inadequate. No guidelines exist, but intakes should be at least appropriate for the proposed energy intake.

Initially weight gain may be rapid, followed by a gradual deceleration until the child's normal centile is reached. Care needs to be taken during the period of catch-up growth in stunted children that carers do not start to limit intake because of fears that the child is becoming obese. Usually weight is regained before an increase in linear growth occurs [3].

Achieving nutritional requirements

The most suitable method of achieving an adequate nutritional intake must be assessed and will depend on the individual needs of the child. The following aspects of feeding need to be considered:

Provision of regular meals and snacks Such provision should include a variety of foods where possible. It will be necessary to devise a regimen consisting of a number of small meals, snacks and nutrient-dense drinks throughout the day if large quantities are not tolerated.

Texture of food Some children may have passed the critical stage in the acceptance of different textures. If children are not given 'lumpy' or textured foods at around 6–7 months of age, they may not accept these textures later [12]. Children with poor oromotor function who are at risk of aspirating liquids may require thickened fluids (page 64). For infants and children who are failing to thrive the use of a starch-based thickener is recommended, as this provides additional energy, rather than the hemicellulose types which have no additional nutrients.

Use of dietary supplements Supplements of protein, fat and carbohydrate can be used to fortify normal foods such as milk, tea, cereal, desserts, soup, yoghurt. Supplements are listed on page 8 and manufacturers generally provide information and recipes for their use. For infants under the age of one year, supplementation of a formula feed may be sufficient (Table 1.9), but they may need supplementation of solid foods in the form of extra sugar, glucose or glucose polymer added to the weaning diet. Older children may need foods supplemented in addition to energy-dense fruit drinks and fortified milkshakes. It is important to re-emphasize that care should be taken to ensure that if energy or protein supplements are used, requirements for vitamins, minerals and trace elements must be met either from the diet or by means of a supplement (Table 1.11).

Use of prepackaged nutrient-dense and energy-dense supplements These consist either of high carbohydrate fruit-based drinks such as Hycal and Fortical or supplemented milk-based drinks in a powder or liquid form. Examples of powdered supplements are Build-Up and Complan; liquid drinks include Fortisip and Fresubin. Milk based nutrient-dense drinks are normally fortified with additional micronutrients, and it is often not necessary to use a separate supplement if sufficient quantities are consumed. Fruit-based high energy drinks are not fortified. These drinks may be prescribable (see below). In addition there are a large number of proprietary fruit drinks and milk shakes on the market, which can also be used, although they are not generally supplemented with micronutrients.

Use of enteral feeding If the child has severe FTT and it is not possible to achieve a reasonable intake orally, enteral feeding (nasogastric or gastrostomy) will be required initially (page 25). The use of overnight continuous feeds is preferred, as this leaves the daytime free for establishing oral feeding.

Although 'failure to thrive' is only recognized as providing grounds for the prescription of starch-based thickening agents, it is usually possible to obtain supplements on prescription if growth retardation is due to organic causes. It may be more difficult to obtain items on prescription for non-organic FTT, and it is important to provide the family doctor with a full explanatory letter to justify such a request.

Other management

Assessment by other members of the multidisciplinary team will help in providing additional guidelines on treatment other than nutrition.

Assessment of oromotor function

Assessment of children with FTT (particularly those with food refusal and neurodevelopmental problems) by a speech and language therapist is important. Such assessments, often in conjunction with videofluoroscopy, will identify children with oromotor dysfunction (i.e. inability to coordinate the suck/swallow reflex) who are likely to aspirate feeds and will require non-oral feeding. They will also detect oral hypersensitivity and be able to help with desensitization programmes.

Assessment by physiotherapist/occupational therapist

Children with failure to thrive who are hypotonic and have poor head control will be helped in their eating if they have seating which offers suitable support for the head and body and also foot support which will allow the child to brace his body.

Behavioural assessment and management

Because in so many cases of FTT the lack of adequate nutritional intake is compounded by behavioural problems, any attempts at improving nutritional intake to achieve catch-up growth should be improved by a behavioural modification programme. Assessment by the clinical psychologist will provide insights into the child's feeding behaviour problems. Observation of the child being fed by his primary caregiver in the normal feeding environment gives information on any abnormal feeding behaviour e.g. methods of food refusal, interaction between child and caregiver.

Abnormal feeding behaviour causing food refusal can be caused by several factors [8], e.g.:

Learned food aversion The child may have had an experience of vomiting which he has associated with ingestion of a particular food, even though the vomiting may not have been caused by the food.

Lack of positive learning experiences with certain foods It is suggested that there may be a sensitive period, possibly between 4–6 months, in which taste preference is acquired through dietary experience. If a child has not been exposed to a wide range of tastes he may refuse to eat a wide variety of foods.

Developmental stage Especially when he is over 12 months of age the child may be exerting more autonomy, such as wanting only to self-feed and so refusing spoonfeeds, and refusing to accept new foods.

Poor parent-child interactions The child needs to control his own behaviour, e.g. needs to signal satiety. If the parent does not respond to these satiety signals the child may then increase behavioural signals by, for example, headturning, screaming, spitting, throwing food, struggling, vomiting. Once a child is showing signs of satiety, i.e. refusing any more food, further attempts to get the child to take more are unlikely to succeed.

Feeding behaviour modification includes:

- no force feeding
- a pleasant atmosphere for feeding – if there are tensions between the child and primary caregiver another person may need to be involved in feeding
- shared mealtimes, unless the child is very young and easily distracted

Table 27.4 Failure to thrive – treatment

Diagnosis and treatment of underlying organic cause
Provision of adequate nutrition for catch-up growth
Provision of appropriate method of nutritional support
Behavioural modification programme
Desensitization programmes for oral hypersentivity

- positive reinforcement of good feeding behaviour; aberrant feeding behaviour should be ignored e.g. by turning the face away from the child
- a time limit for mealtimes
- closely spaced mealtimes are a possibility, to maximize the opportunity for feeding practice and to reduce pressure to eat at any one meal.

In summary there are often multifactorial causes for FTT. The treatment of FTT benefits from a team approach, encompassing diagnosis of any underlying organic cause, assessment of nutritional intake, oromotor function and feeding behaviour. Treatment may need to be multifaceted if the child is to thrive and develop normal feeding behaviour (Table 27.4).

REFERENCES

1 Holt LE *The Diseases of Infancy and Childhood*. New York: Appleton, 1987.
2 Skuse D Failure to thrive: current perspectives. *Current Paediatr*, 1992, 105–110.
3 Frank DA, Zeisal SA Failure to thrive. *Pediatr Clin N Am*, 1988, **35** 1187–1206.
4 Edwards AGK *et al.* Recognising failure to thrive in early childhood. *Arch Dis Childh*, 1990, **65** 1263–1265.
5 Woolston JL *Eating and Growth Disorders in Infants and Children*. Newbury Park CA: Sage Publications, 1991: 21–35.
6 Moy RJD, Smallman S, Booth IW Malnutrition in a UK children's hospital. *J Hum Nutr Diet*, 1990, 3(2) 93–100.
7 Peterson KE, Washington J, Rathburn JM Team management of failure to thrive. *J Am Dietetic Assoc*, 1984, 84(7) 810–815.
8 Harris G, Booth IW The nature and management of eating disorders in pre-school children. In: Cooper P, Stein A (eds) *Monographs in Clinical Paediatrics: Feeding Problems and Eating Disorders*. Switzerland: Harwood Academic Publishers, 1991.
9 Ottenbacher K, Scoggins A, Wayland J The effectiveness of oral sensory-motor therapy with the severely

and profoundly developmentally disabled. *Occupational Therapy J Research*, 1981, **1** 147–160.

10 MacLean WC *et al.* Nutritional management of chronic diarrhoea and malnutrition: primary reliance on oral feeding. *J Paediatr*, 1990, **97** 316–323.

11 Jackson AA Protein requirements for catch-up growth. *Proc Nutr Soc*, 1990, **49** 507–516.

12 Illingworth RS, Lister J The critical or sensitive period, with reference to certain feeding problems in infants and children. *J Paediatr*, 1964, **65** 839–848.

FURTHER READING

Crane S Feeding the handicapped child – a review of intervention strategies. *Nutr Health*, 1987, **5** 109–118.

CHAPTER 28

Children from Ethnic Minorities and those following Cultural Diets

The UK is the home of a multicultural and multi-ethnic society. Immigration occurred mainly during the late 1950s and early 1960s in response to labour shortages and, therefore, the main ethnic minority communities are situated near large industrialized cities. These immigrants have brought with them a wide diversity of cultures, including dietary beliefs and practices, that have to fit into their new lifestyles. Nutritionally adequate diets may be hard to achieve when people suddenly find themselves in an environment very different from their homeland.

Infants and children of any age have special dietary requirements. It is essential, therefore, that religious and cultural attitudes towards diet are known in order to achieve optimal growth and development among these populations. Assessment of intake must be accurate and advice must be relevant to dietary custom so that it is both realistic and achievable.

Children are subject to many outside influences and often start to develop Westernized dietary ideas. With time these ideas are taken home and adopted by other members of the family. The extent of adoption of dietary practices differing from traditional customs is variable and so all diets must be assessed individually.

VEGETARIAN AND VEGAN DIETS

Vegetarianism and veganism are common dietary practices amongst many religious and ethnic groups. In addition, increasing numbers of the indigenous population are also restricting their dietary intake of meat and animal products for either humanitarian, ethical or health reasons. Table 28.1 gives a classification of vegetarian and vegan diets.

Infant feeding

Breast feeding is commonly practised among the indigenous vegetarian and vegan population. Providing the maternal diet is adequate, breast milk will be nutritionally complete for the first 4–6 months of the infant's life. Specific attention must be paid to the mother's vitamin D, calcium and iron intakes, and vegan mothers may require additional supplementation with vitamin B12 [1]. If breast feeding is not the method of choice a suitable infant formula must be chosen (Table 28.2). Infants should not be given home made or unmodified soya milks as these are often deficient in energy, protein, vitamins and minerals [1]. Goats' and ewes' milk are also contraindicated due to their nutritional inadequacy, high renal solute load and questionable microbiological safety [1,2].

Weaning

Breast milk or infant formula will provide sufficient nutrition until the infant is 4–6 months of age [2]. After this period solids should be introduced, gradually increasing flavours and textures (Table 28.3). Fruit, vegetables and pulses should be cooked with the skin on to preserve nutrients. This should then be removed to avoid an excessive fibre intake which adds further bulk to the diet and may also bind certain nutrients inhibiting their absorption [3]. Pulses should be cooked thoroughly to destroy toxins such as trypsin inhibitors and haemaglutinins which may cause diarrhoea and vomiting [1]. As the child gets older he should be encouraged to take 500 mls of full fat cows' or approved soya milk daily or the equivalent in cheese or yoghurt [1].

Table 28.1 Classification of vegetarianism and veganism

	Foods excluded	Protein source		Nutrient at risk of deficiency
Partial vegetarian	Red meat Offal	Poultry Fish Milk Cheese Yoghurt	Eggs Beans Lentils Nuts	Iron
Lacto-ovo vegetarian	Red meat Offal Fish Poultry	Milk Cheese Yoghurt Eggs	Beans Lentils Nuts	Iron
Lacto vegetarian	Red meat Offal Poultry Fish Eggs	Milk Cheese Yoghurt	Beans Lentils Nuts	Iron Vitamin D
Vegan	Red meat Offal Fish Poultry Eggs Milk Cheese Yoghurt	Beans Lentils Nuts		Protein Energy Iron Fat-soluble vitamins Vitamin B2 Vitamin B12 Calcium Zinc

Table 28.2 Infant formulas suitable for vegetarian and vegan children

Milk based	Soya based
Cow & Gate Premium	InfaSoy*
Cow & Gate Plus	Wysoy*
SMA Gold	Prosobee*
SMA White	OsterSoy*
Farley's First Milk	Isomil
Farley's Second Milk	
Aptamil	
Milumil	

Protein hydrolysates (for therapeutic use only)
Nutramigen
Pregestimil
Pepti-Junior
Neocate*

* Suitable for vegans

Table 28.3 Suitable vegetarian and vegan weaning foods [1,8]

3–4 months	Baby rice** Fruit and vegetables purées (cooked)
4–7 months	Rusk** Weetabix Pulse and lentil purées (well cooked) Pulse and vegetable purées Pulse and cereal purées Fruit purées Milk puddings or custards (cows'* or soya milk based)
7–9 months	Introduce lumps to the above foods Wholegrains Bread (white and wholemeal) Pasta and rice Finely ground nuts Dried fruits Cheese e.g. cheese sauces* Eggs e.g. savoury egg custards* Tofu and Quorn

* Suitable for vegetarians only
** Milk-free varieties for vegans

Children

Milk gradually provides less of the total nutrient intake and extra care is needed to ensure nutritional adequacy.

To provide optimal nutrition a vegetarian or vegan diet should be well balanced containing two to three protein foods daily along with cereals, vegetables, fruits and fats (Table 28.4). Vegetable and pulse proteins have a lower concentration and range of essential amino acids than protein from animal or fish sources and, therefore, careful planning of menus with pulse and cereal combinations is necessary to provide sufficient protein of high biological value [1,4]. The intake of energy-dense foods may also be low in the vegan diet which can lead to failure to thrive. The protein and energy content of the diet can be increased by the use of nuts and beans, together with oils for additional energy. Nut butters can be used to increase the energy content of finger foods; however, the nuts should be finely ground to avoid the danger of inhalation [1].

A daily vitamin supplement such as 0.6 mls Abidec is beneficial for both vegetarian and vegan children and should be given from the age of six months to five years [2]. In addition, a daily supplement of $1-2\,\mu g$ vitamin B12 may be required for vegan children [1,4].

Table 28.4 Sample vegetarian or vegan menu plan

Breakfast	Cereal + milk or milk substitute
	Wholemeal OR white bread + margarine + peanut butter OR yeast extract
	Egg*
	Diluted fresh orange juice
Dinner	Bean OR nut based dish OR cheese* based dish
	Vegetables OR salad
	Bread, potato, pasta OR rice
	Fruit OR fruit crumble/pie/sponge* + custard (cows'* or soya milk) OR milk pudding (cows' milk* or soya based)
Tea	Lentil or bean burgers OR bean soup OR baked beans OR egg*
	Bread + margarine
	Fruit OR yoghurt or fromage frais (cows' milk* or soya based)
Snacks	Nuts, toast, biscuits, crisps, fruit, cake

* Suitable for vegetarians only

As the availability of iron from vegetarian and vegan sources may be poor, it is important to give a vitamin C rich food at the same time as this will increase the bio-availability of iron.

When looking at the NACNE and COMA recommendations for dietary fat intake, a vegan diet is often construed as 'healthy' [5,6]. The resultant diet may, however, as well as being low in total energy, contain a poor quality of fat. Docosahexaenoic acid (22:6n-3), which is believed to play an important role in the health of the retina and central nervous system, has been found to be absent from vegan diets. For this reason it has been suggested that vegans should use oils with a low linoleic:alpha-linolenic acid ratio such as soya bean and rapeseed oil [7].

Regular assessment of growth and development is of paramount importance. There have been many conflicting studies examining the dietary intake, growth and development of vegan children [4,7]. In general, the greater the restriction of animal products the higher the risk of nutrient deficiency. Table 28.5 gives sources of nutrients which could be deficient in the diets of vegan children.

Zen macrobiotic diets

The Zen macrobiotic principle originates from Japan and is based on the correct balance between Yin

Table 28.5 Sources of nutrients at risk of deficiency in a vegan diet [8,15]

Nutrient	Vegan sources	
Riboflavin	Wheat germ	Avocados
	Almonds**	Soya beans
	Green leafy vegetables	Fortified soya milk
	Yeast extract* e.g. Marmite Tastex	
Vitamin B12	Fortified cereals	Yeast extracts*
	Fortified soya milk	Tofu
	Soya meat analogues	Quorn
Vitamin D	Fortified margarine	Fortified cereals
	Fortified soya milk	Sunlight
Calcium	Fortified soya milk	Hard water
	Green leafy vegetables	Sunflower seeds**
	Legumes	Sesame seeds
	White bread	Almonds**
	Cashew nuts**	
Iron	Fortified cereals	Nuts**
	Wholegrain cereals	Dried fruit
	Wholegrain bread	Molasses
	Green leafy vegetables	Cocoa
	Pulses	Curry powder
	Legumes	Quorn
	Tofu	
Essential fatty acids	Oils	Nuts**
	Wholegrains	Seeds

* Should be used with care in children under the age of two years due to high salt content
** Should not be given to children under the age of two years unless finely ground

(positive) and Yang (negative) foods. This balance is believed to keep spiritual, mental and physical well-being. The goal is achieved by working through ten levels of dietary elimination. Animal products, fruit and vegetables are gradually removed from the diet until the individual reaches the ultimate goal of consuming brown rice only. Fluids are also severely restricted [8].

This type of diet is nutritionally inadequate for any child. Marked growth retardation associated with muscle wasting and a delay in gross motor and language development, due to lack of energy and protein in macrobiotic weaning diets, has been documented [9,10]. Deficiencies of vitamins B12, D, thiamin and calcium and iron have also been observed [11,12,13,14].

Fruitarian diets

Fruitarian diets are based on fruit and uncooked fermented cereals and seeds. They are nutritionally inadequate for children of any age and can lead to severe protein energy malnutrition, anaemia and multiple vitamin and mineral deficiencies [4].

ASIAN DIETS

The Asian community represent the largest ethnic minority group in the UK. The communities consist of people who migrated directly from India, Pakistan, Bangladesh and those who came via East Africa [16]. Immigration is now strictly limited by legislation. The population, however, continues to expand due to families being born in the UK. Dietary customs are largely based on the religious and cultural beliefs of the three main religious groups (Moslems, Hindus and Sikhs). Great dietary variance is also observed between these groups as the diet in the homeland is affected by income and geographical area [16,17,18].

Hindus

Approximately 30% of the Asian population in the UK are Hindu. The majority come from the Gujarat region of India, although some are from the Indian Punjab and East Africa [16,19,20]. Hindus believe that the soul is eternal and, therefore, in reincarnation.

Dietary customs

The caste system dictates who can prepare and share food [16]. A restriction on eating beef was introduced in 800 BC as Hindus regard the cow as sacred. It is also unusual for them to eat pork as the pig is thought to be unclean, though other meats are acceptable (Table 28.6). Devout Hindus believe in the doctrine of Ahisma (not killing) and are, therefore, vegetarian. Some will eat dairy products and eggs whilst others refuse eggs on the ground that they are a potential source of life. A minority of Hindus practise veganism.

Wheat is the main staple food eaten by Hindus in the UK. This is used to make chapattis, puris and parathas. Ghee (clarified butter) and oil are used extensively in cooking [16].

Most Hindus fast on three days a year to celebrate the birthdays of the Lords Shiva (March), Rama (April) and Krishna (August). In addition to these

Table 28.6 Asian religious groups [16,17,18]

Group	Religion	Language	Staple	Dietary customs
Hindus	Hinduism	Hindi Gujarati	Millet Wheat Rice	No beef Often no pork No alcohol Often vegetarian or vegan
Moslems	Islam	Urdu Bengali Gujarati Punjabi	Rice Millet Wheat	No pork Halal meat No alcohol No fish without scales
Sikhs	Sikhism	Punjabi Hindi	Wheat	No beef Often no pork No Halal meat

days orthodox Hindus may also fast once or twice every week. Fasting lasts from dawn to dusk and varies from avoiding all foods except those considered pure, such as rice, fruit and yoghurt, to total food exclusion [16,19].

Moslems

Moslems comprise approximately 30% of the Asian population in the UK, the majority originating from Pakistan and Bangladesh [16,20]. Moslems practise the Islamic religion, Allah is their god and the prophet Mohammed is his final messenger.

Dietary customs

The Koran provides Moslems with their food laws. The consumption of pork, alcohol, carnivorous animals, fish without scales and some birds is forbidden [16]. These foods which are to be strictly avoided are called Haraam. All meat and poultry must be ritually slaughtered to render it Halal and, therefore, legitimate to eat [16,20]. Wheat, usually in the form of chapattis, is the staple cereal eaten by Moslems from Pakistan, whereas those from Bangladesh eat more rice [16,18]. Cooking oil is used in preference to ghee.

During the lunar month of Ramadan Moslems fast between sunrise and sunset. Children under the age of 12 and the elderly are exempt from fasting. People who are ill, pregnant, menstruating or on a long journey are excused, but are however expected to fast at a later date. Unfortunately, many pregnant women will fast along with the rest of the family during

Ramadan as they find it more convenient [16,19]. The Koran also dictates that children should be breast fed up to the age of two years [16].

Sikhs

The remaining 40% of the Asian population in the UK are Sikh. Sikhism is a relatively new religion originating in the Indian Punjab in the 14th century. Sikhs believe in reincarnation and in one personal god who is eternal, the creator of the universe and the source of all being [16,19]. Devout Sikhs undergo Amarit, a special kind of confirmation where certain practices must be followed. Prayers must be said everyday and Sikhs must not drink alcohol, smoke or eat Halal meat. They must also adhere to a strict ethical code and wear the five signs of Sikhism: Kesh (uncut hair), Kara (steel or silver bangle), Kanga (comb), Kirpa (small symbolic dagger) and Kaccha (special undergarments).

Dietary customs

Most Sikhs will not eat pork or beef, but some will eat lamb, poultry, fish, eggs and dairy produce. Vegetarianism is common, with eggs and dairy produce usually being eaten [16,19].

Wheat and to a lesser extent rice are the main staples eaten, and ghee and oil are used in cooking [16]. Devout Sikhs will fast once to twice weekly, and most will fast on the first day of the Punjabi month or when there is a full moon. This again varies from total food exclusion to eating pure foods only [19].

Common Asian dietary customs

Many of the Asian people in the UK share dietary customs despite their varying religious and geographical background (Table 28.7). Traditional dietary customs have been retained by many members of the Asian community living in the UK, in particular those originating from Pakistan and Bangladesh. There is, however, an increasing consumption of Westernized foods, especially convenience foods. The extent of adoption of these foods is variable, tending to be greater in the younger generations and those who have lived in the UK for some time [16].

At breakfast time chapatti, paratha, bread and occasionally hard boiled or fried eggs are traditionally eaten. The two main meals, usually eaten at lunch time and in the evening, are based around the staple which is served with a curry [17,18,19]. Most curries are based on vegetables, pulses, nuts and seeds and, even if allowed, very little meat, fish or poultry is used. Most foods, including spices are usually fried before being added to the curry, which is then served with homemade chutneys, side salads of tomato and onion, and yoghurt [19,20]. Very little hard cheese is eaten; paneer, an Asian soft curd cheese, is preferred [19]. Meals are usually served with tea which is made with hot milk and sugar, although English tea is becoming more popular [19]. Traditionally Asians rarely eat

Table 28.7 Foods commonly eaten by the Asian population in the UK [21,22,23]

Food	Nutrients	Method of cooking	
Cereals			
Wheat	Energy	Chapatti	Samosa
	B vitamins	Paratha	Pakora
		Popadom	Poori
		Bhagi	
Rice		Boiled	Fried
Semolina		Porridges	
Ground rice		Sweetmeats	
Tubers			
Arvi/colocasia root	Energy	Boiled	
Cassava		Fried	
Taro tuber		Curries	
Yam			
Vegetables			
Ackee Okra	Vitamin A	Boiled	
Bringal Pepper	Riboflavin	Fried	
Cho cho/chayote	Folic acid	Curries	
Fenugreek leaves	Vitamin C	Chutneys	
Bitter gourd/darela	Iron	Pickles	
Kantola	Calcium		
Patra leaves	Fibre		
Spinach			
Peas beans and nuts			
Balor/valor beans	Energy	Curries	
Blackgram/urad gram	Protein	Dahls	
Chickpeas/bengal gram	B vitamins		
Cluster beans/guar	Iron		
Coconut	Calcium		
Red lentils/masur dahl	Fibre		
Mung/moong beans			
Papri beans			
Pigeon peas/red gram			
Lima beans			

Table 28.7 (continued)

Food	Nutrients	Method of cooking
Furits		
Guava, lychee, mango	Vitamin A	Raw
Paw paw/papaya	Vitamin C	Curries
Indian gooseberries	Fibre	Chutneys
Dried fruits		
Meat and fish		
Many types	Protein	Curries
(see Table 28.6)	Fat-soluble	Roast
	vitamins	
	Iron	
Dairy products		
Milk	Energy	Drinks
Yoghurt	Protein	Raw
Cheese/paneer	Vitamin A	Boiled
Eggs	Riboflavin	Fried
	Nicotinic acid	
	Vitamin D	
	Iron	
	Calcium	
Fats and oils		
Ghee/clarified butter	Energy	Frying
Vegetable oil	Essential fatty	Spreading
Margarine	acids	

snacks, although Western snack foods are increasing in popularity. Traditional Asian savoury snacks (usually reserved for celebrations only) are high in fat and the sweetmeats are often very high in refined sugar.

Many Asians believe that foods have heating and cooling effects on the body. These hot and cold foods should be eaten in a correct balance to achieve a healthy state. Certain hot foods may cause symptoms such as constipation, sweating and body fatigue whilst certain cold foods may lead to strength and happiness. Foods may also be used to treat a condition, for example hot foods should be avoided during pregnancy and cold ones avoided when breast feeding [17,19].

Infant feeding

Studies consistently report a lower breast feeding rate among Asians in the UK when compared with the Caucasian population [24,25,26,27] and Asians on the Indian subcontinent [28,29]. Unfortunately, bottle feeding is perceived as the Western ideal and there is

often a lack of education promoting breast feeding [16,24,26]. This problem is compounded by communication difficulties, overcrowded housing and the early return of the mother to work [1].

Higher hospital admission rates for bottle fed Asian babies have been reported. This may be due to difficulties in understanding the instructions on infant formula tins which can lead to poor hygiene and incorrect dilution of feeds [30].

Weaning

Good weaning practice may be compromised by social disadvantage, the varying quality, expense and availability of familiar Asian foods and the pressures of Westernization. Late weaning and prolonged breast feeding are commonly practised in infants who are born on the Indian subcontinent and those who have only been in the UK for a short time [25,26,27, 28,30,31]. On the Indian subcontinent it is considered safer to leave the child on breast milk and wean straight onto adult foods. In the UK late weaning may be partly due to the poor availability of suitable foods and lack of adequate and appropriate advice [32]. Some Asian infants who are born in the UK are weaned earlier [26,27,28,29], but are commonly given sweet proprietary weaning foods which are low in protein and iron [25,26,31]. This mainly occurs because mothers do not know the composition of savoury weaning products and cannot use these foods unless they are vegetarian [16]. There are no proprietary products made from Halal meat at present. Because of these problems mothers should be encouraged to cook savoury weaning foods at home. Suitable homemade Asian weaning foods are given in Table 28.8. The practice of sweetening milk and adding foods such as rusk, honey, Weetabix and baby rice to bottles is also common [16,26] and should be discouraged.

Many Asian infants are given cows' milk from the age of 5–6 months [16]. This practice can lead to a higher saturated fat and salt intake and a reduced vitamin D and iron intake than if breast milk or infant formula were continued [2]. Feeding development is also often delayed with late conversion from bottle to cup and a very late progression onto family foods [16,26,31]. It is not unusual for a two year old to derive the majority of his nutrition from bottles of cows' milk and sweetened fruit drinks.

There are many ways in which infant feeding practices amongst the Asian population can be improved:

Table 28.8 Suitable Asian weaning foods

4–6 months	
Puréed	Cauliflower and potato*
	Cauliflower and pea*
	Pea and potato*
	Aubergine and potato*
	Green vegetable and potato*
	Vegetable and cheese*
	Lentil and rice*
	Chickpea and marrow*
	Porridge
	Fruit purée
6–12 months	
	Introduce small lumps to the above foods
	Mild spices e.g. cumin and coriander may be used
	Introduce finger foods e.g. small pieces of chapatti

* A small amount of meat, poultry or fish may be added if eaten

- the teaching curriculum of all catering and health related training should include ethnic cultures, food and diet, so that effective education on all aspects of infant feeding can be given [31]. This training should be updated regularly [26]
- communication barriers must be overcome. Practical demonstrations, the use of bilingual interpreters and written advice in the Asian languages should be available [16,26,31]
- education promoting breast feeding should reach the parents before pregnancy, and support should be given while breast feeding [26]
- breast or formula milk should be given up to one year of age [26]
- sugary drinks should be avoided [26]
- infants should be weaned at 4–6 months of age [2]
- weaning advice should include the use of appropriate family foods in addition to commercial baby foods [16,26]
- salt, sugar, honey, or hot spices should not be added to bottles or weaning foods [17]
- advice should be given on foods rich in vitamin C, vitamin D and iron, as these nutrients may be at risk of deficiency [26]
- the cup should be introduced at six months to one year of age [26]
- vitamin drops should be given from the age of six months up to two years and preferably up to five years [2].

Further research is required to study nutrient intake and nutritional status of Asian infants, children and adolescents. Studies concerning lifestyle and health perceptions are also required to ensure that nutritional advice is culturally acceptable.

Nutritional problems commonly found in Asian children

Failure to thrive

There are many influences on growth, including diet and to a lesser extent family income, housing standards, maternal education, psychological stress and morbidity [16,25]. Low birthweight has been reported among Asians both in this country and in the country of origin [28,32,33]. Genetic factors and maternal undernutrition may be to blame [16,33]. Birthweight has, however, increased over the last 10 years, suggesting that genetic factors do not have a major influence. Longer birth intervals, fewer teenage pregnancies and improved nutrition are thought to be contributing factors [16].

Despite lower birthweights, some studies show that Asian babies and children appear to grow as well as the indigenous population [16,28,33]. In contrast other workers report that growth failure is common [30,34]. Because of these conflicting observations it is important that growth and the need for nutritional supplementation is assessed for the individual.

Iron deficiency anaemia

Iron deficiency anaemia has been described in Asian infants [30,35,36]. Inadequate dietary intake of iron is commonly related to the early introduction and excessive use of unfortified cows' milk in children who already have low iron stores [16]. There is, however, conflicting evidence regarding the adequacy of dietary iron intakes [25]. It is essential, therefore, that the diets of Asian children are assessed individually. Advice should include information on the use of foods rich in iron and vitamin C.

Megaloblastic anaemia

Megaloblastic anaemia due to vitamin B12 deficiency has been observed in some strict vegetarian and vegan Asians [20]. Education regarding vitamin B12 sources in the vegetarian diet is required and supplementation may be needed for the vegan diet.

Rickets

The steady decline in rickets in the UK was halted in the late 1960s and early 1970s when a number of cases appeared in immigrant families, mainly of Asian origin [30,31,37,38,39]. There is now evidence that the incidence is again in decline following large scale vitamin D supplementation [16]. Conflicting results have been shown from studies comparing vitamin D intakes of Asian and Caucasian children. [4,16,25].

In addition to dietary intake of vitamin D other factors such as low sunlight exposure, skin pigmentation, late weaning, high fibre and high phytate intakes may also contribute to the development of rickets in Asian children [4,16,30]. Until we have more information on the causes of rickets, vitamin supplementation is advisable for both infants and deficient pregnant women to help prevent neonatal hypocalcaemia and rickets [1,16]. The weaning diets of infants should include foods rich in vitamin D such as milk, eggs, oily fish, liver, fortified cereals and margarine [1,15,20].

Dental caries

Traditionally, sugary foods are reserved for celebrations and, therefore, do not play a major role in Asian diets. However, with increasing westernization, over consumption of refined sugar has become a problem. Asian mothers often add sugar to babies' bottles and give sweetened drinks for prolonged periods. These drinks are both laden with sugar and are acidic which can lead to dental decay [26]. Education regarding infant feeding with the restriction of quantity and frequency of sugar intake, the use of fluoride drops and toothpaste and frequent dental visits will all help to reduce the incidence of dental caries.

Obesity

With the increasing consumption of Western high sugar and fat foods the prevalence of obesity is increasing. In addition to restricting these foods advice on Asian foods and cooking techniques must be given. Dietary fat intake can be reduced by avoiding deep fried foods, reducing the oil or ghee used in cooking and restricting or not adding fat to chapattis. Dietary sugar can be reduced by avoiding the popular sweet sugary tea and Asian sweetmeats.

AFRO-CARIBBEAN DIETS

The Afro-Caribbean community is the second largest ethnic minority group in the UK [16,40].

Dietary patterns

The two main meals are taken at breakfast time and in the evening [41,42]. Traditional breakfasts include fried plantain, cornmeal porridge and fried dumplings. However, many dietary practices have now been adopted from British culture and these foods have largely been replaced by cereals and toast. The evening meal is more likely to contain traditional foods, especially with the younger generation who seem keen to retain their identification and culture. Cereals and tubers such as rice, green banana, yam and sweet potato form the main part of the diet [40]. These starchy foods are served with small amounts of meat or fish [41]. Traditionally preserved meat, fish and milk are eaten as the tropical climate in the homeland makes it difficult to keep these foods fresh [40]. Peas, beans, nuts and green leafy vegetables are widely used, often being made into homemade soups and stews which are well seasoned with herbs and spices [16]. Boiling, baking, frying, stewing, steaming and roasting are all commonly used cooking techniques for meat, fish and vegetables [40] (Table 28.9).

Rastafarians

A minority of the Afro-Caribbean population within the UK are Rastafarians. Dietary beliefs are based on laws laid down by Moses in Genesis that state certain types of meat should be avoided. However, many Rastafarians avoid meat completely to obey the commandment 'thou shalt not kill'. Vinegar, raisins, grapes and wine are also avoided by some Rastafarians as the Nazarite law states that fruits of the vine should not be eaten. Dietary restrictions are followed with varying degrees of strictness. The most orthodox are vegans and will eat only 'Ital' (natural) foods; chemicals and additives are thought to pollute the body and soul [40]. In addition, salt and alcohol are also prohibited. Many Rastafarians are socially deprived and often unemployed and are, therefore, unable to provide adequate nutrition for their children within the dietary code [16]. Less orthodox Rastafarians, although accepting the central tenets of 'Ital', will eat dairy prod-

Table 28.9 Foods commonly eaten by the Afro-Caribbean population in the UK [40,43]

Food	Nutrients	Method of cooking
Cereals		
Wheat	Energy	Boiled
Oats	B vitamins	Dumplings
Maize		Porridges
Rice		Bread
Tubers		
Green banana	Energy	Mashed
Sweet potato	B vitamins	Fried
Bread fruit	Vitamin C	Roasted
Yams		Stewed
Cassava		
Plantain		
Peas beans and nuts		
Red peas	Protein	Stews
Pigeon peas	B vitamins	Boiled
Coconut	Calcium	
Almonds	Iron	
Sesame seeds	Fibre	
Black eyed peas		
Broad beans		
Channa		
Cashews		
Pumpkin seeds		
Dark green leafy vegetables		
Cabbage	Vitamin A	Stews
Carrot	Vitamin C	Stir fry
Egg plant	Calcium	
Okra	Iron	
Callaloo		
Dasheen leaves		
Karela		
Pumpkin		
Fruit		
Avocado	Vitamin C	Fresh
Cashewfruit		Stewed
Guava		
Oranges		
Paw-Paw		
Sapodilla		
Mango		
Cane sugar		
Grapefruit		
Oteheite apple		
Passion fruit		
Pineapple		
Soursop		
Coolie		

Table 28.9 (continued)

Food	Nutrients	Method of cooking
Meat and fish		
	Protein	Fry
	Fat-soluble	Steam
Mainly chicken	vitamins	Roast
Many types of fish	Iron	Boil
		Stewed
		Bake
Eggs		
	Protein	Scrambled
	Vitamin A	Cake
	Vitamin D	Fritters
	Iron	Puddings
Fats and oils		
Coconut oil	Essential	Frying
Olive oil	fatty acids	Spreading
Margarine		Baking
Lard		
Vegetable oil		
Butter		
Suet		

ucts, small amounts of fish with scales, sea salt and other seasonings. The nutritional adequacy of these diets is much easier to achieve.

Infant feeding

Information on infant feeding in Afro-Caribbean communities in the UK is scanty; it is mainly influenced by the place of birth, knowledge of traditional practices and advice from relatives. In the homeland above 90% of women breast feed their babies initially. However, even in Africa, this is often short lived and exclusive breast feeding is rare [37]. The large scale marketing of infant formulas and the early return of women to work are implicated. Many Afro-Caribbean mothers avoid giving their babies colostrum and in its place give water, which is thought to cleanse the body before breast milk. This practice may reduce breast milk production and, therefore, also contribute to the low exclusive breast feeding rate both in this country and in Africa.

Table 28.10 Suitable Afro-Caribbean weaning foods

4–6 months	Rice or oat porridge
	Puréed fruit
	Puréed vegetables e.g. yam, peas, okra
	Puréed vegetables and meat or fish
	Puréed rice and vegetable
	Egg custard
7–12 months	Introduce:
	Small lumps to the above foods
	Mashed family foods avoiding highly seasoned foods
	Finger foods e.g. toast, biscuits, fruit

Weaning

Infants are traditionally weaned as early as one month of age and 45% are reported to be receiving food by three months [40,41,42]. In contrast late weaning is commonly observed within the orthodox Rastafarian population [1]. Common weaning solids include high starch foods with a low nutrient density such as cornmeal, oat or rice porridge. This practice may lead to energy, protein, vitamin and mineral deficiencies if continued for a long time [1,19,44,45]. More suitable weaning foods are shown in Table 28.10. There are also many suitable commercial baby foods which are now being used [40]. The common practice of adding thin porridge to bottles should be discouraged as it can lead to a delay in the weaning process. It is also common for infants to be given bush teas (infusions of herbs and leaves) as a cure for minor ailments [41]. Care should be taken that these are not given in preference to milk.

By the age of nine months most children are eating family foods with the diets having both traditional and Western influences [41].

Nutritional problems found in Afro-Caribbean children

Obesity

With the adoption of British dietary customs there has been an increased consumption of high fat and sugar convenience foods and drinks. This has led to an increased prevalence of obesity within Afro-Caribbean children. Advice given should take into consideration both traditional and westernized dietary practice.

Iron deficiency anaemia

Iron deficiency anaemia has been observed in Afro-Caribbean children living in the UK. The main causes are thought to be prolonged bottle feeding, late weaning onto foods with a low iron content and the early introduction and excessive use of cows' milk [16].

Megaloblastic anaemia

There have been reports of megaloblastic anaemia in Rastafarian children living in Jamaica [46,47]. Vegan children may require extra vitamin B12 supplementation.

Rickets

Rickets has been seen in Afro-Caribbean children [16,45]. Advice on dietary sources of vitamin D and calcium, and vitamin D supplementation is beneficial.

Lactose intolerance

There is a high incidence of lactose intolerance because of hypolactasia among the black population. A reduction in, and occasionally the avoidance of, the consumption of milk and other foods containing lactose, such as yoghurt, will usually relieve the symptoms (Table 6.4).

CHINESE DIETS

Chinese people represent the third largest ethnic minority group in the UK [48]. Over 25% are British born, the rest originate from the Caribbean, Hong Kong, Taiwan, China, Malaysia and Singapore [48]. Dietary habits vary according to the country and region of origin. Very few foods are avoided with the exception of pork which is not eaten by the Chinese Moslem population. Northern China has a cool climate favouring the growth of wheat, maize, sorghum and millet. These staples are often made into steamed bread, dumplings, pancakes or noodles [19,48]. Meals are often based on root vegetables such as sweet potato and turnip and very little meat is eaten. In contrast, because of the high rainfall, rice is the staple in Southern China. Fresh vegetables and fruit are also found in abundance [48]. In the East, due to the long coast line, fish and shellfish are plentiful. In the West livestock is reared and, therefore, the consumption of meat, milk and cheese is much higher [48].

Dietary patterns

Traditional breakfasts include rice porridge (congee) served either plain, or with liver, meat, salted fish, salted eggs or Chinese cheese and a soup made from rice and meat [19,48]. These traditional foods are, however, slowly being replaced by Western alternatives. The midday and evening meals consist of boiled rice or noodles and a variety of highly seasoned dishes such as fried or steamed meat and fish and stir fry vegetables. Raw food is rarely eaten as fertilizer in China commonly contains human manure. Meals are usually served with either China tea or a thin soup and are then followed with fruit. Sweet foods are usually reserved for special occasions [19,48].

The main health concerns are the high sodium intake associated with many of the preserved foods and seasonings used and the high fat and refined sugar intake associated with the increased consumption of Western convenience foods, especially by the younger generation [48]. A high incidence of lactose intolerance, due to hypolactasia, is also becoming apparent with the increased consumption of milk and other dairy products [48].

Yin and Yang foods

To Chinese people health is perceived as the maintenance of a sound body and mental state, rather than an absence of disease. Traditional Chinese medicine states that good health relies on the body's balance of two opposite elements, Yin (cold), which represents female energy and Yang (hot), which represents male energy [19,48]. In illness the balance becomes disturbed and the body becomes either too hot or too cold. Tolerance of Yin and Yang increases with age, thus an adult can eat a much wider variety of foods than can a child. The classification of foods varies: in general meat, duck, goose, oily fish, potatoes, coffee, nuts, herbs, spices, alcohol and fats are regarded as hot foods; fish, rice and some vegetables are neutral foods; chicken, certain fruits and vegetables and barley water are cold foods. Boiling and stir frying makes foods colder, steaming neutralizes, and stewing, deep fat frying, grilling and roasting all have a heating effect [19,48].

During pregnancy and after childbirth the woman's body is thought to become colder and, therefore, cold foods are avoided. Alcohol, ice cream, mutton, beef and fizzy drinks are also avoided. In addition, if the woman is breast feeding green vegetables and fruit are avoided because of concern that they may give the baby diarrhoea. As a consequence breast feeding mothers often have a high protein intake [48].

In the UK, Chinese women often return to work soon after childbirth which has led to a decrease in the rate and duration of breast feeding. Because infant formula is regarded as hot, bottle fed babies are often given frequent cooling drinks such as water or barley water. Most infants are weaned at three months of age, traditionally onto rice based porridges but more recently rusks and commercial baby foods are being used [48]. In general, infants and children are thought to have a hot equilibrium and, therefore, neutralizing or cooling foods are considered best for them. It is common practice for children to be given afternoon tea consisting of cooling foods such as bread, biscuits, cake, barley water and herb teas to counteract the heating effect of school meals [48].

VIETNAMESE DIETS

Some 75% of Vietnamese settlers in the UK are ethnic Chinese and, therefore, share many of the Chinese traditions [48].

Food habits

There are no forbidden foods, however certain unfamiliar foods such as lamb, ox liver, tinned or cooked fruit and some root vegetables may be avoided [19]. Rice is the main staple food and is served either boiled or fried with small amounts of meat and fish. Like Chinese food main dishes are often heavily seasoned and vegetables are lightly steamed or stir fried in oil or lard. Very little fresh milk, butter, margarine and cheese are used, due to both their lack of availability in Vietnam and the high incidence of lactose intolerance. Snacks of roasted nuts, sweet potatoes, rice or noodle soup, spring rolls and fresh fruit are frequently eaten. Common beverages include tea, coffee and fruit juice and alcohol is taken on special occasions [19].

The Vietnamese people observe hot and cold food principles similar to the Chinese. In contrast to the Chinese, however, pregnancy is regarded as a hot condition and, therefore, women eat less red meat and fish. A traditional stew called Keung Chow, made from pigs' trotters, boiled egg, vinegar and ginger is given to women after childbirth to help recovery and to celebrate the birth of the child. After childbirth women are encouraged to eat hot foods to regain their strength [19].

Nutrients at risk of deficiency

Calcium

Children are at risk of calcium deficiency especially if little milk and associated products are eaten [19]. The rice traditionally grown in Vietnam is a good source of calcium but is unavailable in Britain. Traditional Vietnamese fruit and vegetables also contain more calcium than British varieties [19].

Vitamin D

Deficiency has been noted in Vietnamese children. For this reason children may need Vitamin D supplementation [18].

REFERENCES

1 Taitz LS, Wardley BL Dietary variants. In: *Handbook of Child Nutrition*, Oxford: Oxford University Press, 1990: 47–56.

2 Committee on Medical Aspects of Food Policy *Present day practice in infant feeding. Report of a Working Party of the Panel on Child Nutrition.* London: HMSO, 1988.

3 British Dietetic Association *Children's Diet and Change.* Birmingham: BDA, 1987: 29–32.

4 Francis D *Nutrition for Children.* Oxford: Blackwell Scientific Publications, 1986. 49–54.

5 National Advisory Committee on Nutrition Education *Proposals for Nutritional Guidelines for Health Education in Britain.* London: Health Education Council, 1983.

6 Committee on Medical Aspects of Food Policy *Diet and Cardiovascular Disease. DHSS Report on Health and Social Subjects.* London: HMSO, 1984.

7 Sanders TAB, Manning J The growth and development of vegan children. *J Hum Nutr Diet,* 1992, **5** 11–21.

8 Vegetarianism and veganism. In: *Manual of Dietetic Practice.* Thomas B (ed.) Oxford: Blackwell Scientific Publications, 1988: 303–306.

9 Dagnelie PC *et al.* Nutritional status of infants aged 4–13 months on macrobiotic diets and matched omnivorous control infants: A population based mixed longitudinal study. 11: Growth and psychomotor development. *Eur J Clin Nutr,* 1989, **43** 325–338.

10 Dagnelie PC *et al.* Do children on macrobiotic diets show catch up growth? A population based cross sectional study in children aged 0–8 years. *Eur J Clin Nutr,* 1988, **42** 1007–1016.

11 Herens MC *et al.* Nutrition and mental development of 4–5 year old children on macrobiotic diets. *J Hum Nutr Diet,* 1992, **5** 1–9.

12 Dagnelie PC *et al.* Nutritional status of infants aged 4–18 months on macrobiotic diets and matched omnivorous control infants: A population based mixed longitudinal study. 1: Weaning patterns, energy and nutrient intake. *Eur J Clin Nutr,* 1989, **43** 311–323.

13 Dagnelie PC *et al.* Increased risk of vitamin B12 and iron deficiency in infants on macrobiotic diets. *Am J Clin Nutr,* 1989, **50** 818–824.

14 Dagnelie PC *et al.* High prevalence of rickets in infants on macrobiotic Diets. *Am J Clin Nutr,* 1990, **51** 202–208.

15 Paul AA, Southgate DAT *McCance and Widdowson's The Composition of Foods,* 4e. London: HMSO, 1978.

16 Health Education Authority *Nutrition in Minority Ethnic Groups: Asians and Afro-Caribbeans in the United Kingdom.* London: HEA, 1991.

17 *Weaning: An Information Pack for those Working with Asian Communities.* Bolton Health Authority Health Promotions Service, 1989. Available from Health Promotion Unit, Bolton HA, Bolton, Lancs.

18 Price SR Observations on dietary practices in India. *Hum Nutr: Appl Nutr,* 1984, **38A** 383–389.

19 Cultural minorities. In: Thomas B (ed.) *Manual of Dietetic Practice.* Oxford: Blackwell Scientific Publications, 1988: 307–312.

20 Hunt S Traditional Asian food customs. *J Hum Nutr,* 1977, **31** 245–248.

21 Holland B *et al. McCance and Widdowson's The Composition of Foods,* 5e. London: Royal Society of Chemistry/MAFF, 1991.

22 Tan SP, Wenlock RW, Buss DH *Immigrant Foods. The Second Supplement to McCance and Widdowson's The Composition of Foods.* London: HMSO, 1985.

23 Jaffrey M *Indian Cookery.* London: BBC Books, 1988.

24 Treuherz J, Cullinan TR, Saunders DI Determinants of infant feeding practice in East London. *Hum Nutr: Appl Nutr,* 1982, **36A** 281–286.

25 Warrington S, Storey DM Comparative studies on Asian and Caucasian children 2: Nutrition feeding practices and health. *Eur J Clin Nutr,* 1988, **42** 69–80.

26 Sahota P *Feeding Baby: Inner City Practice.* Bradford: Horton Publishing, 1991.

27 Goel KM, House F, Shanks RA Infant feeding practices among immigrants in Glasgow. *Brit Med J,* 1978, **2** 1181–1183.

28 McNeill G Birth weight, feeding practice and weight/age of Punjabi children in the UK and in the rural Punjab. *Hum Nutr: Clin Nutr,* 1985, **39C** 69–72.

29 Evans N *et al.* Lack of breast feeding and early weaning

in infants of Asian immigrants to Wolverhamptom. *Arch Dis Childh*, 1978, **51** 608–612.

30 Jivani SKM The practice of infant feeding amongst Asian immigrants. *Arch Dis Childh*, 1978, **53** 66–73.

31 Jones VM Current weaning practices within the Bangladeshi community in the London Borough of Tower Hamlets. *Hum Nutr: Appl Nutr*, 1987, **41A** 349–352.

32 Alvear J, Brooke OG Foetal growth in different racial groups. *Arch Dis Childh*, 1978, **53** 27–32.

33 Warrington S, Storey DM Comparative studies on Asian and Caucasian children. 1: Growth. *Eur J Clin Nutr*, 1988, **42** 61–67.

34 Harris RJ *et al.* Nutritional survey of Bangladeshi children aged under 5 years in the London Borough of Tower Hamlets. *Arch Dis Childh*, 1983, **58** 428–432.

35 Ehrhardt P Iron deficiency in young Bradford children from different ethnic groups. *Brit Med J*, 1986, **292** 90–93.

36 Hunt S The food habits of Asian immigrants. Burgess Hill, West Sussex: Van der Berghs and Jurgens, 1975: 40–41.

37 Hunt SP *et al.* Vitamin D status in different subgroups of British Asians. *Brit Med J*, 1976, **2** 1351–1354.

38 Goel KM *et al.* Reduced prevalence of rickets in Asian children in Glasgow. *Lancet*, 1985, **ii** 405–407.

39 Dunnigan MG *et al.* Prevention of rickets in Asian children: assessment of the Glasgow campaign. *Brit Med J*, 1985, **291**, 239–242.

40 Douglas J *Caribbean Food and Diet*. Cambridge: National Extension College for Training in Health and Race, 1987.

41 Kemm J, Douglas J, Sylvester V Afro-Caribbean diet survey interim report to the Birmingham inner city partnership programme. *Proc Nutr Soc*, 1986, **45**(3) 87A.

42 Kemm J, Douglas J, Sylvester V A survey of infant feeding practice by Afro-Caribbean mothers in Birmingham. *Proc Nutr Soc*, 1986, **45**(3) 87A.

43 Holland B, Unwin ID, Buss DH *Vegetables, Herbs and Spices. The Fifth Supplement to McCance & Widdowson's The Composition of Foods*, 4e. London: Royal Society of Chemistry/MAFF, 1991.

44 Springer L, Thomas J Rastafarians in Britain: a preliminary study of their food habits and beliefs. *Hum Nutr: Appl Nutr*, 1983, **37A**, 120–127.

45 James JA, Clark C, Ward PS Screening Rastafarian children for nutritional rickets. *Brit Med J*, 1985, **290** 899–900.

46 Campbell M, Lofters WS, Gibbs WN Rastafarianism and the vegan syndrome. *Brit Med J*, 1982, **285** 1617–1618.

47 Close GC Rastafarians and the vegan syndrome. *Brit Med J*, 1983, **286** 473.

48 Goodburn PC, Falshaw M, Hughes H *Chinese Food and Diet*. Cambridge: National Extension College for Training in Health and Race, 1987.

Appendices

Manufacturers of Dietetic Products

A full list of drugs appears in the *British National Formulary* (*BNF*), a joint publication of the British Medical Association and the Royal Pharmaceutical Society of Great Britain. Drug manufacturers' addresses may be found in the *Monthly Index of Medical Specialities* (*MIMS*), an independent publication supported by advertising.

Abbott Laboratories Ltd
Abbott House, Moorbridge Road, Maidenhead, Berkshire SL6 8JG.

Alpha Therapeutic UK Ltd
Howlett Way, Thetford, Norfolk, IP24 1HZ.

Bio-Diagnostics Ltd
Upton Industrial Estate, Rectory Road, Upton-upon-Severn, Worcestershire, WR8 0XL.

B Braun Medical Ltd
Braun House, 13–14 Farmborough Close, Stocklade, Aylesbury, Bucks HP20 1DQ.

The Boots Company PLC
Head Office, Nottingham NG2 3AA.

Cadbury Ltd
PO Box 12, Bournville, Birmingham B30 2LU.

Carnation
(See Clintec Nutrition Ltd)

Clintec Nutrition Ltd
Shaftesbury Court, 18 Chalvey Park, Slough, Berkshire SL1 2HT.

Cow & Gate Nutricia Ltd
Trowbridge, Wiltshire BA14 0XG.

Farley Health Products Ltd
Nottingham NG2 3AA.

Fresenius Ltd
6–8 Christleton Court, Stuart Road, Manor Park, Runcorn, Cheshire WA7 1ST.

General Designs Ltd
PO Box 83E, Worcester Park, Surrey KT4 7LX.

Kabi Pharmacia Ltd
Davy Avenue, Knowlhill, Milton Keynes, MK5 8PH.

Larkhall Natural Health Ltd
225 Putney Bridge Road, London SW15 2PY.

E Merck Ltd
Winchester Road, Four Marks, Alton, Hampshire GU34 5HG.

Mead Johnson Nutritionals
Bristol-Myers Squibb House, 141–149 Staines Road, Hounslow, Middlesex TW3 3JA.

Milupa Ltd
Milupa House, Uxbridge Road, Hillingdon, Uxbridge, Middlesex UB10 0NE.

Nestlé
(See Clintec Nutrition Ltd)

Nutricia Dietary Products Ltd
494–496 Honeypot Lane, Stanmore, Middlesex HA7 1JH.

Paines and Byrne Ltd
Bilton Road, Perivale, Greenford, Middlesex UB6
7HG.

Parke-Davis Research Laboratories
Lambert Court, Chestnut Avenue, Eastleigh, Hants
SO5 3ZQ.

Procea Ltd
Alexandra Road, Dublin 1.

Provomel Division
Vandemoortele (UK) Ltd, Ashley House, High Street,
Hounslow, Middlesex.

Ross Laboratories
(See Abbott Laboratories Ltd)

Scientific Hospital Supplies Group UK Ltd
100 Wavertree Boulevard, Wavertree Technology
Park, Liverpool L7 9PT.

Searle Pharmaceuticals
PO Box 53, Lane End Road, High Wycombe, Bucks
HP12 4HL.

SMA Nutrition
Huntercombe Lane South, Taplow, Maidenhead,
Berkshire SL6 0PH.

SmithKline Beecham Consumer Brands
St Georges Avenue, Weybridge, Surrey KT13 0DE.

Sutherland Health Ltd
Turnfields Court, Turnfields, The Moors, Thatcham,
Berkshire RG13 4PT.

UCB (Pharma Ltd)
Star House, 69 Clarendon Road, Watford, Herts
WD1 1DJ.

Ultrapharm Ltd
PO Box 18, Henley on Thames, Oxfordshire RG9
2AW.

Unigreg Ltd
Enterprise House, 181–189 Garth Road, Morden,
Surrey SM4 4LL.

Unisoy Milk 'N' By Products Ltd
Unit 1, Cromwell Trading Estate, Cromwell Road,
Bredbury, Stockport SK6 2RS.

Vitaflo Ltd
6 Moss Street, Paisley PA1 1BJ.

Warner Lambert
(See Parke-Davis Research Laboratories)

APPENDIX II

Dietetic Products

Aglutella	Ultrapharm	Flexical	Mead Johnson
Albumaid XP	SHS	Forceval	Unigreg
Alfare	Nestlé	Fortisip	Cow & Gate
Aminogran Food Supplement	UCB Pharma	Fresubin	Fresenius
		Fructose Formula Galactomin 19	Cow & Gate
Aminogran Mineral Mixture	UCB Pharma	Galactomin 17	Cow & Gate
Aproten	Ultrapharm	Generaid	SHS
Aptamil	Milupa	Generaid Plus	SHS
Boots Follow-on Milk	Boots	Gluco-lyte	Cupal
Build-up	Carnation	Glutafin	Nutricia
Calogen	SHS	Glycerol Trioleate Oil	SHS
Caloreen	Clintec	Human Milk Fortifier	Mead Johnson
Caprilon	Cow &Gate	Hycal	SmithKline Beecham
Casilan	Farley	Hypostop	Bio-Diagnostics
Coffee-mate	Carnation	InfaSoy	Cow & Gate
Comminuted Chicken Meat	Cow & Gate	Instant Carobel	Cow & Gate
Cow & Gate Nutriprem Nutriprem 2	Cow & Gate	Intralipid	Kabi Pharmacia
		Isomil	Abbott
Cow & Gate Nutriprem Breastmilk Fortifier	Cow & Gate	Isocal	Mead Johnson
		Ivelip	Clintec
Cow & Gate Nutrilon Premium	Cow & Gate	Juvela	SHS
		Kindergen PROD	SHS
Cow & Gate Nutrilon Plus	Cow & Gate	Lipofundin	Braun
Dialamine	SHS	Liquigen	SHS
Dioralyte	Rorer	Locasol	Cow & Gate
Duobar	SHS	Lofenalac	Mead Johnson
Duocal	SHS	Loprofin	Nutricia
Electrolade	Nicholas	Lorenzo's Oil	SHS
Elemental 028	SHS	Marvel	Cadbury
Ener-G	General Designs	Maxijul	SHS
Enfamil	Mead Johnson	Maxipro HBV	SHS
Enrich	Abbott	MCT Pepdite 0–2	SHS
Ensure	Abbott	MCT Pepdite 2+	SHS
Eoprotin	Milupa	Metabolic Mineral Mixture	SHS
Farley's First Milk	Farley	Methionine-free amino acid mix (Code 637)	SHS
Farley's Follow-on Milk	Farley		
Farley's Second Milk	Farley	Methionine, threonine,	SHS

valine free and isoleucine low amino acid mix (Code 889)	
Milumil	Milupa
Minafen	Cow & Gate
Monogen	SHS
MSUD Aid III (Code 636)	SHS
MSUD Analog	SHS
MSUD Maxamaid	SHS
MSUD Maxamum	SHS
Neocate	SHS
Nepro	Abbott
Nesquik	Nestlé
Nestargel	Nestlé
Nutramigen	Mead Johnson
Nutrison	Cow & Gate
Nutrison Paediatric	Cow & Gate
Osmolite	Abbott
OsterPrem	Farley
OsterSoy	Farley
Paediasure	Abbott
Paediatric Seravit	SHS
Paediatric Seravit (Flavoured)	SHS
Pastariso	General Designs
Pepdite 0–2	SHS
Pepdite 2+	SHS
Peptamen	Clintec
Pepti-Junior	Cow & Gate
Phenylalanine, tyrosine and methionine free amino acid mix (Code 888)	SHS
PKU 2	Milupa
PKU 3	Milupa
PKU Aid III	SHS
Polycal	Cow & Gate
Polycal Liquid	Cow & Gate
Polycose	Abbott
Portagen	Mead Johnson
Prematil	Milupa
Premcare	Farley
Primene	Clintec
Pregestimil	Mead Johnson
Prejomin	Milupa
Progress	SMA Nutrition
ProMod	Abbott
ProSobee	Mead Johnson
Protein Forte	Fresenius
Protein-free diet Powder (80056)	Mead Johnson

Protifar	Cow & Gate
Provamel	Provamel
Provide	Fresenius
Pulmocare	Abbott
Rapolyte	Janssen
Rehidrat	Searle
Rite-Diet	Nutricia
RVHB Maxamaid	SHS
RVHB Maxamum	SHS
Schar	Ultrapharm
Seravit	SHS
SMA Gold	SMA Nutrition
SMA Lowbirthweight	SMA Nutrition
SMA White	SMA Nutrition
Sno Pro	SHS
Soyacal	Alpha
Step-Up	Cow & Gate
Suplena	Abbott
Thick & Easy	Fresenius
Thixo-D	Sutherland
Tritamyl	Procea
Trufree	Larkhall
Tyrosine and phenylalanine free amino acid mix (Code 726)	SHS
Ultra	Ultrapharm
Unisoy Gold	Unisoy
Vamin	Kabi Pharmacia
Vaminolact	Kabi Pharmacia
Vitajoule	Vitaflo
Vitaquick	Vitaflo
Vitapro	Vitaflo
Wysoy	SMA Nutrition
XMTVI Analog	SHS
XMTVI Maxamaid	SHS
XMTVI Maxamum	SHS
XP Analog	SHS
XP Maxamaid	SHS
XP Maxamaid Bar	SHS
XP Maxamum	SHS
X phen tyr Analog	SHS
X phen tyr met Analog	SHS
X phen tyr Maxamaid	SHS
X phen tyr met Maxamaid	SHS
X phen tyr Maxamum	SHS
X tyr Maxamum	SHS
Code 124 complete amino acid mixture	SHS
Code 767 peptides	SHS

Index

non-starch polysaccharides,
243–4
Familial Hypercholesterolaemia
Association, 244
Familial hyperchylomicronaemia type
I, 240, 241–2
acute episodes, 242
fat restriction, 242
infant feeds, 242
older children, 242
Familial combined
hypertriglyceridaemia type IIb,
240, 241
Familial type III hyperlipidaemia, 240,
241
Familial hypertriglyceridaemia type
IV, 240, 241
Familial hyperlipoproteinaemia type V,
240
Farley's
First Milk, 6, 179, 253, 329, 345
Follow-on Milk, 6, 215, 345
Second Milk, 6, 253, 329, 345
Fat soluble vitamins,
in abetalipoproteinaemia, 239
Fatty acids,
absorption, 146
metabolism in cancer, 269
mitochondrial oxidation, 228–9
odd chain, 200
very long chain, 255–63
Fatty acid oxidation, disorders of,
228–35
Feed making area, 13, 14
bottles, 15
cleaning procedures, 17
legislative requirements, 13
microbiology, 17
pasteurizers and pasteurization, 14,
16
plant and equipment, 14–15
preparation and ingredients, 15–16
staffing, 15
storage area, 13
structural design, 13
wash up area, 14
Feeding difficulties, nutrition for
children with 309–21
causes, 312–13
cerebral palsy, 310, 311
cleft palate, 311–13
Down's syndrome, 310–11
eating and drinking skills, 309
equipment, 318–19
management, 315–20
nutritional assessment, 313–15

nutritional problems, 309–10
Feingold diet, food intolerance, 161
Few food diet
in food allergy and intolerance,
155–7
in nephrotic syndrome, 131
Fibre *see* Non-starch polysaccharides
Flavours, food intolerance, 155
Flexical, 27, 325
Fluid,
in acute renal failure, 128
in chronic renal failure, 136
in gastroenteritis, 64
in nephrotic syndrome, 131
requirements, 6
Fluoride, 183, 187, 199, 212
Follow-on formulas, 10, 215
Food allergy and intolerance, 152–67
antioxidants, 155
artificial colours, 155
benzoate preservatives, 155
double blind placebo controlled
provocations, 159–60
empirical diet, 154–5
few food diet, 155–6
hypoallergenic milk substitutes,
155–7
irritable bowel syndrome, 154
mammalian milks, 154, 157
mechanisms, 152
mother's diet, 157
Nalcrom, 159
nitrite preservatives, 155
open reintroduction of foods, 158
prevention of, 162
radioallergosorbent tests (RAST),
152
salicylates, 155
simple exclusion diet, 154
Food aversion, learned, 82, 270, 326
Food avoidance emotional disorder
(FAED), 279, 280
Food fads, 279, 280
Food intolerance *see* Food allergy and
intolerance
Food Safety Act 1990, 13, 19
Forceval Junior Capsules, 11, 169, 178,
187, 194, 199, 214, 233, 262, 325
Fortical, 325
Fortimel, 216
Fortisip, 94, 128, 252, 300, 306, 325
Fresubin, 94, 252, 300, 306, 325
Fresubin High Energy, 94
Fructosaemia *see* Hereditary fructose
intolerance
Fructose, 7, 103, 210, 222

Fructose-1, 6-bisphosphatase
deficiency, 225–6
emergency regimen, 225
illness, 225
infants, 225
older child, 225
Fruitarian diet, 331
Fulminant hepatic failure *see* Liver
failure

Galactans, 219
Galactokinase deficiency, 221
Galactomin, 17, 19, 65, 68, 219, 253,
325
Galactosaemia, classical, 217–21
alcohol, 220
galactose-1-phosphate levels, 217
galactosides and nucleoproteins,
219, 220
heterozygote mothers, 220–21
milk products and derivatives,
220–21
milk substitutes, 219–20
minimal galactose and lactose diet,
217–21
sources of galactose, 219
Galactosaemia Support Group, 227
Galactose, 210
inborn errors of metabolism, 217–21
Galactosides, 219
Gastric hypersecretion, 86, 112
Gastroenteritis, 64
acute infective diarrhoea, 64
and toddler diarrhoea, 74
dehydration, 64
in breast fed infants, 64
post-enteritis enteropathy, 64, 65
oral rehydration solutions (ORS), 64
regrading feeds, 64
secondary lactose intolerance, 65–6
Gastro-oesophageal reflux (GOR), 63
barium studies, 63
drugs, 83
in cystic fibrosis, 110
in developmental delay, 63
in oesophageal atresia, 83
in the breast fed infant, 63
management, 63–4
Nissen fundoplication, 63, 83
pH monitoring, 63
Gastroschisis, 88
enteral feeding, 88
parenteral nutrition, 88
Gastrostomy feeding, 29
gastrostomy button, 30, 132, 139,
200